Financial Management in Health Care Organizations

Second Edition

Financial Management in Health Care Organizations

Second Edition

Robert A. McLean, Ph.D., CFA
Professor and Director
Master of Health Services Administration Program
Creighton University
Omaha, Nebraska

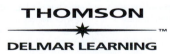

THOMSON

™

DELMAR LEARNING

Australia Canada Mexico Singapore Spain United Kingdom United States

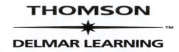

THOMSON

DELMAR LEARNING

Financial Management in Health Care Organizations, Second Edition
by Robert A. McLean

Executive Director
Health Care Business Unit:
William Brotmiller

Executive Editor:
Cathy L. Esperti

Acquisitions Editor:
Maureen Rosener

Technology Project Manager:
Victoria Moore

Executive Marketing Manager:
Dawn F. Gerrain

Developmental Editor:
Darcy M. Scelsi

Editorial Assistant:
Matthew Thouin

Production Editor:
James Zayicek

For permission to use material from this text or product, contact us by
Tel   (800) 730-2214
Fax   (800) 730-2215
www.thomsonrights.com

Library of Congress Cataloging-in-Publication Data

McLean, Robert A.
  Financial management in health care organizations / Robert
  A. McLean--2nd ed.
      p. cm.
  Includes bibliographical references and index.
  ISBN-13: 978-0-7668-3547-4
  ISBN-10: 0-7668-3547-2
    1. Medical economics. 2. Medical care--Finance. 3. Health
  services administration I. Title.

RA410 .M396 2002
362.1'068'1--dc21
                                                    2002073584

NOTICE TO THE READER

Publisher does not warrant or guarantee any of the products described herein or perform any independent analysis in connection with any of the product information contained herein. Publisher does not assume, and expressly disclaims, any obligation to obtain and include information other than that provided to it by the manufacturer.

The reader is expressly warned to consider and adopt all safety precautions that might be indicated by the activities herein and to avoid all potential hazards. By following the instructions contained herein, the reader willingly assumes all risks in connection with such instructions.

The Publisher makes no representation or warranties of any kind, including but not limited to, the warranties of fitness for particular purpose or merchantability, nor are any such representations implied with respect to the material set forth herein, and the publisher takes no responsibility with respect to such material. The publisher shall not be liable for any special, consequential, or exemplary damages resulting, in whole or part, from the readers' use of, or reliance upon, this material.

INTRODUCTION TO THE SERIES

This Series in Health Services is now in its second decade of providing top-quality teaching materials to the health administration/public health field. Each year has witnessed further strengthening of the market position of each of the principal books in the Series, also reflecting the continued excellence of the products. Each author, book editor, and contributor to the Series has helped build what is widely recognized as the top textbook and issues collection of books available in this field today.

But we have achieved only a beginning. Everyone involved in the Series is committed to further expansion of the scope, technical excellence, and usability of the Series. Our goal is to do more for you, the reader. We will add new books in important areas, seek out more excellent authors, and increase the physical attributes of the books to make them easier for you to use.

We thank everyone, the authors and users in particular, who have made this Series so successful and so widely used. And we promise that this second decade will be dedicated to further expansion of the Series and to enhancement of the books it contains to provide still greater value to you, our constituency.

Stephen J. Williams
Series Editor

DELMAR SERIES IN HEALTH SERVICES ADMINISTRATION

Stephen J. Williams, Sc.D., Series Editor

Contents

PART 3 • THE FINANCIAL MARKET ENVIRONMENT 163

Chapter 9 Financial Markets: Institutions, Risk, and Return 165

PART 4 • SELECTING LONG-TERM ASSETS AND PROGRAMS 185

Chapter 10 The Basics of Capital Budgeting 187

Chapter 11 Special Topics in Capital Budgeting 209

PART5 • MANAGING LONG-TERM FINANCIAL ASSETS: THE ENDOWMENT   231

Chapter 12 Managing the Endowment   233

PART 6 • LONG-TERM FINANCING   247

Chapter 13 External Financing: Sources   249

Chapter 14 Procedures for Long-Term Financing   263

LIST OF FIGURES AND TABLES

Chapter 1

Chapter 3

Chapter 4

Chapter 5

Chapter 6

Chapter 7

Chapter 8

Chapter 9

Chapter 10

Chapter 11

Chapter 12

Chapter 13

Chapter 14

Chapter 16

Chapter 17

Chapter 18

Chapter 19

Chapter 20

PREFACE TO THE SECOND EDITION

This second edition of **Financial Management in Health Care Organizations** offers an opportunity to update and revise the 1997 version. Much has happened in health care delivery since the mid-1990s, and this revision is sorely needed.

As was true for the first edition, this text is intended for graduate and undergraduate students in health services administration, public health, and related fields. It is not for the financial specialist, but for the manager for whom financial decision-making is only a part of the position description. Every manager in every health care organization needs a thorough grounding in finance, in order to sit at the table "with the big boys and girls," the senior management team. These pages provide that grounding.

Like the first edition, I have tried to make the material in this edition as easily understandable as possible. I have also tried, particularly in the Continuing Cases, to allow the reader to have as much fun as possible with financial problems.

My move to Creighton University showed me that there really is a Physicians Clinic. The Physicians Clinic of the Continuing Cases is *not* the Physicians Clinic of Omaha, Nebraska. The actors in the Continuing Cases are purely fictitious, although many of their names are borrowed from my friends and family members. I apologize for any unintended confusion. Because some readers found the Continuing Cases to be the most useful parts of the first edition, they remain, except for enlargement, essentially unchanged.

New to This Edition

- Issues arising from managed care are woven throughout the text. This is now mainstream material and every manager needs to think like a managed care manager;

- New accounting standards and terms are incorporated;

- The coverage of cost analysis is substantially expanded. Chapter 7 includes an expanded treatment of Activity Based Costing and a discussion of cost-volume-profit analysis under capitation;

- Data for benchmarking financial statements are updated. These were generously provided by William O. Cleverly, Professor Emeritus of Health Services Administration at the Ohio State University and President of Cleverley and Associates.

- Chapter 20, "Beyond Beancounting," has been substantially revised. The frontiers of the field keep moving and I have added new material in an effort to keep up.

- The Continuing Cases have been expanded, with new attention to the concerns of local health departments.

Acknowledgments

My students at Creighton University, the University of Alabama at Birmingham, the American University of Armenia, and the Czech Republic's Palacky' University have taken entirely too much pleasure in pointing out the typographical errors and logical shortcomings of the first edition. I am grateful, if embarrassed.

My long-time friend and frequent collaborator, Frank Magiera, generously agreed to prepare the Instructor's Manual for this edition. Students always believe that these manuals contain special insight and wisdom. This time they are right.

The months during which I was to revise the text were stressful ones. Darcy Scelsi of Delmar Learning was both tolerant of the inevitable delays and persistent in pressing for completion. I am grateful to her for both.

Sharon, Rob, and Scott allowed me to take over a corner of the basement for many months to complete these revisions. Thanks again.

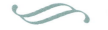

Introduction

Health Care and Finance

Learning Objectives

After reading this introduction, the student should be able to:

1. Explain the nature of the financial management function and distinguish it from accounting.
2. List and explain the major reasons that financial management in health care organizations is unique among industries.
3. Understand the outline and structure of the textbook.

Key Terms

Agency relationship
Capital budgeting
Financial management
Joint Commission for the
   Accreditation of Health
   Care Organizations
   (JCAHO)

Prospective Payment System
   (PPS)
Third-party payors
Working capital management

This is a textbook on the financial management of health care organizations. It is intended for two groups of readers. First, it is intended for students in advanced undergraduate and master's degree programs who seek general management careers in health care organizations and who need to understand the financial management function and the financial way of thinking. Second, it is for clinical health care professionals whose duties, perhaps for the first time, require them to consider financial issues.

This is not a textbook in accounting. Although the reader will have occasion to remember his or her accounting, the accounting function is clearly distinguished from finance throughout the text. The financial manager uses accounting data and must therefore understand how financial statements are constructed. The financial decision rules that managers apply, however, are based on economic principles. Like the study of economics itself, financial management requires the ability to work with complex logical (some would say mathematical) relationships. Although no mathematics beyond basic algebra is required to work through this volume, those who understand mathematical relationships at more advanced levels will enjoy a richer understanding of some of the chapters that follow.

Financial management is the process of selection, financing, and stewardship of the assets of any organization. Assets are the things (tangible or intangible) that organizations own or, under certain circumstances, lease. There are many criteria for selecting assets, including necessity for operation, professional judgment, and legal fiat. In financial management, however, one is concerned with selecting assets according to financial criteria: what assets best serve the financial goals of the organization? Assets, to be acquired, must be paid for (financed). In financial management, one must decide what means of financing is least costly and best balances risk and expected return for the organization as a whole. Once financed and acquired, assets must be cared for. They must be maintained, replaced, abandoned, and in the case of financial assets, their returns reinvested. All of these are the problems of financial management.

Even the smallest health care organizations have professionals (accountants, analysts, bookkeepers, treasurers, planners) who are specialists in financial management (their roles are discussed in Chapter 1). Financial management is also a concern for nonspecialists. Department directors must develop and manage budgets. Directors of operations and nursing administrators must participate in decisions on acquiring equipment. Chief executive officers and trustees take leading roles in decisions about long-term financing and about organizational acquisitions. Broadly conceived, financial management is not a task for specialized managers, but is a special approach to what all managers do.

HEALTH CARE IS DIFFERENT/
HEALTH CARE IS THE SAME

First and foremost, the financial management of health care organizations *is* financial management. Health care organizations must generate cash flows, acquire assets, and put those assets to work, just as do manufacturing, retailing, and banking organizations. The decision-making rules that health care organizations should use are based on the same economic principles as those of any other type of enterprise. To understand financial management in health care settings, one must first master the fundamentals of finance.

Financial management in health care organizations is, however, different from financial management in other settings. The most important difference between financial management in health care and elsewhere is the abundance and importance of **agency relationships** in health care organizations. In an agency relationship, one party (the agent) acts in behalf of another party (the principal). If the agent acts out of any degree of self-interest, the principal may suffer a loss. Physicians are agents for patients; administrators are agents for trustees; health care providers are agents for the providers of capital; and third-party payors are agents for those who pay insurance premiums. The financial effects of agency relationships on health care providers (and on the health care system as a whole) are profound. These are discussed in detail in Chapter 2.

Second, in the United States, health care is delivered by a complex mixture of government, private not-for-profit, and investor-owned organizations. That these types of providers coexist and compete with one another has curious origins (beyond the scope of this text) and creates confusion for many consumers. Providers who offer the same services in the same market may have very different motivations for so doing. County health departments have different expectations of their home health agencies than do investor-owned home health firms and will act differently because of them. The rich pluralism that is the result of this mixture of organizational and ownership types provides an abundance of choices for those consumers with the financial wherewithal (or the insurance coverage) to seek out the types of care they choose. That pluralism also means that managers making financial decisions must consider the type and goals of the organizations for which they work, as well as the nature of the problem at hand.

Third, health care services are provided in a regulatory environment that is both different from and more comprehensive than that affecting almost any other industry. Capital investment in most health care settings is not merely a matter of making a financial decision but, in many cases, must also be approved by certificate-of-need regulators. Organizational structure and staffing patterns are issues to be evaluated for controlling costs, but they are also issues that will be evaluated by the **Joint Commission on the Accreditation of Healthcare Organizations** and involve decisions that must be made in compliance with state professional licensure acts. Hospitals must report their financial data in the usual formats, but they must also report their costs to the U.S. Centers for Medicare and Medicaid Services.

Fourth, a wider range of financing options exists for health care organizations than is true in other industries. Not-for-profit hospitals can enjoy tax-exempt bond financing, can use mortgage financing for their physical plants, can borrow from commercial banks, can act as general partners in limited partnerships, or can form for-profit subsidiaries that issue common stock. Both not-for-profit and investor-owned health care firms can sell their patient accounts receivable.

Fifth, closely related to the agency cost issue just discussed, most of the revenues that health care organizations receive pass through **third-party payors** rather than coming directly from clients. The role of third-party payors (Blue Cross/Blue Shield, commercial insurance companies, health maintenance organizations, and federal and state governments) reduces the degree to which providers of care can manage the collection of patient accounts. In addition, the effective prices of various services are subject to constant negotiations with cost-conscious insurance carriers. The most powerful of the third parties, the federal government, has been able to introduce an innovative basis for making payment, the so-called **Prospective Payment System**, for a very large share of total patient volume.

Finally, the health care system is growing much more rapidly than almost any other sector of the U.S. economy. The share of gross domestic product accounted for by health care spending has risen from 7.3 percent in 1970 to 13.4 percent in 1997 (U.S. Department of Health and Human Services, 2000). That growth is not bad in itself; it may represent only an increased concern for good health by an increasingly affluent society. That health outcomes have not improved commensurately with increased spending, however, suggests that health care managers need to focus on cost control and efficiency now as never before.

All of the unique features of health care organizations and of the health care industry notwithstanding, health care providers face the same basic financial management problems as any other independent economic entity. Health care organizations must select assets and operate them so as not to require external subsidies (or they must secure those subsidies). That selection and operation constitutes the basic problem of **capital budgeting**. Health care organizations face greater problems of **working capital management** than do other types of firms because so much of their accounts receivable are owed by third-party payors and because of the potentially life-threatening situations that can arise because of inventory "stockouts." Health care organizations that cannot access external sources of capital to finance the acquisition of new technology are likely to fall behind in services provision and be driven out of business. Not-for-profit health care organizations that hold endowment funds are just as concerned with portfolio management as any pension plan or mutual fund. The financial management *of* health care organizations is financial management (in the broadest sense) *in* health care organizations.

PLAN OF THE TEXT

Part I of this text sets the stage for all of the chapters that follow by placing health care financial management in its environmental context and (in Chapter 2) explaining the defining financial characteristic of health care organizations: the large number and complexity of the agency relationships within them. Part II presents tools for the financial manager and for the general manager faced with financial problems. Part III introduces the reader to financial markets and to the important relationship between risk and expected return. Parts IV and VI deal with long-term assets and programs. These assets and programs must be identified and selected (Part IV) and paid for (Part VI). The focus here is on financial, rather than clinical, criteria. Part V stands alone within the text; it deals with the management of one particular type of long-term asset: the endowment. Some instructors may wish to omit discussion of Part V, whereas others will want to supplement its relatively brief treatment. Part VII deals with short-term assets and liabilities. The material in those chapters makes up the day-to-day business of most financial managers. Part VIII discusses emerging issues in health care financial management, some of which are only now making their way into professional practice.

SUMMARY

In the United States, the health care sector exhibits unique features, distinguishing it from virtually all of the rest of the economy. Organizations within that sector, however, require the same management functions and the same level of management expertise as do organizations in any other sector. The chapters that follow are an introduction to the practice of financial management in health care organizations. This knowledge is essential to meet the challenges of providing health care services in the twenty-first century.

Discussion Questions

1. Many financial management professionals in health care took their early training and experience in accounting. What sorts of competencies must they have developed to move from accounting to senior financial management?

2. In the United States, health care services are provided by government-owned, private not-for-profit, and investor-owned organizations. What sorts of differences would you expect to find between the organizational and financial goals of those three types of organizations? Would you expect to find homogeneity of goals within each of the three ownership types? Explain.

3. Explain what an agency relationship is. What are some of the principal-agency relationships in health care delivery organizations? In other business settings (e.g., retailing)? In family life?

4. Most health care services are paid, at least in part, by third-party payors. What incentives do third-party payors have in promoting, denying, and regulating patients' access to care?

5. Is health care "just another industry?" Is it an industry at all? Explain.

CONTINUING CASES

In the chapters that follow, the reader will observe three organizations, Physicians' Clinic, Lone Star Home Health Services, and the Clearwater County Health Department as they come to grips with the financial issues involved in operations, survival, and growth. These organizations are entirely fictitious; they, and the city and county in which they are located, are the products of imagination. Although they and their decision problems are simplified to highlight the financial issues under review, these imaginary organizations and the problems they face are similar to those of many real health care organizations.

Clearwater County

The organizations in the continuing cases are based in Jamestown, the county seat of Clearwater County, Texas. Jamestown is a medium-sized city (350,000 population in 2000) in central Texas, about 125 miles southwest of Fort Worth. A widely scattered rural population and two small crossroads municipalities bring the total population for the county to 450,000 (in 2000). Jamestown has the only hospitals in the county. St. Mary's Hospital (125 licensed beds, 115 staffed) enjoys strong support from local Catholic physicians. It offers a wide range of services, but its medical staff refer patients to a large Catholic hospital in Dallas (150 miles away) for most tertiary services. St. Mary's carries a substantial burden of uncompensated care for the region's Hispanic agricultural workers. Clearwater County Memorial Hospital (250 licensed and staffed beds) is owned by the Clearwater County Hospital Authority, created by the county in 1983. Memorial is the hospital at which most of the county's physicians practice. In fact, every member of the Clearwater County Medical Society is a member of Memorial's medical staff. Memorial's services, once nearly comprehensive, have recently been under review, as the average daily occupancy rate has fallen below 50 percent.

Physicians' Clinic

Physicians' Clinic is the home of 53 health care professionals and operates a small (15 licensed and staffed beds) inpatient facility in a suburban Jamestown neighborhood. The professional practices in the clinic include a group of three dentists; a psychiatric social worker (MSW) specializing in the treatment of children and adolescents; 15 primary care physicians each in solo practice; four small single-specialty group practices; and one large multispecialty group practice, the Jackson Group. The physicians who rent office space in the clinic all have admitting privileges there, although most of the clinic's specialists practice at Memorial. A few of the clinic's physicians admit only at St. Mary's. The building (including the inpatient facility) belongs to Physicians' Clinic, Inc. (PCI, Inc.).

PCI, Inc., is an investor-owned corporation with 10 shareholders, all providers renting space in the clinic. The clinic is PCI's only subsidiary. Roger Jackson, MD, managing partner of the Jackson Group, is the largest shareholder of PCI and chairs its board of directors. Henry Kirk, MHA, is the president and chief operating officer of PCI and president and chief executive officer of the clinic, positions he has held for the past 5 years. Kirk came to the clinic with 12 years of hospital operating experience. At the corporate (PCI, Inc.) level, a comptroller, Janet Fowler, CPA, and a director of marketing and planning, report to Kirk. Fowler is also the chief financial officer of the clinic. A director of patient accounts (currently unfilled) reports to her. The professional practices that rent space in the clinic have their own staffs.

Lone Star Home Health Services

Lone Star Home Health Services (LSHHS) is a not-for-profit organization providing a variety of services in Jamestown and Clearwater County. Originally organized by the regional bishop of the United Methodist Church, the LSHHS's board is now quite diverse, with 27 members drawn from the local charitable and business leadership. Billy Bob Ferguson, a retired bank lending officer, serves as the full-time, salaried director. The Reverend Jason Cooper, a Baptist minister, was recently elected to a 3-year term as chairman of the board.

Mr. Ferguson, with one secretary, handles all administrative matters. Alice Ferguson, RN, Billy Bob's wife, hires and directs the nurses and aides who deliver services. Most of the nurses use their own cars and are reimbursed for mileage. Meals-on-Wheels has been the most important generator of cash for LSHHS over the years, supplemented by a visiting nurse service. Home infusion therapy is a growing line of business. Most of the Meals-on-Wheels clients pay their own bills. For the past few years, about 35 percent of LSHHS's revenue, including virtually all of the revenue for visiting nurse services, has come from a contract with the Clearwater County Health Department.

Clearwater County Health Department

Clearwater County's Department of Health survives on funding from the county, the State of Texas, and a couple of small federal programs. Originally an inspector of restaurants and septic systems, it has, under Director Jolene Garza, MD, MPH, taken on responsibilities for home health (contracted out to Lone Star Home Health Services) and for the Children's Health Insurance Program (CHIP). Its funding, however, remains slim.

The physicians on the staff of Memorial Hospital rotate (as volunteers) in the county's CHIP clinic. Mary Turner, RN, directs the clinic's day-to-day operations, with the help of three part-time nurses. Joleen's principal assistant, Tom Carter, is one semester short of a degree in accounting from Tarleton State University in nearby Stephenville (a condition in which he has been for almost 20 years). Joleen, Tom, and a part-time secretary share quarters in what was once a barbershop, located in a blue-collar neighborhood of Jamestown. Ben Reilly, the Department's sanitarian (i.e., inspector) has a desk in the office, but is seldom there. That list is the sum total of Clearwater County's public health staff.

The Board of Health, consisting of five members (two physicians and three members of the community at large), supervises the Health Department. Never a glamorous job, Board membership has become progressively more burdensome, and Clearwater County's physicians have to be cajoled into accepting it. Two of the three community members have each served for more than 20 years.

Joleen Garza grew up in Jamestown, older child and only daughter of John Garza, owner of three Texaco stations in and near Jamestown. Joleen's only brother, John (Little John to most), is now the President and Chief Operating Officer of Garza Oil Co. Joleen graduated from the University of Texas at Austin and from the University of Texas Medical School at San Antonio. After a residency in pediatrics in Fort Worth, concern for community issues led her to Tulane's School of Public Health and Tropical Medicine and to a Master of Public Health degree. At Tulane, she met Alex McEuen, a doctoral student in history, whom she would marry. The McEuen-Garzas returned to Jamestown in 1982, when Joleen was offered the directorship of the Health Department. Alex, now Dr. McEuen, commutes to a teaching job a Tarleton State. Although both Joleen and Alex hold positions with relatively low pay, their combined incomes, including Joleen's 20 percent stake in Garza Oil, provide a comfortable living for them and their daughters, Courtney and Whitney.

Joleen is a perfectionist, dedicated to improving the health of Clearwater County's population. Some local physicians and administrators find it difficult to work with her, a fact not lost on the Board of Health, to which she reports. She does not suffer fools gladly, and says what she thinks (perhaps a bit too quickly). She has had several bitter arguments with Roger Jackson over Physicians' Clinic's (and the Jackson Group's) refusal to accept Medicaid patients.

REFERENCES

U.S. Department of Health and Human Services, Public Health Service. (2000). *Health, United States, 2000, with Adolescent Chart Book.* Washington, DC: U.S. Government Printing Office.

SELECTED READINGS

Brealey, R.A. & Myers, S.C. (2000). *Principles of corporate finance,* (6th ed.). New York: McGraw-Hill.

Healthcare Financial Management, monthly journal of the Healthcare Financial Management Association. Two Westbrook Corporate Center, Suite 700, Westchester, IL 60153.

Stevens, R. (1999). *In sickness and in wealth.* (revised) New York: Basic Books.

PART

1

Introduction to Health Care and Finance

CHAPTER

1

Financial Management In Health Care Organizations

Learning Objectives

After reading this chapter, the student should be able to:

1. Explain the relationship between the financial management function and other functions of management.
2. Explain the placement and structure of financial management in the organization chart of a typical health care organization.
3. List and explain the four concerns shared by all financial managers.
4. List and explain the five conceptual pillars of financial management practice.
5. Explain how managed care contracts affect health care providers' financial incentives.

Key Terms

Arbitrage profit	Internal auditor
Capital	Law of one price
Cash	Managed care
Cash flow	Maximizing behavior
Chief financial officer (CFO)	Opportunity cost
Chief information officer (CIO)	Risk aversion
Comptroller (or controller)	Treasurer
Conservation	Time value of money
Costs	
Generally accepted account- ing principles (GAAP)	

Although every manager is a financial manager to the extent that he or she considers asset selection or is responsible for a budget, a few professionals in every large organization are specifically charged with financial analysis and stewardship. Figure 1-1 shows a simplified organization chart for a hospital financial services division. The details of such charts vary from organization to organization, and in small organizations several of the separate functions shown may be performed by one individual. In all but the largest physicians' practices, all of the financial functions are performed by one or two staff, with the help of an outside accountant. In health maintenance organizations and other insurance carriers, the financial function is more complex and highly differentiated than that shown in the figure.

Supervising the financial management function is a **chief financial officer (CFO)**, who may report to the chief operating officer, or may report directly to the chief executive officer. The CFO, in turn, supervises two distinct realms. First, the CFO supervises the **comptroller** (always pronounced, and often spelled, *controller*). The comptroller is charged with the accounting and reporting functions, the generation of periodic financial reports, and the cost analysis and budget functions.

The other major branch of the financial services division is the realm of the **treasurer**, who is charged with stewardship of the organization's financial resources. This area is responsible for commercial bank relations, cash management, lease-versus-purchase analysis, management of any pension or endowment funds, and the management of obligations under long-term debt. Because of their effect on cash, the treasurer is also responsible for accounts payable and patient accounts.

Most large organizations have an **internal auditor**. The internal auditor, a staff position reporting to the CFO, ensures that the accounting and reporting functions are performed in accordance with **Generally Accepted Accounting Principles (GAAP)**. The internal auditor cannot perform the function as watchdog over the reporting function without independence from the comptroller. If the internal auditor is doing his or her job properly, visits from external auditors and relationships with third-party payors are much less stressful.

In some organizations a new function, that of **chief information officer (CIO)**, is becoming critical. The CIO is responsible for the departments, the equipment, and the processes that move information within the organization. A hospital CIO (who may report to or who may be an equal of the CFO) supervises the medical records, data processing, telecommunications, admitting, and, sometimes, quality management departments.

The financial management functions shown in Figure 1-1 correspond closely to the academic disciplines of fiscal management as organized in Figure 1-2. Indeed, if academic fields didn't correspond closely to the arenas of practice, it would be time for the professors to make a visit to the real world. Although the treasurership function and the academic field of financial management are not identical in their concerns, this text is, largely, a treatment of the treasury function.

THE UNIVERSAL CONCERNS OF FINANCIAL MANAGEMENT

Figure 1-3 depicts the four C's, the four categories of issues with which all financial managers are concerned. Those four sets of issues are *costs, cash, capital,* and *conservation.*

In an era of resource constraints, the identification and control of **costs** is a paramount issue in financial management. One of the principal functions of the financial department in any health care organization is the identification of operating costs. From 1965 (the introduction of Medicare) to 1983 (the introduction of the Prospective Payment System), the Health Care Financing Administration (now the Centers for Medicare and Medicaid Services) and most private payors paid ("reimbursed") hospitals on the basis of allowable costs per unit of service. In that era, the purpose of cost finding was to allocate the greatest possible cost to the patients covered by the most generous payor. The objective of cost finding was "revenue

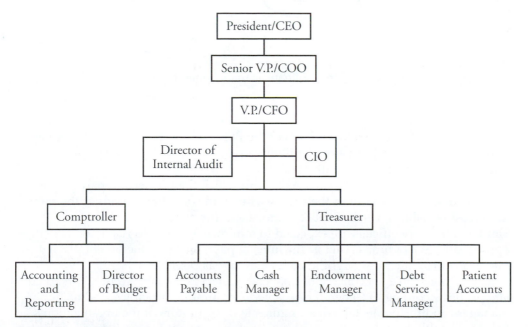

Figure 1-1 Typical hospital financial services division

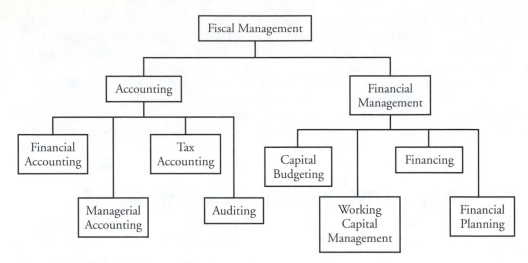

Figure 1-2 The disciplines of fiscal management

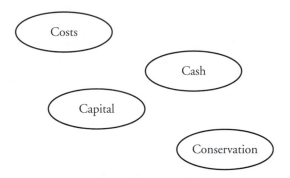

Figure 1-3 The universal concerns of financial management

maximization." Since the introduction of the PPS, and the virtual end of cost-based reimbursement, the objective of identifying operating costs has been to provide information to enhance the control of costs.

Operating costs are not the only costs with which the financial department is concerned. One of the roles of the treasury function is to obtain funds at the minimum cost possible, given market conditions and the organization's level of risk. Similarly, treasury officials are expected to minimize (subject to risk tolerance) the opportunity cost of funds. That is, the interest payments forgone by not placing idle funds in another use ought to be kept as low as possible.

The second universal concern of financial managers is **cash**. Accountants calculate profits according to Generally Accepted Accounting Principles, and naive managers and the public take those figures to be indicators of the organization's financial health. In fact, as discussed in Chapter 3, accounting profits will change as the accountants' assumptions change. Cash, on the other hand, is unambiguous, available to pay obligations, and necessary. It is only the organization's cash holdings that are available to meet the payroll, and employees and creditors accept only cash for compensation.

Some health care analysts have suggested that access to **capital** is the principal determinant of organizational success and viability. Lack of access to capital is often cited as one of the major reasons that hospitals close. New technology can be introduced only by those organizations that have the funds to acquire it. Access to financial capital and the stewardship of the funds acquired are always functions delegated to the financial division.

Conservation, as used here, refers to the financial manager's obligation to preserve the asset base of the organization. Organizations that liquidate themselves (through unwise investments, inappropriate capital acquisitions, or inability to control costs) do not survive. The minimum condition for organizations success is survival. Survival requires attention to the other three concerns of financial management.

THE FIVE PILLARS OF FINANCIAL PRACTICE

If financial managers are concerned with the four C's (cost, cash, capital, and conservation), they approach those concerns with five basic tools, the five pillars of financial practice. These basic building blocks are the understanding of primacy of **cash flows**, recognition of **maximizing behavior**, **risk aversion**, the **time-value-of-money**, and control of **opportunity cost**. These are elaborated in later chapters, but they are important enough to deserve introduction here.

As financier Donald Trump says, "Cash is king." Hyperbole aside, it is cash, not accounting profits, that pays bills. When considering capital investment alternatives, it is the asset's ability to generate cash that determines whether or not that project is feasible. The financial viability of the organization as a whole depends on the organization's generation of cash. Measures of profits based on accrual accounting conventions do not capture, without further arithmetic manipulation, the generation of cash. Cash flow measures, however, will be the principal indicators of financial performance used throughout this text.

Economic actors tend to act as if they were maximizing their well-beings. That is, investors seek out the highest rates of return they can find at the levels of risk they have chosen. Employees seek out the highest levels of total compensation they can achieve, given their training and experiences, at a given level of workplace amenities. Users of capital seek out the lowest cost sources of funds they can find, given the levels of risk they display to the providers of funds. Some actors are driven only by self-interest (e.g., commercial banks), whereas some are required by law to act as maximizers (e.g., those charged with fiduciary responsibility for endowments). The large number of participants in most financial markets, and the impersonal nature of interaction in them, make the prices determined in those markets act as if they are set by true maximizing behavior, by the search for the best possible price.

Virtually all economic actors are risk averse. Intuitively, one is risk averse if one prefers $5, with certainty, to a bet whose average payoff is $5. The ubiquity of risk aversion in economic life spills over into financial markets. For a risk-averse investor to make a risky investment, he or she must expect compensation, in the form of enhanced expected return, over and above what he or she expects for a risk-free investment. Thus risk aversion, coupled with investors' maximizing behavior, generates a market price for risk. The market price for risk is that addition to the risk-free rate of return that investors demand for accepting a unit of market risk.

The value of money to those who would hold it depends on when it is to be received. If one is offered $1,000 today, one can invest it to earn interest. If the interest rate is 10 percent, at the end of a year one would have $1,100. If one is offered $1,000 to be received 1 year from today, one loses the possibility of earning a year's interest. At any positive rate of interest, then, one should prefer $1,000 today to a promise of $1,000 at the end of a year. That preference, and the interest-paying process that causes it, is known as the time value of money and is independent of both the rate of inflation and the riskiness of the offer. The time value of money drives much of financial practice, including capital investment decisions, the pricing of bonds and other securities, and cash management decisions.

The time value of money is caused by actors' desire to exploit opportunities to earn interest (and other forms of return). If one cannot earn interest because funds have not yet arrived, one is poorer than if one had earned the interest. The effect of not earning $100 in interest is exactly the same as if one had earned the $100 and then had incurred a $100 cost. Benefits not received are a special type of cost: opportunity cost. The opportunity cost of investing in a bond yielding 6 percent is the income forgone by not investing in a bond yielding 7 percent. Financial actors seek to avoid opportunity costs with the same zeal that they seek to avoid out-of-pocket costs.

Maximizing behavior and the desire to avoid opportunity costs lead to a fundamental economic law that has powerful implications in financial markets: the **law of one price**. The law of one price says that in a given market, without transportation costs, in which information is freely available, only one price can prevail for any given good or service (assumed to be of uniform quality). The law applies everywhere the conditions are met, whether considering the price of cherry tomatoes at the various stalls of a local farmers' market or the price of a given bond as quoted by various securities dealers.

When the law of one price is violated, opportunities for **arbitrage profit** occur. That is, if a share of stock in XYZ Corporation is selling for $15 on the New York Stock Exchange and for $25 on the Chicago Stock Exchange, one can buy in New York and sell in Chicago simultaneously. If one's broker will lend the $15 for the purchase, one can earn an infinite rate of profit ($10 profit on a $0 investment). Individuals and corporations exploit arbitrage opportunities very quickly. Thus deviations from the law of one price are very short-lived.

If a widely traded 30-year corporate bond, in the risk class denoted AAA by a rating service, yields 8 percent, then the law of one price says that all other corporate bonds of the same term to maturity, risk class, and trading frequency must also yield 8 percent. If an equivalent bond yielded only 7 percent, investors would perceive an opportunity cost in purchasing it. To eliminate that opportunity cost, they would sell a 7 percent bond to purchase the 8 percent bond. Mass selling of the 7 percent bond would drive down its price and (due to the inverse relation between price and yield) drive its yield up. The selling would stop when all of the bonds in the class in question provided the same yield.

The law of one price is as important, and as limiting, for financial management in health care as in any other sector of the economy. Absent charity, the cost of capital is determined in capital markets, with one price prevailing for all borrowers in a given risk class. Opportunities for gain through short-term investments are determined in the money market, with one set of short-term rates prevailing for all. Health care financial management is financial management in the health care sector, with the same economic and financial constraints faced by financial managers everywhere.

THE MANAGED CARE CHALLENGE

Television's fictional crime boss, Tony Soprano, once taunted Dr. Jennifer Melfi, his beautiful, long-suffering psychiatrist, by asking, "What's wrong? Still upset about the coming of managed care?" *The Sopranos* is famous for its characters' clever one-liners, but that one rings truer than many. Dranove estimates that more than 80 percent of working Americans were enrolled in some form of managed care in 2000 (Dranove, 2000, p. 67).

"**Managed care**" refers to any of many arrangements in which a health plan assumes the responsibility and (to varying degrees) the financial risk for the health of the members of a defined population, its "covered lives." The health plan is a type of third party payor, and may be distinct from the providers who sign contracts with it and provide care. Managed care has dramatically changed the financial incentives for health care providers, and, by so doing, has significantly reduced the total expenditure on health care.

Once (at least in an enduring myth) patients "presented" illnesses to health care professionals, who then provided curative services. The patients, or their insurance carriers, then paid the providers' charges (or some negotiated payment different from actual charges). Under managed care, covered lives contract for care (most commonly through their employers) with health plans. Health plans, in turn, make contracts with providers (individually, or organized into contracting groups) to provide care. The providers may receive a negotiated fee for each service, or may assume some part of the financial risk of care by accepting some form of "capitation" payment.

Typically, a single provider (the primary care physician, or PCP) becomes each covered life's gatekeeper to health care services, the initial point of contact and only authorized source of referrals. Covered lives go "out of plan" only with some financial penalty, if at all. In the most restrictive form of managed care (the true health maintenance organization, HMO), the covered life is covered only for referrals made by the PCP to specialists within the HMO's panel. In the least restrictive form (the point of service plan or preferred provider organization) the covered life has insurance coverage for covered services, no matter who provides them, but has an incentive to use physicians within a particular panel.

The exact arrangements for payment for care are specified in the covered lives' contracts with their health plans, and vary widely. The exact incentives for providers are laid down in their contracts with health plans, and also vary widely. Any individual provider may have contracts with multiple health plans, each offering different incentives. So, why was the fictional Dr. Melfi concerned about managed care?

Managed care places a new organization, the health plan, between the patient and the physician. Some services that physicians might provide (even some services deemed medically necessary) may not be covered by the patient's contract with the health plan. The patient is free to pay out of pocket for those services, but the health plan will not do so. A national health system, like that of the United Kingdom, is managed care writ large.

Where once the provider's incentive was to provide any and all medically justified services, under managed care the provider's financial incentive is to provide only covered services. If the provider has accepted financial risk for care, his or her incentive is to provide only those services necessary to keep the covered life from requiring more costly services in the future. The financial incentive, in that case, is at odds with the provider's medical instincts.

The inevitable conflicts over what services are covered and appropriate must be resolved through some form of adjudication. Calls for a Patient's Bill of Rights and the right of patients to sue their health plans in court (rather than to take disputes to a plan-dominated review board) reflect fear that cost concerns will dominate medical decisions. Each of the chapters that follow will explore the effects of managed care on providers' decisions and financial health.

SUMMARY

Financial managers have some concerns in common in every organization: these are cost, cash, capital, and conservation. Managers in health care are no less concerned with these issues than managers in manufacturing. Finance departments perform a wide variety of functions: comptrollership, treasurership, internal auditing, and, in many organizations, information services. The CFO orchestrates all of these activities within the organization.

The financial environment, outside the CFO's control, puts important constraints on any organization. The behavior of financial actors in financial markets acts to eliminate the possibility of arbitrage profits, constraining health care organizations' access to capital and strategic opportunities.

Discussion Questions

1. Explain the differences between the duties of the comptroller and the duties of the treasurer.

2. What the time value of money? Why would there be a time value of money even if there were no possibility of inflation?

3. Why is cash flow a better measure of an organization's financial viability than profit, as recorded according to Generally Accepted Accounting Principles?

4. What is risk aversion? Are all financial actors equally risk averse? Explain.

5. Is the law of one price ever violated? Give an example and explain what circumstances made the violation of that law possible.

CONTINUING CASE

Henry Kirk and Janet Fowler were having a rare moment of quiet contemplation over lunch at Wong's, Jamestown's only good Szechuan restaurant. "Janet, I can't keep all of this straight. You're controller for the corporation and CFO for the clinic. When you tell me we have a cash flow problem, which organization are you speaking for?" Fowler had just informed Kirk of an impending cash flow shortfall.

"The corporation's and the clinic's cash situations are closely linked, so I'm speaking for both. I get confused when Dr. Jackson (Roger Jackson, largest shareholder in PCI, Inc., and lead partner of the clinic's largest tenant) treats corporation, clinic, and private practice money as if they were all his own. None of us works for the Jackson Group, but last week Dr. Jackson insisted I work up a spreadsheet to divide up his practice's earnings for the first quarter." Fowler's frustration was evident from her tone. "I did it, but I didn't like it."

"We're big enough to sort these things out. Janet, why don't you draw up organization charts for the corporation's and the clinic's financial offices, and we'll meet next week to sort out who does what, and what the overlapping areas are?"

"I can draw charts, Henry, but my name will be in every box."

That evening, after serving dinner, cleaning up, and helping Jeff and Ronnie with their homework, Janet sat down to draw organization charts. "Can't put people's names in the boxes, just the names of functions."

CASE QUESTIONS

1. What functions belong on the organization chart for the corporation (PCI, Inc.) and what functions belong on the organization chart for the clinic? (Remember that Ms. Fowler's task is to chart financial management functions only.)

2. At which organizational level do some of the basic functions (cost accounting, reporting, tax, patient accounts and billing, accounts payable) belong? What problems might arise if those functions are placed at the wrong level?

3. What is the proper relationship between the financial functions of the corporation and clinic on the one hand and those of the Jackson Group on the other?

REFERENCES

Dranove, D. (2000). *The economic evolution of American health care*. Princeton, NJ: Princeton University Press.

SELECTED READINGS

DeLew, N., Greenberg, G., & Kinchen, K. (1992, Fall). A layman's guide to the U.S. health care system. *Health Care Financing Review, 14*(1), 151-169.

Dranove, D. (2000). *The economic evolution of American health care*. Princeton, NJ: Princeton University Press.

Unland, J.J. (1991). *The trustee's guide to understanding hospital business fundamentals*. Westchester, IL: Healthcare Financial Management Association.

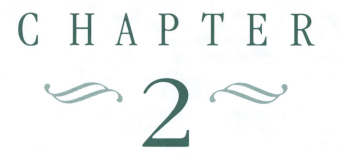

CHAPTER

2

Agency Problems and Agency Costs

Learning Objectives

After reading this chapter, the student should be able to:

1. Define agency relationships and agency costs.
2. Explain how agency relationships can generate agency costs.
3. List and explain some of the common agency relationships that exist in health care settings, and recognize them in health care settings.
4. Explain the special agency problems that managed care contracts create.
5. Explain how health care organizations can ameliorate their agency costs.

Key Terms

Agency cost

Agency problem

Agency relationship

Financial engineering

Hospital revenue bond

One visits a physician (or dentist or physical therapist) because one trusts her to deliver healing or preventive services in the patient's, and only the patient's, interest. One expects a hospital to have the range of services one needs, without regard to whether or not each of those services is profitable. One expects one's insurance carrier to pay one's bills quickly and without argument. Those are not the expectations one has about relationships with plumbers and mechanics.

The principal distinguishing features of health care organizations are the number, complexity, and importance of the **agency relationships** that exist within those organizations. Agency relationships, more than anything else, are what distinguish financial management in health care organizations from financial management in other settings (Arrow, 1963).

An agency relationship exists when one party, an agent, acts on behalf of another party, a principal (McLean, 1989). A physician acts as her patient's agent when prescribing some treatment or when admitting the patient to a hospital. An insurance carrier acts as the patient's agent when processing payment for services rendered. A medical group's administrator acts as an agent for the physicians in the group when negotiating a contact with a medical supply firm or health plan (Dranove & White, 1987). The agent need not be an employee of the principal. Generally, an agency relationship exists when any party can pursue his or her own interest while contractually obligated to represent the interests of another.

Agency relationships offer the opportunity for the agent to act in his own self-interest. Those opportunities, whether exercised or not, are known as **agency problems** (Barnea, Haugen, & Senbet, 1985). A physician can order tests that have no diagnostic value but for which she will collect a fee. An insurance carrier can refuse (or substantially delay) payment by interpreting the terms of the insurance contract at substantial cost to the patient. A hospital chief executive officer can take advantage of the absence of the board of trustees to consume perquisites on the job, such as leasing a large automobile rather than an equally serviceable, but smaller, one.

Agency costs are losses in market value (or health status) due to the presence of agency problems. If a physician orders a test whose outcome has no diagnostic value, the loss in the patient's wealth (being unmatched by any gain in the patient's health) is an agency cost to the patient. If an insurance carrier's slowness in paying claims causes physicians to bill directly those patients insured by that carrier, the interest costs to those patients (from having their funds tied up while awaiting reimbursement) is an agency cost to the patients. If lenders demand an interest premium for fear that the hospital's cash flows are diverted to managerial perquisites, the additional interest payments incurred are agency costs to the hospital.

TYPES OF AGENCY PROBLEMS

Economic and financial theory identifies five types of agency problems (Barnea, Haugen, & Senbet, 1985). First, agents may take advantage of their situations to enjoy excessive perquisites at the expense of their principles. The administrator who leases a Cadillac when a Chevrolet would do, or who takes home floppy disks for private use because no one is counting is generating such a problem. The first type of agency problem is most often found when the agent has much to gain and when the agent's behavior is difficult to monitor. Health care organizations provide both potential gains and monitoring difficulties. Indeed, in private, not-for-profit organizations, there may be no one with an incentive to monitor administrators' use of resources. Boards of trustees are seldom present to monitor management. Also, in not-for-profit organizations the trustees, unable to receive any share of profit, have little incentive to monitor management or staff. Monitoring physicians is notoriously difficult because it is hard for nonphysicians to determine which tests and treatments are appropriate and which are not.

The second class of agency problems includes situations in which equity holders decide to undertake projects that are "too risky," that is, projects whose risks will not be adequately rewarded. The rationale for this type of agency problem lies in option pricing theory. Equity holders have the equivalent of an option to buy (a call option) the full value of the firm from lenders. The option can be exercised by paying off the face value of the firm's outstanding debt. The option expires on the day the outstanding debt matures (the day the outstanding principle and debt are due). Option pricing theory says that call option values rise when the riskiness of the underlying assets rises (Black and Scholes, 1973). Thus equity holders can increase the values of their shares by undertaking risk in excess of that which the market will reward. Further, because the holders of debt securities will bear at least some of any losses that the equity holders' risky decisions produce, it is the firm's bondholders who bear this type of agency cost. This type of agency problem is most likely to appear when shareholders are in control of the organization's management, and when there is a substantial amount of debt outstanding. Such a situation is typical of a medical group practice that has borrowed to finance equipment and facilities or of for-profit organizations that are closely held (have few shareholders) and are deeply in debt.

In a third type of agency problem, stockholders reject potentially profitable investments. Chapter 10 will develop the proposition that the organization should undertake any investment whose net present value is greater than zero. Organizations that have substantial amounts of debt, like many health care organizations, will not always do that. If the value of debt claims exceeds the net present value of assets, bondholders will gain a share of the increase in value from any investment. Because shareholders will not receive all of the gain from an investment, some profitable projects will be ignored. The result may be, especially for hospitals in financial distress, socially undesirable reluctance to invest.

A fourth type of agency problem occurs when organizations are in sufficient financial distress to enter formal bankruptcy proceedings. Some of the claimants to a share of the organization might, out of concern for "getting their share," demand legal proceedings and liquidation. Those proceedings and the liquidation process reduce the value of the organization that can be realized by all claimants.

The last type of agency problem is due to informational asymmetry. If managers have information that others do not, several undesirable outcomes can occur. In some cases, managers can benefit at the expense of stakeholders by acting on their superior information (as in selling securities just before public announcements of bad news). In other cases, when managers cannot inform other stakeholders of the desirability of some course of action, desirable actions may be forgone. That is, the cost of providing (for example) trustees with enough information for the trustees to know that a new product line is justified may be so high as to eliminate the benefit of a new product line. In health care organizations, important expert knowledge is not widely shared. Trustees typically have less knowledge of market conditions and of emerging technologies than do managers and physicians. That informational asymmetry may cause important projects to be abandoned.

COST CONTROL AND AGENCY PROBLEMS

A hospital, like any production unit, must control its costs. Failure to keep costs within the limits implied by revenues causes losses that, if continued, mean bankruptcy and closure. When the federal government imposed fixed reimbursement rates for each diagnosis-related group (DRG) for patients covered by Medicare beginning in 1983, the pressure to control costs intensified as never before. A set of important agency relationships severely limits the ability of any hospital to control its costs.

Although cost control is usually considered a financial concern, operating decisions actually determine the majority of hospital costs. In hospitals, who is responsible for the decisions that determine the level of most operating costs? In the hospital, then, several agency relationships can lead to cost control difficulties. Management's consumption of perquisites is difficult to monitor. Not only can physicians consume perquisites; they can, with the same effect, use the resources of the organization to perform tests and procedures beyond what is medically "necessary." Physicians' behavior and the outcomes of tests and procedures are notoriously difficult to monitor. Physicians have strong incentives to engage in cost-inflating practices, both to serve their patients' needs (at the hospital's expense) and to avoid legal liabilities.

AGENCY PROBLEMS IN HEALTH CARE FINANCE

There are many agency problems in health care organization beyond cost control. Some of these have serious financial repercussions. Consider first the familiar relationship between the physician and the patient. The physician acts as the patient's agent in a variety of ways. The patient, because of legal restrictions and lack of expert knowledge, can neither diagnose his or her ailments nor prescribe his or her medication. The patient contracts with the physician to perform those services. The physician *can* use this relationship to perform (and to charge for) unnecessary services. The present value of all of the unnecessary services for any given patient is the agency cost to that patient. In any particular physician-patient relationship, that agency cost can vary from zero to some extremely high number. It is no surprise to those who understand agency theory that when the physician is liable for the cost of the services provided, as in the case of a physician-owned health maintenance organization, the utilization of some services decreases.

The physician is also the agent of the patient in selecting a hospital and in prescribing hospital services. Although the physician will receive no direct compensation for the services provided by the hospital, those services can enhance the physician's own productivity and can reduce the probability of the physician's being subject to a professional liability suit. Thus the physician may overprescribe in this aspect of the relationship as well.

Not only is the physician the patient's agent in the selection of a hospital and in ordering hospital services, but the physician is also an agent for the hospital in managing the utilization of the hospital's resources (Pauly, 1980). The medical staff make decisions as to resource utilization: for admissions, for tests, for the use of operating suites, even for the delivery of special dietary services. Whereas trustees and management may determine what product lines are offered, within product lines the staff physicians command the organization's resources. Except in rare cases, staff physicians are not hospital employees but are independent contractors (Harris, 1977). The implications for cost control and for the profitability of hospitals is profound. Cost control will be more rigorous either when physicians are employees (as in the military and in the Department of Veterans Affairs) or when physicians own a stake in the hospital (as in so-called proprietary hospitals).

In their own practices, however, managed care has given some physicians strong incentives to alter their behavior. McLean (1989) argues that the cost-saving incentives for HMO panel members are due to their becoming principles, as well as agents, in their treatment relationships. Consider the physician who agrees to accept $50 per month to act as primary care physician (PCP) for Patient X. He is responsible for all medical services to that patient and (typically) suffers a penalty for all referrals to specialists. Patient X then "presents" with unusual or conflicting symptoms. What are the physician's incentives with regard to referrals, costly tests, and continuous monitoring? The patient relies on the physician to ignore the financial incentives, and to act in his best interest. Loss of wealth and deteriorating health status are (potentially) the agency costs to the patient. But, by ordering such tests, the physician potentially loses wealth.

In the same situation, the health plan is also both principal and agent, agent to the patient, and principal in its own sphere. Consider the case in which the PCP refers Patient X for surgery, for which the plan is obligated to pay. What is the plan's incentive? Feldstein (1998, especially Chapter 9) argues that competition among health plans will ameliorate the possible agency costs. To be effective in that, however, the competition must be at the level of choice of the consumer, or that of an employer that is a perfect agent for its employees.

The management of a hospital acts as the agent of the equity holders of the hospital. Managers have varying degrees of opportunity to consume perquisites at work at the expense of the bottom line. The Cadillac rather than the Chevrolet, for the chief executive officer, the club membership, or the lavish continuing education budget all represent situations in which management may be imposing agency costs on the equity holders. In investor-owned organizations, the threat of corporate takeover can discipline managements and prevent extravagant perquisite consumption. In private, not-for-profit hospitals, on the other hand, there is no threat of corporate takeover and little incentive for the trustees who represent the (nonexistent) equity holders to police management's perquisite consumption. Agency costs due to management perquisite consumption ought, then, to be greater in the not-for-profit than in the investor-owned sector.

Equity holders and managers are, at various times, the agents of bondholders. Many health care organizations have very high ratios of debt-to-equity financing. Equity holders, then, have strong incentives to undertake risky activities, which have the possibility of enriching equity and have the possibility of wiping out the claims of bondholders. The financing decisions, the project selection (capital budgeting) choices, and the risk level (strategic financial management) choices of health care organizations, then, are affected by this type of agency problem.

RESOLVING AGENCY PROBLEMS

Health care organizations are rife with agency relationships and potential agency costs. Agency costs are the reductions in the market value of the organizations that are the result of investors' reluctance to invest in organizations in which agency relationships are important. When investors are aware of agents' (especially managements') abilities to pursue their own interest, the organization can acquire outside financing only at high cost, if at all. When agency relationships threaten to undermine the value of an organization or to interfere with the access to financial capital, principals and their agents can arrange complex contracts to shift incentives to eliminate those agency costs. These contracts are designed to make principals' and agents' incentives coincide. Those contracts can change the agents' incentives to prevent their doing what investors fear. Health care organizations have developed several complex contracts to alleviate the agency costs that are so common in the health care sector. Some of these complex contracts are so familiar that their role in reducing agency costs is not obvious.

In investor-owned organizations, the resolution of some types of agency problems is relatively simple. Paying professionals and managers for their performances (the determination of which, one must recognize, requires effective monitoring), profit sharing (not allowed in not-for-profit organizations), and partial ownership are all means of aligning the interests of agents and principals. A fairly recent innovation in the compensation of medical practice managers, for example, is the inclusion of the managers as partners in the practice's net income.

Financial engineering is the term applied to the formation of contracts that have unusual cash flow patterns (Financial Management Association, 1988). Mortgage pass-through securities, in which the investor receives a monthly payment based on receipts of payments against a pool of mortgages, were among the first popular examples of financial engineering. More recently, securities whose periodic payments to investors are based on collections of hospital patient accounts have been engineered into the marketplace. Most of the examples of financial engineering that health care organizations (and their financial advisers) have introduced are intended to alleviate investors' fears of agency costs and thus to reduce the cost of capital to the issuing organization.

In many parts of the United States, hospitals owned by units of local government receive only a small amount of their resources from the public treasury. Rural hospitals owned by county governments in many states, for example, receive little or no assistance from county tax revenues. When these organizations need external financing to acquire long-term assets, they can go to several sources. Local banks are one source of external financing. Another is mortgage financing, with a mortgage loan secured by the asset in question (an off-site clinic or a mobile piece of equipment, for example). The municipal bond market usually offers financing at lower cost than either bank or mortgage loans due to the tax advantages that holding municipal debt confers on the investor. Municipalities *could* issue general obligation bonds (municipal bonds whose payment obligations are backed by the general tax revenues of the issuing unit of government) to finance public hospital capital needs; in fact, they almost never do so.

In place of general obligation financing, almost all municipal bonds issued to support hospital facility construction and equipment purchases are **hospital revenue bonds**. Hospital revenue bonds are guaranteed only by the revenues of the hospital for whose benefit they are issued. General obligation bonds would carry much less default risk (less risk that the hospital would not meet in principal and interest payments) than hospital revenue bonds. After all, they would be backed by local tax revenues *and* by hospital revenues. Why then are hospital revenue bonds almost always the preferred financing mechanism?

The answer lies in the agency relationships that surround municipally owned hospitals. The senior managements of those organizations are agents of the units of government that own them. Were those managers relieved of the duty of meeting their debt obligations by the taxing authority's promising to pick up the tab, they would be free to make the "wrong" capital investment decisions. They could invest in pet projects (their own or those of their medical staffs) that would not generate sufficient cash flows to meet their debt obligations. Were general obligation bonds used to fund hospital projects, hospital managements would not be subject to the discipline of the capital market.

Note that this special type of financial contract, the hospital revenue bond, is only necessary in organizations like public hospitals. Other public projects (street improvements, for example) can be funded by general obligation bonds, as city and county governments do not expect streets to generate revenues. Investor-owned health care corporations do not need to issue bonds for specific projects because the firm as a whole is under the discipline of the financial marketplace, and managers who ignore the need to generate cash flows can be fired. It is the agency relationships in public organizations that generate the need for hospital revenue bonds.

SUMMARY

One of the distinguishing characteristics of health care organizations is the multiplicity of agency relationships that exist within them. In health care organizations, unlike other types of firms, financial agency relationships are complicated by agency relationships in the market for the service provided. Thus in health care, as in any setting, managers are agents of equity holders and equity holders and managers are both agents of debt holders. In health care organizations, however, physicians are agents of patients, as are third-party insurance carriers.

The professional relationships that are so important in the delivery of health care create complicated agency relationships of their own. Nonphysician professionals (nurses, medical technologists, the various allied health therapists who deliver much of hospital care) all become agents of physicians in the delivery of care. Managers and boards of trustees become agents of the medical staff in their selection of product lines and equipment, even though the medical staff are not actually principals in any meaningful way in the hospital.

All of these agency relationships (and all of the agency costs they can generate) have profound implications for financial management and for the financial aspects of the strategic management of health care organizations. Obtaining external financing often requires financial engineering to alleviate investors' fears of agency costs. Capital acquisition decisions are often conditioned by complex interprofessional agency relationships. Beginning with Part Three, agency relationships will dominate many of the topics that follow.

Discussion Questions

1. Define *agency relationship*. In what agency relationships are you now involved?

2. Can there be agency relations in which there are no agency problems? Explain.

3. What is the role of monitoring in ameliorating agency costs? What are some of the difficulties involved in monitoring the behavior of managers and health care professionals?

4. How has the ability to issue hospital revenue bonds changed the risk/return position of hospital lenders? Of hospital borrowers?

5. Cite an example of financial engineering (from health care or any other business setting) and explain how it helped resolve an agency problem.

6. Explain how managed care contracts change agents' incentives to control costs. What agency costs are eliminated, and what new ones are created?

CONTINUING CASE

Most mornings, Henry Kirk is happy to go to work. Mr. Kirk is both the chief executive officer of Physicians' Clinic and chief operating officer of its parent, PCI. He has performed well for his employer over the years and hopes someday to convince the board of PCI that he should be allowed to purchase shares and should be promoted to CEO. For the time being, however, Mr. Kirk is well paid to see that the clinic is properly managed and that its interests are represented in local affairs.

After breakfasting with Kate, his wife of 20 years, Henry drives to work in the Buick Park Avenue that the clinic provides him. It was 3 years ago that he convinced the executive committee that he needed a company car for his trips about town and that the Chevrolet Impala that Dr. Whatley's brother offered to sell to PCI would not be adequate for the task. Kate has recently suggested, several times, in fact, that when the lease on the Park Avenue expires (next month) a Ford Expedition sport-utility vehicle would be a nice replacement. Not only does Henry sometimes need to pick up office and medical supplies for the clinic ("they would fit so nicely in the back of a big SUV, dear"), but the large vehicle would be more comfortable for Henry, Kate, the two boys, and Sasha (their intimidating, but good-natured, German shepherd) on their annual vacation.

After a 10-minute drive to the clinic, Henry settles into his comfortable office. A check of e-mail on his Palm Pilot reveals nothing, and he decides to read the *Wall Street Journal* and to scan this week's issue of *Modern Healthcare*. The rollers on his big leather chair have an annoying tendency to sink into the pile carpet ("make a note to have Jerry in maintenance get a plastic floor pad for me"), and Henry spends a few seconds adjusting his seating. A memo from Dr. Jackson is on top of *Modern Healthcare*, and Henry's pulse quickens when he sees it again. It's been festering on the desk for several weeks, and the executive committee will want a response soon.

Dr. Jackson is both the largest single shareholder in PCI and the senior-most partner in the clinic's largest tenant. When Dr. Jackson speaks or writes a memo, Henry Kirk listens. Jackson's most recent idea could make all of the shareholders in PCI rich (again, Henry thinks how good it would be to be the first nontenant shareholder in PCI). He wants PCI to enter into a joint agreement with the Jackson Group. PCI would borrow heavily from a big Dallas bank that has been trying to drum up high-quality loan business in Clearwater County. With the funds, PCI would open a fully equipped outpatient imaging center on the site of a defunct convenience store, one block from Memorial Hospital.

The Jackson Group would put up none of its own capital for the imaging center but would staff it 16 hours per day. The gist of Dr. Jackson's memo is that there is little risk to PCI, as the bank loan would be secured by the equipment in the center. If things don't work out, PCI could walk away from the assets, its local reputation and credit rating intact. "Stick it to those Dallas bankers," is how Dr. Jackson put the matter privately.

Henry is not so sure about the limited risk exposure of PCI. Dr. Jackson has responded that he would not put PCI at risk, as he holds the largest single interest in the holding company. Henry is unaccustomed to thinking about creative finance, but the executive committee wants a response. It's enough to worry about for most of the morning.

Lunch offers a nice diversion. PCI holds a corporate membership in the Clearwater Golf Club, and Henry often eats there. The buffet is excellent, and Henry uses the time to visit with his broker.

After lunch, Henry meets with Janet Fowler, the controller of PCI and of the clinic. There's a problem with rent collections again, and this time the situation is very delicate. The Jackson Group has been slow with its rent check. Dr. Jackson says that he's instructed his office manager to hold cash as long as possible and that he wishes Janet would learn to do the same. Besides, why should Jackson take money out of his Jackson Group pocket to put into his PCI pocket? If the Group doesn't pay today, the clinic will have to tap its line of credit at CCB Bank to meet the week's payroll. Henry agrees, reluctantly, to call the Group's office manager. He also tells Janet to alert the bank; no use taking chances.

CASE QUESTIONS

1. Identify the agency problems that PCI and Physicians' Clinic need to resolve.

2. Identify the agency costs that PCI shareholders suffer.

3. How might some of those agency costs be reduced?

4. What agency problems will be involved if PCI goes though with the joint venture that Dr. Jackson has proposed?

5. What sort of financial contracts might the Dallas bankers require of PCI so that they don't suffer the agency costs that Dr. Jackson is willing to impose on them?

REFERENCES

Arrow, K.J. (1963). Uncertainty and the welfare economics of medical care. *American Economic Review, 53*(5), 941-973.

Barnea, A., Haugen, R.A., & Senbet, L.W. (1985). *Agency problems and financial contracting.* Englewood Cliffs, NJ: Prentice-Hall.

Black, F., and M. Scholes (1973). The pricing of options and corporate liabilities. *Journal of Political Economy, 81*(3), 637-654.

Dranove, D. & White, W.D. (1987). Agency and the organization of health care delivery. *Inquiry, 24*(4), 405-415.

Feldstein, P.N. (1998). *Health care economics* (5th ed.). Clifton Park, NY: Delmar.

Financial Management Association. (1988). *Financial management* (special symposium on financial engineering), 17(4).

Harris J.E. (1977). The internal organization of hospitals: Some economic implications. *Bell Journal of Economics, 8*, 647-682.

McLean, R.A. (1989). Agency costs and complex contracts in health care organizations. *Health Care Management Review, 14*(1), 65-71.

Pauly, M.V. (1980). *Doctors and their workshops*. Chicago, IL: University of Chicago Press.

SELECTED READINGS

Barnea, A., Haugen, R.A., & Senbet, L.W. (1985). *Agency problems and financial contracting*. Englewood Cliffs, NJ: Prentice-Hall.

Jensen, M.C. & Meckling, W.H. (1976). Theory of the firm: Managerial behavior, agency costs, and ownerstructure. *Journal of Financial Economics, 3*(4), 305-360.

McLean, R.A. (1989). Agency costs and complex contracts in health care organizations. *Health Care Management Review, 14*(1), 65-71.

Smith, C.W., Jr., & Smithson, C.W. (Eds.). (1990). *The handbook of financial engineering*. New York: Harper Business.

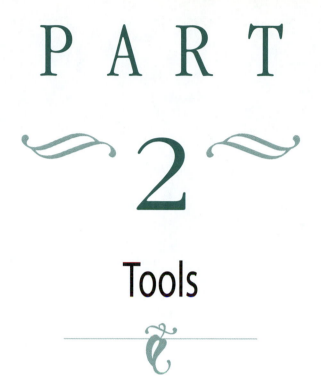

PART

2

Tools

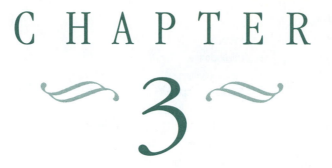

Accounting and Cash Flow Analysis

Learning Objectives

After reading this chapter, the student should be able to:

1. Explain basic accounting rules under the accrual principle, including how accrual results differ from results under cash accounting.
2. Interpret the individual items in financial statements.
3. Define major accounting terms.
4. Make simple bookkeeping entries.
5. Begin the study of financial statement analysis in Chapter 4.

Key Terms

Accelerated depreciation

Accounting cycle

Accrual principle

Asset

Auditors

Auditor's opinion

Balance sheet

Basic accounting equation

Budgeting

Cash flow statement

Certified Healthcare Finance
   Professional (CHFP)

Conservatism

Contra-asset

Cost of goods sold (CGS)

Credit

Current assets

Current liabilities

Debit

Deferred tax liability

Depreciation

Diagnosis-related group (DRG)

Fellow of the Healthcare
   Financial Management
   Association (FHFMA)

Financial accountant

Financial Accounting
   Standards Board (FASB)

Financial reporting

First in–first out (FIFO)

Footnotes

Full disclosure

Fund accounting

Generally Accepted
   Accounting Principles
   (GAAP)

Going concern

Government Accounting
   Standards Board (GASB)

Healthcare Financial
   Management Association
   (HFMA)

Historical costs

Income statement

Internal audit

Journal entry

Last in–first out (LIFO)

Liability

Managerial accountant

Modified accelerated cost
   recovery system (MACRS)

Monetary terms

Net assets

Owners' equity

Post

Straight-line depreciation

Systems design

Trial balance

Variance analysis

Financial management involves the selection, financing, and stewardship of an organization's assets. In practicing financial management, one's decisions must have a logical basis; they must be defensible. To find the course of financial action that maximizes the well-being of the organization's stakeholders, the manager has to calculate. He or she must look to the actual records of the organization to determine how things have worked in the past. He or she must calculate the potential effects of alternative courses of action. He or she must be able to determine the costs and benefits of possible actions through analysis of data.

This chapter and the remainder of Part Two, are about calculations. In this chapter the basics of financial accounting are explored, and accounting numbers are compared to figures based on cash flows. Accounting numbers and cash flow data tell quite different stories about the financial health of any organization, and both are important for the financial decision maker. This chapter, although adequate to follow Chapter 4, is no substitute for serious study of accounting.

Accounting numbers such as revenue, expenses, net income, assets, liabilities, and owners' equity (which may go by several names in various health care organizations) are the "raw material" for financial decisions. It is in accounting records that the firm's transactions, and its cash inflows and outflows, are recorded. The only genuine record of the firm's financial health is in its accounting records and statements.

WHY LEARN ACCOUNTING?

Financial management is so dependent on accounting records that many people, including many financial professionals, believe that financial management *is* accounting. Many hospitals, for example, hire accountants, and only accountants, to perform their treasury functions. Although accountants have the "inside track" on the use of financial data (they are, after all, the experts in recording and summarizing those data), one need not be an accountant to make correct, careful decisions about selecting, financing, and caring for the firm's assets. However, every financial manager, and every manager who deals with financial decisions, must know at least the rudiments of accounting.

Accounting is, first, the language of business. Business records are kept by accountants. Organizations communicate their financial health to lenders, regulators, and potential partners in accounting terms. Ignorance of the difference between net patient revenue and net income can lead to terrible decisions. Accounting is a language that every manager needs to master.

Second, the clearest picture of the *past* financial health of the firm is that presented in its financial statements. The income statement, the balance sheet, and the cash flow statement provide, for the trained reader, detailed information about the firm's financial strength and success in previous periods. To read and understand financial statements, one must understand the accounting rules according to which they were constructed. Serious misinterpretations of financial health are inevitable for the reader who does not understand how the entries in the financial statements were calculated.

Finally, knowledge of financial accounting is important for the manager who is involved in cost analysis and budgeting. Virtually every manager, in health care and elsewhere, has to prepare a budget. To prepare a budget, the manager must know how his or her department's costs change over time and as service volume changes. Information about costs is embedded in accounting data on expenses. The manager who does not have at least a passing understanding of accounting has ceded leadership to the firm's accountants.

FIELDS OF ACCOUNTING PRACTICE

Just as health care managers specialize (in long-term care, hospitals, or medical group management), accountants specialize as well. Seldom does an accountant perform the full range of accounting services, either for his employer or for clients. Rather, accountants, either in public practice or in private employment, tend to concentrate their attention in one of five areas: financial, managerial, auditing, tax, and systems.

The **financial accountant** is usually employed by an operating organization, such as a hospital or clinic. The financial accountant designs procedures for the recording of transactions, supervises that record-keeping function, and is responsible for summarizing those records in financial statements. An organization's financial accountants are responsible for the **financial reporting** function within the comptroller's department.

The **managerial accountant** (once known as the cost accountant) is also employed by an operating organization. Her job is to take information about the costs of doing business from the financial records. Once those cost data are captured, the managerial accountant analyzes them to find out how costs change with changing volume and how well management is doing at controlling costs. The managerial accountant plays important roles in **budgeting** and in **variance analysis.** Accountants employed by operating organizations are not required by law to achieve the Certified Public Accountant (CPA) designation (although some employers may require that designation for professional advancement). Those who wish can earn a special designation, Certified Management Accountant (CMA).

Auditors can work either for operating organizations or for public accounting firms. In public practice, auditors are charged with verifying that the firm's financial statements are prepared in accordance with **Generally Accepted Accounting Principles (GAAP)**. Securities law requires that every organization whose shares are sold to the public at large have its financial statements audited. Lenders, third-party insurance carriers, and regulators also require audits of health care organizations' financial statements. An acceptable external audit can be made only by a CPA who has no financial ties to the organization he is auditing.

Many operating organizations, including most hospitals, have developed **internal audit** capability. The internal auditor's job is to ensure that adequate records, both financial and operating, are maintained to support the financial statements that the organization presents. The internal auditor tries to make sure that all of the assertions that the firm will make about itself are supported by documentation and that the financial accountant's record-keeping procedures are followed. The internal auditor may also be responsible for assuring that internal financial control procedures are followed. Internal auditors may be CPAs but need not be. Those who perform this function have developed a testing and certification program of their own, leading to designation as a Certified Internal Auditor (CIA).

Partially as a result of the growing importance of computers and of distributed data entry (many persons entering financial and other data at widely separated terminals), a growing field of accounting is **systems design**. The systems designer creates and installs computer hardware/software combinations to serve the needs of organizations' financial and managerial accountants. Most of those who practice accounting information systems design are consultants, offering their services to many organizations. Given the size of the health care industry, it is no surprise that several consulting firms provide those services exclusively to health care organizations.

Accounting (and other aspects of financial management practice) in health care organizations requires specialized knowledge. In recognition of that fact, the **Healthcare Financial Management Association (HFMA)** has established its own education and professional certification programs. A financial professional employed in a health care organization (or in related consulting and educational organizations) can seek designation first, as a **Certified Healthcare Finance Professional (CHFP)**, and, later, as **Fellow of the Healthcare Financial Management Association (FHFMA)**. Although many senior financial professionals in health care organizations do not hold them (and do quite well professionally), these designations are widely recognized as certifying high levels of professional training and competence.

ACCOUNTING PRINCIPLES: WHAT ARE THEY AND WHO MAKES THEM UP?

Modern financial accounting emerged from double-entry bookkeeping, the recording of transactions as self-balancing entries. Financial accounting, however, is more than merely making two book entries per transaction. It is based on a set of underlying principles, GAAP, that guide both the nature of the bookkeeping entries made and their interpretations.

An assumption that underlies all of financial accounting is that the entity (or organization or firm) is that of the **going concern**. That is, the entity is assumed to exist in the current time period and to continue to exist for the foreseeable future. One consequence of the going concern assumption is that the entity's assets and obligations must balance. The **basic accounting equation** must hold now and at all times in the future. The basic accounting identity is

$$\text{Assets} = \text{Liabilities} + \text{Owners' equity}$$

Assets are all of the things, tangible and intangible, that the entity owns. Most of those assets are tangible, such as beds, syringes, and cash on hand. Some of those assets, however, are intangible; they cannot be seen, touched, or picked up. Among intangible assets are goodwill, prepaid expenses, and accounts receivable. Assets that will cease to exist within one accounting period, usually a year, are **current assets**. Many current assets, such as accounts receivable, are intangible. However, inventory, a very tangible asset, is also a current asset. Cash, which may remain on hand for a long time, is also a current asset.

Liabilities are all of the items that the entity owes to others. Accounts payable (expenses already incurred but not yet paid), interest payable (interest expense incurred but not yet paid), and long-term debt are examples of the organization's liabilities. Liabilities that are due within the current accounting period, usually a year, are called **current liabilities**.

The difference between the value of the entity's assets and its liabilities is its **owners' equity**. Owners' equity is a residual account. There is nothing tangible that one can identify as belonging to the organization's shareholders, partners, or government. Owners' equity is also something of a fiction. In principle, it is what the owners could claim were the entity to be liquidated. In fact, the market values of assets are seldom equal to the values at which they are recorded in the accounting records (their book values). There is no guarantee that owners could actually receive an amount equal to the owners' equity account balance.

In not-for-profit organizations and in government organizations, there are neither shareholders nor partners to claim the owners' equity account. As a result, that account is identified as the **net assets**. Until the early 1990s, that entry was called "fund balance," a term derived from the type of accounting that these organizations do, **fund accounting** (Seawell, 1992, Chapter 15; Hay & Wilson, 1992, Chapters 2–5).

The two sides of the fundamental accounting identity are usually called the **debit** side (left-hand side) and the **credit** side (right-hand side). The two terms have no meaning in this context other than left-hand and right-hand. There is nothing honorific associated with credit accounts and no negative connotation associated with debit accounts. One can rewrite the fundamental accounting equation as follows:

$$\text{Debits} = \text{Credits}$$

In order for the basic accounting identity to be met at all times, debits must equal credits for every transaction. Figure 3–1 shows how various transactions are classified as debits (abbreviated as *dr*) or credits (abbreviated as *cr*).

Another basic accounting principle is **conservatism**. Most assets should be valued conservatively, usually at their **historical costs**. When, for example, land is purchased and held for long periods of time, the value recorded in the asset accounts is not to be increased to show changes in the land's market value. Rather, the land remains on the books at its historical cost as long as it is there. Some assets whose market values are easily observable are exempt from this standard. Marketable securities (stocks and bonds, for example) are recorded at their current market value.

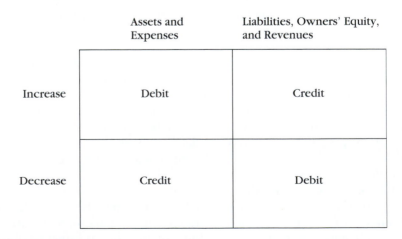

	Assets and Expenses	Liabilities, Owners' Equity, and Revenues
Increase	Debit	Credit
Decrease	Credit	Debit

Figure 3-1 Rules for debit and credit entries.

An accounting principle so basic that its importance is easily overlooked is that all information must be recorded in **monetary terms**. Some of the most interesting problems for financial accountants arise from the need to record not "one light-weight red pickup truck with an air conditioner and automatic transmission," but a monetary value.

Accounting reports may not conceal relevant information. If they did, they would not be useful to those who rely on them: investors, lenders, regulators, and internal management. Thus financial statements are to present a complete picture of the entity's financial position, "warts and all." That is, accounting statements must represent **full disclosure**.

The **accrual principle** requires that revenues be recorded in the period in which the associated service is performed, and that expenses be recorded in the period in which they are incurred, regardless of whether or not cash has changed hands. The accrual principle is intended to make financial accounting records show the flow of resources, rather than the flow of cash, through the entity. It also creates the need for such accounts as accounts payable and accounts receivable and requires the measurement of depreciation expense.

If some of the principles underlying financial accounting are controversial (the accrual principle introduces substantial room for ambiguity in the financial records), one must ask from whence those principles come. Who determines which organizations must adopt accrual accounting? Are the principles outlined above immutable, or do they and their interpretations change from time to time?

The principal rule-making body in financial accounting in the United States today is the **Financial Accounting Standards Board (FASB)**, chartered for that purpose by the U.S. Congress in 1973 (Miller & Redding, 1988). The FASB took the standard-setting authority that had previously been exercised by the Accounting Principles Board (APB) of the American Institute of Certified Public Accountants (AICPA). Unless they have been specifically modified by the FASB, all AICPA-APB pronouncements remain in force.

Governmental entities, including health care organizations owned by agencies of government, are governed by another accounting group, the **Governmental Accounting Standards Board (GASB)**, formed in 1984 (Hay & Wilson, 1992, pp. 1–6). The jurisdictions of the GASB and the FASB are not always as clearly defined as they seem, and conflicts of rules do occur (Garner & Grossman, 1991). Those organizations whose securities (stocks and bonds, other than municipal bonds) are sold to the public at large are also subject to accounting oversight by the United States Securities and Exchange Commission, a federal regulatory body (Pointer & Schroeder, 1986).

Current financial reporting standards require three basic financial statements. The **balance sheet** shows the balance between assets and liabilities plus owners' equity. The balance sheet shows a snapshot of the entity at the end of the reporting period.

The **income statement** (statement of profit and loss, operating statement, or statement of revenues and expenses) shows the revenues, expenses, and net income of the entity over the course of the reporting period. The income statement is like a videotape of the entity *calculated in accrual terms*. The **cash flow statement**, on the other hand, shows the flow of cash into and out of the entity over the course of the reporting period. It is like a videotape of the entity *in cash flow terms*. The three statements, interpreted properly, tell much about the performance and the health of the organization for the reporting period.

An integral part of the accounting statements are the accompanying **footnotes**. These explain and elaborate such issues as the dollar value of uncompensated care, the method of calculating pension fund expense, and any pending legal actions that could generate liabilities in the future. A full analysis of the financial statements requires a careful reading of their footnotes.

THE ACCOUNTING CYCLE

Every transaction, every monetary or physical exchange, between the entity and the outside world generates two bookkeeping entries. That is the essence of double-entry bookkeeping. From those double entries come budget information, cost data, and, ultimately, financial statements for auditors' examination. The steps that lead from the original bookkeeping entries to financial statements constitute the **accounting cycle**. Figure 3–2 summarizes the accounting cycle.

The first step in the cycle is the **journal entry**. Equal debit and credit entries are made in the organization's general journal. Samples of those entries, for several key types of transactions, are illustrated in the next section. Entries in the general journal are the raw data for all further accounting calculations.

At regular intervals, perhaps daily or weekly, journal entries are **posted** to account ledgers. Computerized accounting makes automatic and instantaneous posting possible. Separate accounts are maintained for each major revenue and expense item and for each major class of asset, liability, and equity. Asset accounts, if a positive amount of the assets are held, have debit balances. A revenue account, if positive amounts of that revenue item have been received, has a credit balance.

After posting, a **trial balance** is computed. The trial balance is a test for the consistency and accuracy of the bookkeeping process. All of the debit account balances are totaled, as are all of the credit account balances. If the transactions have been recorded in the books properly, and if the posting process has been done accurately, the total of the debit balances will exactly equal the total of the credit balances.

At longer, but regular, intervals, the account ledgers are summarized in the three basic financial statements. At this point, the books must balance. That is, in

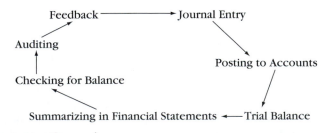

Figure 3-2 The accounting cycle.

the balance sheet, assets must equal the total of liabilities plus owners' equity (or of liabilities plus net assets). Further, the period's net income (profit, or excess of revenues over expenses), less any distribution of profit to shareholders, must equal the period's net change in owners' equity.

SOME BASIC ACCOUNTING ENTRIES

The following series of transactions illustrates the use of the general journal and the manner in which the entries are made. In this section, a set of entries are made under the accrual principle. In the section that follows, the same transactions are recorded on a cash flow basis.

Consider Home Health Services Corporation (HHSC), an investor-owned organization, established to provide home health care services in a suburban market. In Table 3–1, the initial investors provide $100,000 in cash to start HHSC. Because cash is an asset, a debit entry for $100,000 is made and labeled as "Cash" to indicate the account ledger to which the amount will later be posted. To maintain the balance of the fundamental accounting identity, a credit entry is necessary. The initial $100,000 establishes the shareholders' claim against the organization, so the appropriate credit entry is an owner's equity entry, "paid-in capital."

Now capitalized, HHSC is ready to begin offering its services. Prior to beginning operations, HHSC was awarded a contract to provide home health visits on behalf of its county's health department. The terms of the contract are for visits to be compensated at the fixed rate of $50 per visit. The county insists that it pay HHSC for the visits made in each quarter only at the end of the quarter.

In its first month of operation, January, HHSC provided 120 home health visits for the county. Because January is only the first month of the quarter, the county makes no cash payment to HHSC. In fact, HHSC will receive no cash for January's visits until early April. The 120 visits were provided, however, and the management of HHSC is reasonably certain that payment will be made (the County Health Director signed the contract, after all), so the accrual principle requires that HHSC record (recognize or book) the associated revenues in January.

Table 3–2 shows the general journal double entries for recognition of January's revenues. Notice that the entries make no mention of cash, which is unaffected. Rather, a different asset, *accounts receivable*, increases with a debit entry of $6,000. The corresponding credit entry, required to maintain balance in the fundamental accounting identity, is to increase *revenues* by $6,000.

Three nurses make home health visits for HHSC. HHSC pays them as independent contractors at the rate of $35 per visit. At the end of January, checks are written to the nurses for a total of $4,200. As the checks deplete HHSC's cash hold-

Table 3-1 Initial contribution of capital

Date	Transaction	dr	cr
1/1/20XX	Cash	$100,000.00	
	Paid-in capital		$100,000.00

Table 3-2 First revenues received

Date	Transaction	dr	cr
1/31/20XX	Accounts receivable	$6,000.00	
	Revenue		$6,000.00

ings, the cash account must be decreased with a credit entry. The balancing debit entry is an expense, labeled "nursing service expense." Table 3–3 illustrates this entry.

In January, management decided to purchase a personal computer system to use in managing HHSC's accounts. The cost to purchase and install the system was $6,000. That purchase involved an exchange of one type of asset (cash) for another (computing equipment). HHSC's accountant debited "computing equipment" and credited "cash." Because the benefits of the purchase of the computer will be enjoyed over several accounting periods, the accrual principle dictates that the purchase not be treated as an expense in the month of purchase. Rather, the "computing equipment" (asset) account is increased with a debit entry, and the cash (asset) account is decreased with a credit entry, each for $6,000. Table 3–4 illustrates this entry.

Clearly, the addition of the computer system involves an expense of some type at some time for HHSC. The accrual convention requires that the expense of the system be recognized not at the time of purchase (the time of the cash flow), but as the benefits of the use of the system are enjoyed. That is, an expense is recognized in each period during the useful life of the asset. That periodic expense is known as **depreciation**.

Depreciation

In common usage, *depreciation* means "loss of value." One might say, for example, that a new automobile depreciates the moment it is driven off the sales lot. Engineers say that a piece of equipment depreciates as it is used up or worn out. In accounting,

Table 3-3 Nursing service expense incurred

Date	Transaction	dr	cr
1/31/20XX	Nursing service expense	$4,200.00	
	Cash		$4,200.00

Table 3-4 Purchase of computing equipment for cash

Date	Transaction	dr	cr
1/15/20XX	Computing equipment	$6,000.00	
	Cash		$6,000.00

depreciation has a very different meaning. Depreciation expense is neither a measure of the using up of an asset nor an indication of its loss of market value. Accounting depreciation is *only* an expense item that allocates the historical cost of an asset to the years of its useful life. The selection of the means of allocating that cost need not correspond to the actual loss of market value of the asset over its life.

The simplest means of allocating the historical cost of an asset over its useful life is **straight-line depreciation**. Under straight-line depreciation, one begins with the full historical cost of the asset: its purchase price plus the other costs (delivery, installation) associated with bringing it into service. From that historical cost, one subtracts the expected salvage value at the end of the asset's useful life. The remainder is the basis for calculating depreciation. That basis is then divided by the number of years in the asset's useful life. The quotient is the asset's annual depreciation expense.

HHSC's computer system, for example, had a purchase price of $6,000 and no other historical costs. Personal computer systems are typically considered to have useful lives of 3 years. If the expected salvage value of the system is zero, then the system's annual depreciation expense is $2,000. Table 3–5 shows these calculations. Note that by adjusting the expected salvage value, one can increase or decrease the periodic depreciation expense.

Table 3–6 shows the entries that HHSC's bookkeeper should make in the general journal at the end of the computer system's first year of operation. First, an expense item, depreciation expense, is increased with a debit entry of $2,000. Note that no cash changes hands when that entry is made. Depreciation is a *noncash expense*. Instead, a new type of account, a **contra-asset**, accumulated depreciation, is established to receive the matching credit entry.

Contra-asset accounts are accounts that adjust the values of assets. They are increased with credit entries, just as are liabilities. As each year's depreciation expense is recognized, the accumulated depreciation account grows. Each year's balance sheet shows the value of assets as "assets less accumulated depreciation." Thus, at the end of an asset's useful life, its accumulated depreciation will equal its historical cost minus its salvage value, and only the anticipated salvage will remain on the books.

Table 3-5 Calculating straight-line depreciation

Historical cost of asset	$6,000.00	
Minus salvage value	0.00	
Depreciable basis		$6,000.00
Divided by estimated useful life		3
Annual depreciation expense		2,000.00

Table 3-6 Recording annual (straight-line) depreciation expense

Date	Transaction	dr	cr
1/31/20XX	Depreciation expense	$2,000.00	
	Accumulated depreciation		$2,000.00

Organizations that are subject to income taxation will not want to use straight-line depreciation for income tax reporting. Because depreciation is an expense that is deducted from net income for calculating income tax liability, those organizations that are subject to income taxation can lower their tax bills by increasing their annual depreciation expense. Because there is no cash outflow associated with depreciation expense, increasing depreciation expense and lowering income tax liability actually increases the net cash flow of a taxable organization.

The United States Internal Revenue Code allows the use of **accelerated depreciation** for organizations that want to increase their depreciation expense, and lower their tax liabilities, in the early years of the life of an asset. For assets put into place after 1986, the code mandates the use of the **Modified Accelerated Cost Recovery System (MACRS)** tables. Those tables specify, for assets of various useful lives, what proportion of the depreciable base can be deducted as depreciation expense each year. Table 3–7 shows those percentages for assets purchased, such as HHSC's computer system, in the first quarter of the year. Note that, under MACRS, HHSC

Table 3-7 Annual depreciation percentages under the modified accelerated cost recovery system: Assets placed in service in the first quarter. Reproduced with permission from CCH 2000 Depreciation Guide published and copyrighted by CCH Incorporated, 2700 Lake Cook Road, Riverwoods, IL 60015 (1-800-TELL-CCH)

Recovery Year	Recovery Period					
	3 Years	5 Years	7 Years	10 Years	15 Years	20 Years
1	58.33	35.00	25.00	17.50	8.75	6.563
2	27.78	26.00	21.43	16.50	9.13	7.000
3	12.35	15.60	15.31	13.20	8.21	6.482
4	1.54	11.00	10.93	10.56	7.39	5.996
5		11.01	8.75	8.45	6.65	5.546
6		1.38	8.74	6.76	5.99	5.130
7			8.75	6.55	5.90	4.746
8			1.09	6.55	5.91	4.459
9				6.56	5.90	4.459
10				6.55	5.91	4.459
11				0.82	5.90	4.459
12					5.91	4.460
13					5.91	4.459
14					5.91	4.460
15					5.90	4.459
16					0.74	4.460
17						4.459
18						4.460
19						4.459
20						4.460
21						0.557

Reproduced with permission from *CCH 2000 Depreciation Guide* published and copyrighted by CCH Incorporated, 2700 Lake Cook Road, Riverwoods, IL 60015 (1-800-TELL-CCH).

would be able to take more than half of the total historical cost of its computer system (58.33 percent) as depreciation expense in the first year.

Some organizations are torn between the desire to lower their tax bills by using accelerated depreciation and the desire to report high profits to shareholders by using straight-line depreciation. These groups need have no alarm. The code allows the use of two methods of depreciation, one for tax purposes and the other for reports to shareholders and others. The difference in tax lability between the two methods is placed in a liability account, **deferred tax liability**.

Table 3–8 shows the calculation of the first year's annual depreciation expense for HHSC's computer system under MACRS. Table 3–9 shows the entries HHSC would make in its general journal for that year's MACRS depreciation expense.

Inventory

Inventory consists of goods purchased or made and held for resale. Most health care organizations carry only a small proportion of their total assets as inventory, as they exist to provide services rather than to sell goods. Pharmacies and medical supply firms, however, carry substantial inventories, some items of which are very expensive. Providers of home infusion services and meals-on-wheels also hold substantial inventories.

Inventory is difficult to value. Consider a clinic that uses 100 1-cc syringes per day. Every few days, a clerk opens several boxes of syringes and dumps their contents into plastic bins, one bin for each size and type of syringe. To value the syringes on hand accurately, one would have to know on what day each syringe was dumped into its bin. Imagine a time of very rapid inflation, in which the historical cost of syringes (the market prices at which the syringes are purchased) rises by 10 percent per week. Are the syringes on hand the most recent ones purchased (are old syringes always used before new ones)? If so, the inventory is quite

Table 3-8 Calculating first-year depreciation under MACRS

Historical cost of asset	$6,000.00	
Minus salvage value	0.00	
Depreciable basis		$6,000.00
Multiplied by the first-year MACRS proportion*		0.5833
Annual depreciation expense		3,499.80

*This proportion depends on the useful life of the assset, the recovery year, and the quarter in which the asset is put into service.

Table 3-9 Recording annual (MACRS) depreciation expense

Date	Transaction	dr	cr
12/31/20XX	Depreciation expense	$3,499.80	
	Accumulated depreciation		$3,499.80

valuable. Or are the syringes on hand the oldest ones purchased (are new syringes dumped on top of old ones so that new syringes are used first and older, lower cost, syringes are always on hand)? If so, the inventory was purchased at a relatively low price and has a relatively low value.

The valuation of inventory has to be presented in dollar terms. One cannot report a holding of "400 1-cc disposable syringes with attached 12-gauge needles." But the historical cost of the 400 syringes depends on whether inventory is handled on a **first in–first out (FIFO)** basis or on a **last in–first out (LIFO)** basis. The choice of FIFO or LIFO affects not only the value of inventory reported on the balance sheet but also the **cost of goods sold**, an expense that affects net income. One's choice of FIFO or LIFO inventory valuation does not imply any difference in the physical treatment of inventory.

In practice, organizations may select whether they wish to use either the FIFO or the LIFO basis of inventory valuation. In either case the expense reported for cost of goods sold for the accounting period is defined as follows:

Cost of goods sold = Beginning inventory + Net purchases − Ending inventory

That is, beginning inventory and net purchases (the cost of purchases minus discounts and returns) equals the value of goods available for sale. Goods available for sale minus what is left at the end of the period (ending inventory) is the cost of the items sold.

Return to the case of HHSC, discussed earlier. When HHSC opened for business on January 2, it had no inventory (beginning inventory = $0). On January 5, HHSC purchased, for cash, 200 frozen meals to be resold to its clients. These meals were purchased for $2.50 each. On January 20, HHSC purchased 200 more meals, but by that time the unit price had risen to $3.00. At the end of January, a visit to the freezer found 100 meals on hand. What was HHSC's end-of-the-month inventory value, and what was its cost of goods sold for January?

Table 3–10 shows the necessary calculations for inventory value and cost of goods sold using the FIFO convention. Under FIFO, the first meals sold were the first ones purchased. Therefore the 100 meals on hand at the end of the month are assumed to be from the last group purchased. Thus the ending inventory value of the meals is $300 (100 meals at $3.00).

Table 3-10 Determining cost of goods sold; first in-first out inventory method

Date	Quantity	Price per Unit	Total Value
January 5, purchase	200	$2.50	$500.00
January 20, purchase	200	3.00	600.00
Available for sale in January	400		1,100.00
Minus January 31, inventory on hand	100		
Sold in January	300		800.00
200 @ $2.50			
+100 @ $3.00			
January 31, inventory on hand	100		300.00
(100 @ $3.00)			

Under FIFO the cost of goods sold is $800 (200 meals at $2.50 plus 100 meals at $3.00). The first order of meals was purchased for $500 and the second for $600. The value of goods available for sale in January, then, was $1,100. Because ending inventory was $300, cost of goods sold was $800.

Table 3–11 shows the calculation of inventory value and cost of goods sold under the LIFO convention. Under LIFO, the most recently purchased goods are assumed to be sold first. Now the 100 frozen meals remaining at the end of the month are assumed to be from the first order. Thus the value of the ending inventory is $250 (100 meals at $2.50). Following the necessary calculation, the cost of goods sold for January is $850 under the LIFO convention, compared to $800 under FIFO.

In periods of rising prices, use of the LIFO convention will produce lower inventory values and higher costs of goods sold than will the use of the FIFO convention. During the 1960s and early 1970s, many organizations subject to income taxation switched from FIFO to LIFO. Why? Because, with prices rising steadily, use of LIFO increased cost of goods sold (an expense) and decreased taxable income. Use of LIFO may have depressed the income reported to shareholders, but it reduced the cash necessary to pay taxes. Note that the switch from FIFO to LIFO did not change anything real; no different handling of inventory was necessary. Also, although the switch reduced reported income, it did not involve any increase in cash outflows. In fact, for the taxable organization, after-tax net cash flows increased due to the change from FIFO to LIFO. Unlike the choice of depreciation method, firms must use the same method to value inventory for tax purposes as for reporting to shareholders.

Technological advances have made continuous inventory monitoring, identifying exactly which items from exactly which purchase lots are sold, quite easy. Bar coding of individual items allows organizations to track which items are used, when they are used, and which items remain on hand. Note, however, that for accounting purposes (and for the calculation of income tax liability), organizations can use LIFO inventory evaluation, even if they monitor their stocks continuously.

Table 3–12 shows HHSC's total revenues, total expenses, and net income for January, its first month of operation, under FIFO and LIFO. Note that no deprecia-

Table 3-11 Determining cost of goods sold; last in-first out inventory method

Date	Quantity	Price per Unit	Total Value
January 5, purchase	200	$2.50	$500.00
January 20, purchase	200	3.00	600.00
Available for sale in January	400		1,100.00
Minus January 31, inventory on hand	100		
Sold in January	300		850.00
200 @ $3.00			
+100 @ $2.50			
January 31, inventory on hand	100		250.00
(100 @ $2.50)			

Table 3-12 Revenues, expenses, and net income for January

First In–First Out		Last In–First Out	
Revenues		Revenues	
Sales of services	$6,000	Sales of services	$6,000
Expenses		Expenses	
Nursing services	4,200	Nursing services	$4,200
Cost of goods sold	800	Cost of goods sold	$850
	5,000		$5,050
Net income	1,000	Net income	$950

tion was recorded for January, as that entry is left until year-end. Under FIFO, January's net income is $1,000. Under LIFO, cost of goods sold is higher, and net income is $950.

CASH FLOW ACCOUNTING

Table 3–13 shows all of the transactions for HHSC for the month of January in cash flow terms. The investors' initial contribution of capital is the same as under accrual accounting but now is recognized as a source of cash. Under cash flow accounting, HHSC had no other revenue (no other source of cash inflow) for the month of January.

Nursing service expense involved a cash outflow of $4,200 in January and is recognized under cash flow accounting, just as it is under accrual accounting. The purchase of the computer system was treated as the acquisition of an asset, generating subsequent annual depreciation expense, under accrual accounting. Under cash flow accounting, however, the entire purchase price is regarded as a cash outflow at the time the purchase was made. Note that HHSC could have delayed that cash outflow by making the purchase on credit. On a cash flow basis, the choice of FIFO and LIFO is irrelevant. Cash out for inventory was $1,100 (200 meals at $2.50 and 200 meals at $3.00).

Thus HHSC's net cash flow for January is $94,700. That figure is quite different from $1,000 or $950 (depending on inventory valuation method) net income shown under accrual accounting. Why the difference? One difference is timing. Under

Table 3-13 Cash flows for January

Cash inflows	
Contribution of equity	$100,000
Revenues	0
	100,000
Cash outflows	
Nursing services	4,200
Inventory purchases	1,100
	5,300
Net cash flow	94,700

cash accounting, only cash transactions matter. Under accrual accounting, revenues and expenses are matched to the events that produce them.

The second difference between cash and accrual accounting is the treatment of the equity contribution. It is a cash inflow, but it is not revenue. Note that, without that extraordinary item, January's net cash flows would be grim indeed.

FUND ACCOUNTING

Government entities, including hospitals, clinics, and public health departments, have a special record-keeping need. Rather than being revenue based, depending on the sale of services for their survival, they are appropriation based, depending on appropriations from the public purse for their operating and capital funds. To maintain adequate records to demonstrate that they use their (publicly appropriated) funds in the manner in which they were intended, government entities developed a bookkeeping system known as *fund accounting*. Private, not-for-profit organizations often use fund accounting to demonstrate stewardship of their assets in the manner in which donors and trustees intend.

Although fund accounting is tedious and can be cumbersome, most specialists in governmental accounting recommend it for all government entities. Indeed, the GASB mandates the use of fund accounting for those entities subject to its rule-making authority (Hay & Wilson, 1992, pp. 17–18). Despite encouragement to drop the practice, fund accounting is still common in the private, not-for-profit sector.

Under fund accounting, the entity is divided into artificial subentities called *funds*. These funds need not correspond to any organizational units. A fund does not typically have its own staff. A fund need not even have its own separate bank account. Rather, each fund maintains its own set of internally balanced books (debits equal credits within each fund; a debit entry in one fund must be matched by an equal credit entry *in the same fund*).

Typically, there is a general fund to which are debited most of the entity's assets and which, in most cases, conducts all of the transactions between the entity and the outside world. There may also be a capital fund; one or more special-purpose funds; a fund for debt service; and enterprise funds, one for each revenue-producing enterprise (or subsidiary) within the entity. Moving cash from a special purpose fund to the general fund, in anticipation of a transaction with outsiders, requires an interfund transfer. The balance sheet of an entity that uses fund accounting shows the assets, liabilities, and net assets of each of the entity's funds.

Table 3–14 shows the purchase of an incubator by Clearwater County Memorial Hospital (from the Continuing Case at the end of the chapter). Memorial is owned by a hospital authority, established by the county. As such, it is obliged to use fund accounting. To facilitate managerial control, all transactions with outsiders must be made through the general fund.

Some years ago, Mrs. Beulah Smith bequeathed $250,000 (virtually all of her estate) to Memorial to provide care for newborn infants. The endowment (Mrs. Smith's fund) still exists and provides new and replacement assets for Memorial from time to time.

Table 3-14 Purchase of incubators by Mrs. Smith's fund

	Journal entries for Mrs. Smith's fund		
Date	**Transaction**	**dr**	**cr**
2/1/20XX	Due from other funds	$5,000.00	
	Cash		5,000.00
2/15/20XX	2 incubators	5,000.00	
	Due from other funds		5,000.00

	Journal entries for Mrs. Smith's general fund		
Date	**Transaction**	**dr**	**cr**
2/1/20XX	Cash	$5,000.00	
	Due to Mrs. Smith's fund		5,000.00
2/10/20XX	2 incubators	5,000.00	
	Cash		5,000.00
2/15/20XX	Due to Mrs. Smith's fund	5,000.00	
	2 incubators		5,000.00

As shown in Table 3–14, Memorial's trustees have authorized, at the request of a committee of pediatricians, the purchase of two incubators ($2,500 each) with money from Mrs. Smith's fund. Mrs. Smith's fund is classified as a *restricted fund* because its assets can be used only for specified purposes. Note that, for the purchase to take place, entries must be made in the general journals of both Mrs. Smith's fund and the general fund.

First, $5,000 must be transferred from Mrs. Smith's fund to the general fund. The financial office accomplishes this on February 1. Cash, an asset, is decreased in Mrs. Smith's fund (a credit entry decreases an asset), while "Due from other funds," also an asset, increases in that fund. The debit and credit entries balance within Mrs. Smith's fund, as the principles of fund accounting require. The general fund must also recognize the interfund transfer. Cash must increase, with a debit entry for $5,000. To balance that entry within the general fund, "Due to other funds," a liability, increases by an equal amount. The debit and credit entries balance within the general fund.

Now the incubators may be purchased. As the purchase is a transaction with an outside party, only the general fund's general journal is involved. "Incubators," an asset, is increased by $5,000 through a debit entry on February 10. To offset that entry, and to actually make the purchase, cash, an asset is decreased by $5,000 through a credit entry. Again, the debit and credit entries balance on the books of the general fund.

Finally, ownership of the two incubators must be transferred to Mrs. Smith's fund. The general fund's liability, "Due to other funds," is decreased by a debit entry on February 15. To balance, the general fund's holding of the asset class "Incubators" decreases by $5,000 through a credit entry. Mrs. Smith's fund increases its holdings of "Incubators" through a debit entry. To balance, Mrs. Smith's fund's holding of "Due from other funds" decreases through a credit entry.

When all of the transactions are completed, Mrs. Smith's fund has traded $5,000 in cash for $5,000 in incubators. The general fund is unaffected. The transaction flowed through the general fund but left its assets and liabilities unchanged.

Why all of the fuss? Why the elaborate transfer of assets from fund to fund? Ultimately, the purpose of maintaining the integrity of Mrs. Smith's fund is to keep faith with the late Mrs. Smith. Fund accounting is a means of demonstrating the stewardship of Mrs. Smith's bequest. Why force all transactions through the general fund? One reason is to make internal control easier. If one fund and one bank account are used for all purchases, control of those purchases is easier than if many subentities deal with the outside world.

Fund accounting is not required of private, not-for-profit institutions, and in recent years many such organizations have dropped the practice. Similarly, many not-for-profit hospitals have adopted, under FASB prodding, other aspects of GAAP, such as the depreciation of fixed assets. It is still difficult, given the differences in their accounting practices, to compare the accounting records of not-for-profit institutions with those of investor-owned entities (Sherman, 1986).

THE SPECIAL CASE OF HOSPITAL REVENUES

Measuring revenues has always been a problem for hospitals. When a hospital service is provided, a bed-day in an adult medicine unit, for example, the provider often has no way of knowing exactly how much revenue it will eventually receive from the patient or from a third-party payor.

As a first approximation, the hospital's patient accounts office can record the *charge* for the service. The charge is the standard fee assessed for the service before any adjustments are made. The charge need be tied neither to the cost of providing the service nor to the actual cash the hospital will eventually receive.

Over time, the differences between charge-based gross revenue and what the hospital is likely to receive have grown huge. Some patients are objects of charity. Their care will never be compensated. Other patients are admitted with a promise to pay but never do. Their accounts become uncollectible as bad debts. The total of charity care and bad debts (measured in some consistent way) is known as uncompensated care.

Many third-party payors exert pressure on hospitals to reduce what the payor must render for services. The difference between the charge for a bed-day in the adult medicine unit and the amount that the hospital has agreed to accept from the patient's insurance carrier is a contractual allowance. Preferred provider organizations (PPOs) and health insurance firms with substantial shares of local markets (Blue Cross, for example) are able to negotiate substantial contractual allowances.

Under the Prospective Payment System (PPS), the federal Health Care Financing Administration (HCFA), the administrator of the Medicare program, has *imposed* a system of contractual allowances on most of the hospitals in the United States. For Medicare-eligible patients, HCFA pays a fixed amount *per admission* based on the patient's **diagnosis-related group (DRG)** (Grimaldi, 1991; Russell,

1989; Torchia, 1992). DRGs are categories of diagnoses upon admission based on the International Classification of Diseases (Karaffa, 1993). The difference between charges and the DRG-based reimbursement is a contractual allowance and is often substantial.

Medicaid reimbursement, covering a portion of medically indigent patients, varies from state to state. In every state in which the program operates (every state except Arizona, which has a substitute program), the difference between the Medicaid reimbursement rate for any given service and the provider's charge constitutes a contractual allowance.

Prior to 1990, standard hospital accounting practice was to record the total of charges for all services as *gross revenue* for the period in which the services were rendered. Uncompensated care (charity care plus bad debt valued at charges, not cost) and contractual allowances were deducted from gross revenue on the income statement to obtain a net revenue figure. Net revenue, then, became the starting point for the other calculations that went into the income statement and the basis for well-informed financial statement analysis.

In 1990 the American Institute of Certified Accountants (AICPA) issued its *Audits of Providers of Health Care Services*, changing the way hospitals record and account for their revenues (American Institute of Certified Public Accountants, 1990; Bitter & Cassidy, 1992). Under the new rules, charity care does not generate revenue because the provider has no expectation of payment, but is to be described in detail in footnotes to the financial statements. Bad debts are to be treated as an expense, as is the practice in other industries. No gross revenue figure is to be presented, but net revenue (now the starting point on the income statement) is to be net of all contractual allowances.

AUDITING: THE MISUNDERSTOOD ART

Most users of financial statements pay little or no attention to the **auditor's opinion** that accompanies the reports themselves. Many users misunderstand the role of the audit, attributing to it meaning that it does not have. An audit does not guarantee the financial soundness of the organization. An auditor's opinion does not guarantee that the reporting organization will not be bankrupt by the end of the following year.

The auditor's opinion guarantees only that the statements were prepared according to Generally Accepted Accounting Principles. That is, the statements mean what an accountant understands them to mean for the period they cover. The next period may be different from the last, but for the reporting period the statements are a fair representation of the organization's position, if they are interpreted according to the logic of GAAP.

Privately owned organizations (whether not-for-profit or investor-owned) are audited, if so required, by independent accounting firms. Government-owned organizations may be audited by independent CPAs or, in some situations, by governmental agencies.

Auditors check a sample of transactions records, the organization's accounting procedures, and the basis for the accounting decisions represented in the financial statements. On that basis, they issue an opinion. The auditor's opinion may be unqualified (these statements fairly represent the financial position of the organization, according to GAAP), qualified (these statements fairly represent the financial position of the organization, except that . . .), or unfavorable (these statements do not fairly represent . . .).

The opinion includes several sections. Especially important are the Scope section, in which the auditors spell out what statements their opinion covers, and the Opinion section, in which the auditors state their opinion in detail. Figure 3–3 shows the auditor's opinion for recent financial statements of Tenet Healthcare Corporation.

SUMMARY

Accounts have developed a set of rules and procedures for recording the financial transactions of health care organizations. Those rules are known as Generally Accepted Accounting Principles, and their requirements are far from commonsensical to most managers. First, every transaction required two entries, a debit and a credit. Second, revenues and expenses must be recorded not when cash flows in and out but when promises are made, or at (arbitrary) points in the lives of assets.

These rules, and the financial statements produced under them, constitute the language of the health care business. Those who would use accounting data to make financial decisions must understand what those data mean. The ambiguities of accounting language make interpreting financial statements (the subject of Chapter 4) a challenging task.

Discussion Questions

1. Which is the better accounting basis for a large hospital, accrual or cash? For a one-physician medical practice? For a household? Explain.

2. What are some anomalies that would be introduced into financial statements by a conversion from accrual to cash accounting?

3. What are some ambiguities introduced by the use of accrual accounting?

4. "We know they're a good, sound outfit. Look, their auditor signed off on their financial statements." Why is the speaker mistaken? Explain.

5. *Debit* and *credit* have neither honorific nor pejorative meaning in accounting. Explain.

The Board of Directors
TENET HEALTHCARE CORPORATION:

We have audited the accompanying consolidated balance sheets of Tenet Healthcare Corporation and subsidiaries as of May 31, 1999 and 2000, and the related consolidated statements of income, comprehensive income, changes in shareholders' equity and cash flows for each of the years in the three-year period ended May 31, 2000. These consolidated financial statements are the responsibility of the Company's management. Our responsibility is to express an opinion on these consolidated financial statements based on our audits.

We conducted our audits in accordance with auditing standards generally accepted in the United States of America. Those standards require that we plan and perform the audit to obtain reasonable assurance about whether the financial statements are free of material misstatement. An audit includes examining, on a test basis, evidence supporting the amounts and disclosures in the financial statements. An audit also includes assessing the accounting principles used and significant estimates made by management, as well as evaluating the overall financial statement presentation. We believe that our audits provide a reasonable basis for our opinion.

In our opinion, the consolidated financial statements referred to above present fairly, in all material respects, the financial position of Tenet Healthcare Corporation and subsidiaries as of May 31, 1999 and 2000, and the results of their operations and their cash flows for each of the years in the three-year period ended May 31, 2000, in conformity with accounting principles generally accepted in the United States of America.

As discussed in Note 15 to the consolidated financial statements, effective June 1, 1999, the Company changed its method of accounting for start-up costs.

KPMG LLP

Los Angeles, California
July 25, 2000

Figure 3-3 Auditor's report. Source: Tenet Corporation, Annual Report, 2000.

CONTINUING CASES

Henry Kirk and Janet Fowler are sitting across the desk from Tom Land, PCI's loan officer at CCB Bank (once known as Clearwater County Bank, the bank now aspires to compete with the major regional banks for commercial loan business in this part of the state). They have come to ask for a 90-day, $100,000 note (loan), as they have many times in the past. The request should be routine. In fact, PCI's 90-day loans are one of the mainstays of CCB's business.

This time, however, Tom asks some embarrassing questions about PCI's flagging profits. Janet Fowler, as the only accountant present, has supported PCI's request with a couple of special arguments. She says PCI is in better shape than it appears. Profits are low because the clinic's recent purchase of a third-generation lithotripter generated a big expense in the last quarter. Also, LIFO valuation has made inventories, actually a healthy item on the balance sheet, look artificially low. Besides, she says, if there is any trouble with current cash flows over the next 90 days, PCI can always pay off the note out of its substantial retained earnings.

CASE QUESTION

Evaluate the case Ms. Fowler makes to Mr. Land.

REFERENCES

American Institute of Certified Public Accountants. (1990). *Audits of providers of health care services*. New York: Author.

Bitter, M.E. & Cassidy, J. (1992). Perceptions of new AICPA audit guide. *Healthcare Financial Management, 46*(11), 38.

Garner, M. & Grossman, W. (1991). Consistency endangered by FASB-GASB dispute. *Healthcare Financial Management, 45*(2), 62–72.

Grimaldi, P. (1991). Capital PPS: Trekking through the labyrinth. *Healthcare Financial Management, 45*(11), 72–87.

Hay, L.E. & Wilson E.R. (1992). *Accounting for governmental and nonprofit entities* (9th ed.). Homewood, IL: Richard D. Irwin.

Karaffa, M.C. (Ed.). (1993). *ICD-9-CM, international classification of diseases, 9th revision, clinical modification, 4th revision*. Los Angeles: Practice Management Information Corporation.

Miller, P.B.W. & Redding, R.J. (1988). *The FASB: The people, the process, and the politics* (2nd ed.). Homewood, IL: Richard D. Irwin.

Pointer, L.G. & Schroeder, R.G. (1986). *An introduction to the Securities and Exchange Commission*. Plano, TX: Business Publications.

Report to the Audit Committee, Massachusetts General Hospital, September 30, 1989.

Russell, L.B. (1989). *Medicare's new hospital payment system: Is it working?* Washington, DC: Brookings Institution.

Seawell, L.V. (1992). *Introduction to hospital accounting* (3rd ed.). Dubuque, IA: Kendall/Hunt for the Healthcare Financial Management Association.

Sherman, H.D. (1986). Interpreting hospital performance with financial statement analysis. *Accounting Review, 61*(3), 526–550.

Torchia, M.M. (1992). Capital PPS 10-year transition up and running. *Healthcare Financial Management, 46*(4) 21–38.

White, G.I., Sondhi, A.C., and Fried, D. (1994). *The analysis and use of financial statements*. New York: J. Wiley.

SELECTED READINGS

American Institute of Certified Public Accountants. (1990). *Audits of providers of health care services*. New York: Author.

Davidson, S., Stickney, C.P., & Weil, R.L. (1985). *Financial accounting*. Chicago, IL: Dryden.

Freeman, R.J., Shoulders, C.D. & Lynn, E.S. (1988). *Governmental and nonprofit accounting* (3rd ed.). Englewood Cliffs, NJ: Prentice-Hall.

Hay, L.E. & Wilson, E.R. (1992). *Accounting for governmental and nonprofit entities* (9th ed.). Homewood, IL: Richard D. Irwin.

Seawell, L.V. (1992). *Introduction to hospital accounting* (3rd ed.). Dubuque, IA: Kendall/Hunt Publishing Company for the Healthcare Financial Management Association.

CHAPTER 4

Organizational Diagnostics: Financial Statement Analysis

Learning Objectives

After reading this chapter, the student should be able to:

1. Use an organization's financial statements to evaluate its past liquidity.
2. Use an organization's financial statements to evaluate its past asset utilization.
3. Use an organization's financial statements to evaluate its past financial leverage (capital structure and debt service coverage).
4. Use an organization's financial statements to evaluate its past profitability.
5. Make recommendations to management on how to improve diagnosed deficiencies in liquidity, asset utilization, leverage, and profitability.

Key Terms

Asset/equity ratio	Liquidity
Capital structure	Long-term debt to equity
Cash flow coverage	Performance (or asset utiliza-
Collection period	tion)
Common-size	Profitability
statement	Ratio analysis
Coverage ratio	Return on assets (ROA)
Current ratio	Return on equity (ROE)
Financial leverage	Times interest earned
Financial statement analysis	Total asset turnover
Inventory turnover ratio	Total margin

Chapter 3 introduced the accounting rules under which organizations, including health care organizations, prepare financial statements. The methods for using accounting records to diagnose an organization's financial health are known, collectively, as **financial statement analysis**. The statement analyst uses the end products of the accounting cycle (the financial statements: income statement, balance sheet, and cash flow statement) to make inferences about how viable the organization is and how profitable it has been. Managers who do not understand accounting rules can make serious mistakes when interpreting a firm's financial health. After studying this chapter, the reader should be able to make a detailed analysis of an organization's financial health using information from its financial statements.

USING FINANCIAL STATEMENTS

Financial statement analysis is useful for decision makers in a variety of settings. Consider the small proprietary hospital in this text's continuing case, Physicians' Clinic. The *managers* of Physicians' Clinic need the information that the financial statements provide. How are they doing? What is their rate of profit? Are they managing their inventories and accounts receivable as efficiently as they should? Answers to all of those questions are embedded in the financial statements. The *board of directors* as representatives of the stockholders of the parent corporation (PCI, Inc.) are interested in the organization's profitability as well as in its overall risk/return profile. Is its mix of debt and equity financing appropriate? What is the quarter-to-quarter variability of its revenues? Those questions can be answered with financial statement analysis. In not-for-profit organizations, the *trustees*, as representatives of the community and donors, are just as interested in the answers to those questions as are the directors of an investor-owned firm.

Lenders (banks or bond buyers) are concerned that their interest and principal can be paid on schedule. *Equity owners* want assurance that, after paying lenders, there will be something left either to reinvest for growth or to pay out as dividends. Those coverage questions can be answered through attention to the financial statements. In the health care sector, both *regulators* and *third-party payors* want to know what rate of profitability their rules and rates of reimbursement offer to providers.

Financial statement analysis is an art that has evolved over a long period of time. Originally, financial reporting was simpler, there were fewer bits of information to process, and no research existed to indicate what types of financial statement information was actually useful. The art evolved to include a variety of measures (ratios), each of which, originally, was to be compared to a standard, a "magic number," that indicated the presence or absence of sound managerial practice. Today, financial analysts know that, when practiced well, good management can lead to a variety of ratio values, not to a single magic number. There is also a large body of research demonstrating what information is useful (Foster, 1978) and how to calculate it (White et al, 1997).

That health care financial statements are compiled under different rules from those in other industries was discussed in Chapter 3. Those differences in accounting procedure require the financial analyst to compute some ratios differently for health care organizations than she would for other types of organizations. Failure to recognize those differences can lead to serious misunderstanding by the analyst and by those who use her analyses (Cleverly and Cameron, 2002; Cleverly & Rohleder, 1985; Coyne, 1985; McCue, 1991; Sherman, 1986).

Fortunately, there are several sources of financial statement data available for comparison purposes, some of them unique to health care. Standard & Poor's Corporation publishes *Industry Surveys* that are rich in comparison data and in discussion. S&P provides a survey for the health care sector. That report, updated regularly, includes information on hospital and on nonhospital sectors. S&P's data are, however, limited to the investor-owned sector. Several private vendors also offer health care-specific comparison data. Those analyzing health maintenance organizations can acquire the Group Health Association of America's *HMO Industry Profile*. Each of these sources has its own uses and limitations, and analysts should know the characteristics of their comparison data (Johnsson, 1992).

Figure 4–1 shows the 2000 financial statements for Tenet Healthcare Corporation (an investor-owned corporation operating acute care hospitals throughout the United States).

FINANCIAL STATEMENT ANALYSIS: ITS POWER AND LIMITATIONS

The financial statements of any organization summarize all of that organization's transactions with outside parties during the reporting period. Every exchange of goods and services (whether buying or selling), every conversion of accounts receivable or payable into cash, and the depreciation of each piece of capital equipment is reflected in the financial statements. Thus the statements summarize an enormous amount of information and, properly analyzed, can reveal a great deal about the health and performance of the organization. Using appropriate comparison data, the organization's health, relative to some reference group, can be determined.

Figure 4-1 2000 financial statement for Tenet Healthcare Corporation.

Source: Tenet Healthcare Corporation (2000). Annual Report, 2000. Los Angeles.

CONSOLIDATED FINANCIAL STATEMENTS   **May 31**

Consolidated Balance Sheets
Dollars in Millions

Assets	1999	2000
Current Assets:		
Cash and cash equivalents	$ 29	$ 135
Short-term investments in debt securities	130	110
Accounts receivable, less allowances for		
doubtful accounts ($287 in 1999 and $358 in 2000)	2,318	2,506
Inventories of supplies, at cost	221	223
Deferred income taxes	196	176
Assets held for sale or disposal, at the lower of carrying		
value or fair value less estimated costs to sell or dispose	655	132
Other current assets	413	312
Total current assets	**3,962**	**3,594**
Investments and other assets	569	344
Property and equipment, net	5,839	5,894
Costs in excess of net assets acquired, less accumulated		
amortization ($339 in 1999 and $421 in 2000)	3,283	3,235
Other intangible assets, at cost, less accumulated		
amortization ($70 in 1999 and $80 in 2000)	118	94
	$13,771	**$13,161**

Liabilities and Shareholders' Equity

	1999	2000
Current Liabilities:		
Current portion of long-term debt	$ 45	$ 9
Accounts payable	713	671
Employee compensation and benefits	390	383
Accrued interest payable	163	155
Other current liabilities	711	694
Total current liabilities	**2,022**	**1,912**
Long-term debt, net of current portion	6,391	5,668
Other long-term liabilities and minority interests	1,048	1,024
Deferred income taxes	440	491
Commitments and contingencies		
Shareholders' Equity		
Common stock, $0.075 par value; authorized 700,000,000		
shares; 314,778,323 shares issued at May 31, 1999		
and 317,214,748 shares issued at May 31, 2000	24	24
Additional paid-in capital	2,510	2,555
Accumulated other comprehensive income (loss)	77	(70)
Retained earnings	1,329	1,627
Less common stock in treasury, at cost, 3,754,708 shares		
at May 31, 1999 and 2000	(70)	(70)
Total shareholders' equity	**3,870**	**4,066**
	$13,771	**$13,161**

See accompanying NOTES TO CONSOLIDATED FINANCIAL STATEMENTS. (continues)

Years Ended May 31

Consolidated Statements of Income

Dollars in Millions, Except Per Share Amounts

	1998	1999	2000
Net operating revenues	$ 9,895	$10,880	$11,414
Operating Expenses:			
Salaries and benefits	4,052	4,412	4,508
Supplies	1,375	1,525	1,595
Provision for doubtful accounts	588	743	851
Other operating expenses	2,071	2,342	2,525
Depreciation	347	421	411
Amortization	113	135	122
Impairment and other unusual charges	221	363	355
Operating income	**1,128**	939	**1,047**
Interest expense	(464)	(485)	(479)
Investment earnings	22	27	22
Minority interests in income of consolidated subsidiaries	(22)	(7)	(21)
Net gains (loses) on disposals of facilities and long-term investments	(17)	—	49
Income from continuing operations before income taxes	**647**	**474**	**618**
Income taxes	(269)	(225)	(278)
Income from continuing operations, before discontinued operations, extraordinary charge and cumulative effect of accounting change	**378**	**249**	**340**
Discontinued operations, net of taxes	—	—	(19)
Extraordinary charge from early extinguishment of debt, net of taxes	(117)	—	—
Cumulative effect of accounting change, net of taxes	—	—	(19)
Net income	**$ 261**	**$ 249**	**$ 302**

Earnings (Loss) per Common and Common Equivalent Share:

	1998	1999	2000
Basic:			
Continuing operations	$ 1.23	$ 0.80	$ 1.09
Discontinued operations	—	—	(0.06)
Extraordinary charges	(0.38)	—	—
Cumulative effect of accounting change	—	—	(0.06)
	$ 0.85	$ 0.80	$ 0.97
Diluted:			
Continuing operations	$1.22	$0.79	$1.08
Discontinued operations	—	—	(0.06)
Extraordinary charges	(0.38)	—	—
Cumulative effect of accounting change	—	—	(0.06)
	$ 0.84	$ 0.79	$ 0.96

Weighted Shares and Dilutive Securities Outstanding (in thousands):

	1998	1999	2000
Basic	306,255	310,050	311,980
Diluted	312,113	313,386	314,918

See accompanying NOTES TO CONSOLIDATED FINANCIAL STATEMENTS.. (continues)

Figure 4-1 (continued)   2000 financial statement for Tenet Healthcare Corporation.

Years Ended May 31

Consolidated Statements of Comprehensive Income
Dollars in Millions

	1998	1999	2000
Net Income	**$ 261**	**$ 249**	**$ 302**
Other Comprehensive Income (Loss):			
Unrealized gains (losses) on securities			
held as available for sale:			
Unrealized net holding gains (losses)			
arising during period	(56)	51	(142)
Less: reclassification adjustment for gains			
included in net income	(40)	—	(92)
Foreign currency translation adjustments	—	(5)	(1)
Other comprehensive income (loss),			
before income taxes	**(96)**	**46**	**(235)**
Income tax benefit (expense) related to items			
of other comprehensive income	36	(19)	88
Other comprehensive income (loss)	(60)	27	(147)
Comprehensive income	**$ 201**	**$ 276**	**$ 155**

See accompanying NOTES TO CONSOLIDATED FINANCIAL STATEMENTS.

Financial statement analysis does not, however, "tell all" about organizational health and performance. Statement analysis is, by its very nature, backward looking. It provides information about the accounting period for which the statements were produced. That period is, necessarily, in the past. Statement analysis is not predictive. Knowing the net income of an organization for each of the past 5 years *does not* provide information as to what net income will be next year. To know that, one would have to have knowledge about economic conditions, third-party payor decisions, federal and state regulations, and technological changes to come. That sort of foreknowledge is not contained in the financial statements. A substantial body of research shows that financial statements are not good tools for predicting performance or for revealing continuing "trends" (Foster, 1978, pp. 107–111). Financial statement analysis is a *diagnostic tool*, but not a *predictive tool*.

Financial statement analysis can only be as good as the financial statements, and therefore the accounting practices, on which it is based. The accounting scandals of 2002; involving Enron Corporation, WorldCom, and others; highlight this limitation. Further, health care statement analysis can be only as good as the analyst's understanding of the accounting practices used in the health care sector. Continuous study of accounting and of industry practice is the price one must pay to become and to remain a good financial statement analyst.

Years Ended May 31

Consolidated Statements of Changes in Shareholders' Equity
Dollars in Millions, Share Amounts in Thousands

	Outstanding Shares	Issued Amount	Additional Paid-In Capital	Accumulated Other Comprehensive Income (Loss)	Retained Earnings	Treasury Stock
Balances, May 31, 1997	302,825	$ 23	$ 2,311	$ 110	$ 819	$ (39)
Net Income					261	
Other comprehensive loss				(60)		
Issuance of common stock	997		26			
Stock options exercised	5,468		138			(31)
Balances, May 31, 1998	309,290	23	2,475	50	1,080	(70)
Net income					249	
Other comprehensive income				27		
Issuance of common stock	1,044		22			
Stock options exercised	690	1	13			
Balances, May 31, 1999	311,024	24	2,510	77	1,329	(70)
Net income					302	
Other comprehensive loss				(147)		
Issuance of common stock	1,222		20			
Stock options exercised	1,214		25			
Redemption of shareholder rights					(4)	
Balances, May 31, 2000	313,460	$ 24	$ 2,555	$ (70)	$ 1,627	$ (70)

See accompanying NOTES TO CONSOLIDATED FINANCIAL STATEMENTS. (continued)

Figure 4-1 (continued)   2000 financial statement for Tenet Healthcare Corporation.

Consolidated Statements of Cash Flows
Dollars in Millions

	1998	1999	2000
Cash Flows from Operating Activities:			
Net income	**$ 261**	**$ 249**	**$ 302**
Adjustments to Reconcile Net Income to			
Net Cash Provided by Operating Activities:			
Depreciation and amortization	460	556	533
Provision for doubtful accounts	588	743	851
Additions to reserves for impairment and			
other unusual charges	221	363	355
Deferred income taxes	131	101	2
Gain on sales of facilities and			
long-term investments	—	—	(49)
Discontinued operations	—	—	19
Extraordinary charges from early			
extinguishment of debt	117	—	—
Cumulative effect of accounting change	—	—	19
Other items	38	17	33
Increases (Decreases) in Cash from Changes			
in Operating Assets and Liabilities,			
Net of Effects from Purchases of			
New Businesses and Sales of Facilities:			
Accounts receivable	(988)	(1,347)	(1,139)
Inventories and other current assets	(100)	(114)	51
Accounts payable, accrued expenses and			
other current liabilities	143	197	(15)
Other long-term liabilities and			
minority interests	(83)	(108)	17
Net expenditures for discontinued operations,			
impairment and other unusual charges	(385)	(75)	(110)
Net cash provided by operating activities	**403**	**582**	**869**
Cash Flows from Investing Activities:			
Purchases of property and equipment	(534)	(592)	(619)
Purchases of new businesses, net of			
cash acquired	(679)	(541)	(38)
Proceeds from sales of facilities, long-term			
investments and other assets	170	72	764
Other items, including expenditures related			
to prior-year purchases of new businesses	(40)	(86)	(143)
Net cash used in investing activities	**(1,083)**	**(1,147)**	**(36)**

(continues)

Cash Flows from Financing Activities:

Proceeds from borrowings	3,349	5,634	1,298
Repayments of borrowings	(2,762)	(5,085)	(2,085)
Proceeds from exercises of stock options	80	13	25
Proceeds from sales of common stock	17	23	20
Other items	(16)	(14)	15
Net cash provided by (used in)			
financing activities	**668**	**571**	**(727)**
Net increase (decrease) in cash and			
cash equivalents	(12)	6	106
Cash and cash equivalents at beginning of year	35	23	29
Cash and cash equivalents at end of year	**$ 23**	**$ 29**	**$ 135**

See accompanying NOTES TO CONSOLIDATED FINANCIAL STATEMENTS.

A FIRST APPROACH: COMMON-SIZE STATEMENTS

Consider the data shown for Tenet Healthcare Corporation in Figure 4–1. The bottom line of the Statements of Income indicates that Tenet produced net income of $302 million in its 2000 fiscal year. Is that $302 million enough to satisfy the worries of its creditors? Is it excessive? Somehow, that $302 million must be placed in an appropriate context in order to know the answers to those questions.

To make judgements about financial performance, one must *normalize* financial statement data. To say that Billy Bob Ferguson of Lone Star Home Health Services (in the continuing case) weighs 250 pounds is to provide little information. To say that Mr. Ferguson weighs 250 pounds and is five feet three inches tall is to provide much more; "250 pounds and six feet two inches tall" tells a very different story. With weight normalized by height, one can make an inference about Mr. Ferguson's health, appearance, and, perhaps, self-esteem. If one can normalize profit information in some way, one can make comparisons over time and across organizations.

One way of normalizing financial statement data is by the construction of **common-size statements**. In a common-size statement, each of the items in the statement is presented as a percentage of some base. Balance sheet items are shown as percentages of total assets. Income statement items are shown as percentages of total revenue. Cash flow statement items are shown as percentages of net change in cash. The term *common-size* refers to the fact that, on the balance sheet, for example, total assets are a common size, 100 percent, for every organization.

Table 4–1 shows the common-size statements for Tenet Healthcare Corporation for 2000. With common-size statements, one can compare Tenet's net income, as a percent of total revenue, to that of any other corporation. One can also examine the composition of assets and liabilities. For example, on May 31, 2000, more than 19 percent of Tenet's total assets were in the form of accounts receivable (representing care for which patients were billed, but for which no cash had been collected).

Most financial analysts find common-size statements to be interesting, but seldom used, tools. By far, the more useful tool is ratio analysis, discussed in the following section.

Table 4-1 Common-size statements, Tenet Healthcare Corporation, 2000

Tenet Healthcare Corporation
Common-Size Statements, 2000

Balance Sheet

Assets	
Current Assets	
Cash and cash equivalents	1.0258%
Short-term investments	0.8358%
Accounts receivable	19.0411%
Inventories	1.6944%
Deferred income cases	1.3373%
Assets held for sale	1.0030%
Other current assets	2.3707%
Total current assets	27.3080%
Investments and other assets	2.6138%
Property and equipment	44.7838%
Costs in excess of net assets acquired	24.5802%
Other intangible assets	0.7142%
Total Assets	**100.0000%**
Liabilities and Shareholders' Equity	
Current Liabilities	
Current portion of long-term debt	0.0684%
Accounts payable	5.0984%
Employee compensation	2.9101%
Accrued interest payable	1.1777%
Other current liabilities	5.2732%
Total Current liabilities	14.5278%
Long-term debt, net of current portion	43.0666%
Other long-term liabilities	7.7806%
Deferred income taxes	3.7307%
Commitments and contingencies	0.0000%
Total shareholders' equity	30.8943%
Total Liabilities	**100.0000%**

THE POWER APPROACH: RATIO ANALYSIS

Construction of common-size statements is useful for some purposes, but most financial analysts devote most of their attention to another approach, **ratio analysis**. Ratio analysis consists of computing ratios (one number divided by another) from an organization's financial statements and comparing those ratios to the average for some relevant comparison group or to some ideal or standard.

Ratios are useful devices. Standard & Poor's Corporation, for example, uses ratio analysis when rating the bonds of hospitals and other organizations (Standard & Poor's, 1989). What do the ratios do that common-size statements do not? They normalize financial statement data. For example, rather than looking at the Tenet's profits ($302,000,000), one can look at profits normalized by the value

Table 4-1 Common-size statements, Tenet Healthcare Corporation, 2000 (continued).

Tenet Healthcare Corporation
Common-Size Statements, 2000

Income Statement

Net Operating Revenues	**100.0000%**
Operating Expenses	
Salaries and benefits	39.4954%
Supplies	13.9741%
Provision for doubtful accounts	7.4558%
Other operating expenses	22.1220%
Depreciation	3.6008%
Amortization	1.0689%
Impairment and other unusual charges	3.1102%
Operating Income	**9.1729%**
Interest expense	-4.1966%
Investment earnings	0.1927%
Minority interests	-0.1840%
Net gains on disposals	0.4293%
Income from continuing operations before income taxes	**5.4144%**
Income taxes	-2.4356%
Income from continuing operations before	
discontinued operations	**2.9788%**
Discontinued operations, net of taxes	-0.1665%
Cumulative effect of accounting change	-0.1665%
Net income	**2.6459%**

of total assets that it has in place ($13,161,000,000). The resulting ratio, called *return on assets*, shows profits normalized by asset base (2.29 percent). Not only do ratios normalize financial statement data; they also provide a way of summarizing a great deal of information in a very few numbers. Those who are practiced in financial statement analysis can discern a great deal about an organization by looking at only a few ratios.

What do financial ratios tell the analyst? Ratios provide information about four dimensions of organizational performance. First, they provide information about **liquidity**. Liquidity, in this sense, means how quickly an organization can raise cash to meet its short-term obligations. Second, ratios provide information about **performance or asset utilization**. A wide variety of ratios indicate how well the organization is using its assets to generate revenue, how quickly the organization is collecting cash, and how well the organization is controlling and managing its asset base.

Third, ratios provide information about **financial leverage**. Financial leverage, simply put, is the use of other people's money. Organizations increase their financial leverage whenever they borrow. Leverage has two sides, and there are two types of leverage ratios. **Capital structure** ratios show the extent to which the organization has borrowed. **Coverage ratios** show to what extent the organization can meet the financial obligations (interest and principle) it has incurred by borrowing. Finally, **profitability** ratios provide information about the extent to which the organization can reward shareholders (in investor-owned organizations) or can provide services to stakeholders (not-for-profit organizations).

One can divide any financial statement number by any other financial statement number, but so doing does not necessarily generate a useful ratio. Of the very many ratios that analysts have developed (and that finance textbooks present), only a few are genuinely useful.

LIQUIDITY RATIOS

Liquidity, in moderation, is a good thing to have. A hospital with a great deal of cash and marketable securities is very liquid. A home health agency all of whose assets are tied up in vehicles and pharmaceutical inventory is not. Liquidity is defined only in relative terms. That is, how liquid an organization is depends on the size of its current obligations, as well as on its current assets.

The assets that can be turned into cash quickly are easy to spot on the financial statements (and in real life). Current assets (those that are expected to be held for 1 year or less) are generally considered to be liquid assets. Those include cash, marketable securities, accounts receivable, inventory, and prepaid expenses. The current liabilities that form the denominator of any liquidity measure are those liabilities that will fall due (require a cash outflow) within 1 year. Those include accounts payable, wages and salaries payable, interest payable, taxes payable, and the portion of the principle of long-term debt that is due within the year.

The most commonly used liquidity ratio is the **current ratio**. That ratio is defined as the dollar value of current assets divided by current liabilities. For Tenet 2000, that ratio is 1.8797. To arrive at that number, add the value of cash, receivables, investments, and other current assets. Is 1.9 (approximately) a "good" liquidity ratio or a poor one? It certainly represents a high measure of liquidity. In the "magic numbers" days of financial statement analysis, a liquidity ratio of 2.0 or higher was considered good. In 1994 the median current ratio for all acute care hospitals was 2.07. Table 4–2 summarizes some comparison data for 1999. It is clear, then, that Tenet was about median in its liquidity in 2000.

Was it too liquid? Holding assets in very liquid form involves an opportunity cost; those assets could have earned higher returns in another form.

ASSET UTILIZATION RATIOS

The second dimension about which ratio analysis provides information is asset utilization (or performance). Asset utilization ratios provide information about how effectively the organization is using its assets to generate revenues and cash. Several of these ratios fall into the category of turnover ratios. The **inventory turnover ratio**, for example, show how many times, on average, the organization's total volume of inventory turns over, or changes, during an accounting period. Computed as total revenues plus net nonoperating gains divided by ending inventory, a high value means that a small investment in inventory is generating a large

Table 4-2   Ten useful financial ratios

	Median for All U.S. Acute Care Hospitals, 1999
Current ratio	2.07
Inventory turnover	50.35
Total asset turnover	1.01
Days in accounts receivable (collection period)	74.26
Debt financing percentage	43.66
Long-term debt to equity (percent)	31.16
Times interest earned	2.37
Cash flow to total debt (percent)	15.48
Return on assets	2.01
Return on equity	5.46

Source: Cleverly and Associates, Columbus, Ohio

volume of sales. Because inventories of goods for sale are such a small part of the assets of most health care service providers, the inventory turnover ratio is of little use for most hospitals, clinics, nursing homes, and group practices, but it is important for pharmacies, medical supply vendors, and home health providers.

A more important turnover ratio for health care providers is **total asset turnover**. No one supposes that total assets actually change (or turn over) during the accounting period, but total asset turnover does indicate the extent to which assets produce revenues. Defined as total revenue plus nonoperating gains divided by total assets, a high value indicates effective revenue generation from the asset base.

Consider the 2000 total asset turnover for Tenet Healthcare. To find the numerator for the ratio, divide operating revenues ($11,414,000,000) by total assets ($13,161,000,000). The resulting total asset turnover ratio is 0.8673.

An acute care hospital in the United States can expect to have a total asset turnover of about 1.00 (in 1999 the reported median was 1.01 (see Table 4–2)). There is no theoretical reason for that number to be so common as a total asset turnover; it is only an empirical regularity.

A desirable value for total asset turnover depends on the nature of the organization and on the nature of the services it provides. For example, a health maintenance organization (HMO) can expect to have a total asset turnover ratio much greater than 1.00. The HMO collects revenues (premiums) that it will distribute to its participating providers. Except in a minority of cases, the HMO itself will own very few assets, so its total asset turnover can be 6.0 or higher.

Another indicator of performance is the organization's success at turning accounts receivable into cash. The **collection period** (or days in accounts receivable) indicates how long, on average, accounts receivable remain uncollected. The longer that time, the greater is the strain on the organization's cash reserves and on its line of credit.

The collection period shows how many days of revenues are "tied up" in accounts receivable. Its definition is net patient accounts receivable divided by net patient service revenues per day. To calculate the ratio, first divide patient service revenue for the period by 365 (to obtain revenue per day). Then divide that quotient *into* net patient accounts receivable to obtain the average time (in days) needed to collect each patient's account.

For Tenet in 2000, the collection period is 80.1376 days. In most health service organizations, the collection period (days in accounts receivable) is dictated by the payment practices of third-party payors, the most important of whom is the regional Medicare intermediary. Collection periods of between 60 and 90 days are quite normal. HMOs and other types of health insurers, on the other hand, receive most of their premiums from employee payroll deductions and employers' matching payments. For those organizations, then, collection periods of (almost) exactly 30 days are the norm.

LEVERAGE RATIOS

Organizations must finance their assets. That is, in order to purchase assets, they must obtain funds. As shown in the basic accounting identity in Chapter 3, assets are financed by a combination of liabilities and owners' equity. Any organization's relative degree of debt financing (borrowing and leasing) is called financial leverage.

Financial leverage has two important aspects. First, it involves a choice of the mix of debt and equity financing. The results of that choice determine the organization's capital structure. Second, financial leverage involves a choice of how much interest to pay. A consequence of that decision is, given the organization's earnings and cash flows, the extent to which interest obligations are covered or can be met. There are two types of leverage ratios, capital structure ratios and coverage ratios.

The most basic and most useful capital structure ratio is the **asset/equity ratio**. That ratio is defined as total assets divided by owners' equity (or, in not-for-profit organizations, net assets). For Tenet the ratio is derived by dividing total assets ($13,161,000,000) by shareholder's equity ($4,066,000,000) to obtain 3.2368. Thus, in book value terms, every dollar of Tenet's equity controlled $3.24 of total assets.

To the extent that assets are held in excess of the value of equity (or fund balance), the organization has incurred debt. Thus an asset/equity ratio above 1.00 means that the organization has gone into debt. The presence of debt financing alone is neither good nor bad. If the organization is able to meet its debt obligations, the use of debt increases the return to equity holders. It is good to use other people's money.

The connection between the asset/equity ratio and other capital structure ratios is close and direct. Asset/equity contains the same information as many of the related ratios. Asset/equity is the inverse of the equity funding ratio (equity/assets). Asset/equity is equal to 1 plus the debt equity ratio (asset/equity = 1 + [debt/equity]). The analyst who knows any one of those ratios can compute any of the others.

Not containing the same information as asset/equity is **long-term debt/equity**. That ratio's formula is embedded in its name. For Tenet for 2000, long-term debt/equity was 1.3940.

A high degree of debt financing is not a problem for organizations that can meet their debt obligations. Ratios that assess ability to meet debt obligation measure coverage. A traditional coverage ratio goes by the cryptic name of **times interest earned**. The times interest earned ratio answers the question, "How many times your interest obligation did you earn?" It measures the accounting (accrual basis) profits available to pay each dollar of interest and is defined as net income plus interest expense plus income tax divided by interest expense. The numerator of that expression is known as *earnings before interest and taxes* (EBIT).

That interest expense should be the denominator of this ratio is clear. It is income to cover interest expense that is to be measured. The numerator is less obvious. Net income is certainly available to pay interest. Net income is profit that was available, but was not necessary, to meet interest payments. The cash used to pay interest expense was available to pay interest expense; indeed, that is the way those resources were used. In the United States, interest is an income tax–deductible expense. Thus resources used to pay income tax were potentially available to meet interest obligations. Therefore the best measure of the accounting profits available to meet interest expense is profit plus interest expense plus income tax expense, or EBIT.

Tenet's asset/equity ratio was 3.2368 at the end of its 2000 fiscal year. Its times interest earned ratio will provide a first look at its ability to service that much leverage. Dividing Tenet's EBIT by its interest expense yields a times interest earned of 2.2109. In the "magic numbers" approach to ratio analysis, analysts understood a timed interest earned ratio of 3.00 to be safe. Cleverly and Associates computed a 1999 median times interest earned ratio of 2.37. Tenet, although able to cover its interest obligations, was below most benchmark figures for this ratio.

Analysts have come to realize, sometimes from hard experience, that times interest earned is not by itself an adequate measure of ability to cover debt obligations. An organization can have positive accrual profits while, as accounts receivable accumulate, little or no cash is generated. Because cash is necessary to meet debt obligations, some measure of the organization's cash generation compared to its debt obligation is necessary. The ratios that provide that measure fall into the class known as **cash flow coverage**. There are several ways to define cash flow coverage, each valid for its own purposes. Perhaps the most commonly used definition of cash flow coverage (although not the cash flow to total debt ratio that Cleverly provides) is EBITDA/interest expense. EBITDA (often pronounced "ebit-da") is "earnings before interest, taxes, depreciation, and amortization." Depreciation and amortization, being non-cash expense, are added back to give an approximation of the cash flows available to service debt. For Tenet, at the end of fiscal year 2000, that ratio was 3.3236.

PROFITABILITY RATIOS

The bottom line for any organization, at least in financial terms, is its ability to generate profits. Profits go by many names: net income, net earnings, excess of revenues over expenses, and (in one self-conscious not-for-profit hospital) "overage." Profits are, in accrual terms, the resources that the organization generated above those necessary to meet its obligations. Profits must be reinvested in the organization; used as a cushion against bankruptcy in the future; or, in investor-owned organizations, distributed to shareholders. To survive, an organization must be profitable.

Several ratios provide information about profitability. None of them is completely satisfactory. Perhaps the most often used is the **total margin**, the ratio of profit to the sum of revenues and nonoperating gains (Cleverly and Cameron, 2002, p. 159). That ratio indicates the amount of profit earned per dollar of revenue. It says nothing about the economic return on assets in place or the organization's ability to pay the required return to its equity holders. In fact, margin ratios (operating or total, pretax or after-tax) say more about an organization's ability to keep its unit prices above cost than about its ability to generate economic return. For Tenet for 2000, the total margin was 0.0265.

The second most commonly used profitability ratio is the **return on assets (ROA)**, or return on investment. That figure is profit divided by total assets. ROA measures the amount of profit per dollar of assets in place and indicates the ability of the organization to pay a return to its investors. There is, however, substantial controversy as to whether or not return on assets is an adequate measure of economic performance (Anthony, 1986; Fisher & McGowan, 1983; Long & Ravenscraft, 1984; Salaman, 1985). For Tenet for 2000, that figure was 0.0229.

The third profitability measure is **return on equity (ROE)**. That ratio also measures the organization's ability to pay a return to its equity holders and is defined as net income divided by owners' equity (or fund balance). For Tenet for 2000, ROE was 0.0743.

ROE can be decomposed into several parts. Doing so highlights the various components of economic performance. The basic decomposition of ROE begins with its definition:

$$ROE = \text{Net after-tax income}/\text{Owners' equity}$$

Algebraically, one can simultaneously multiply and divide one side of an equation by the same number without disturbing the equality. It follows, therefore, that

$$ROE = (\text{Net after-tax income}/\text{Total assets}) \times (\text{Total assets}/\text{Owners' equity})$$

That equation shows that ROE consists of ROA (net after-tax income/total assets) multiplied by the asset/equity ratio. Thus one of the effects of financial leverage is to multiply a modest ROA into a larger ROE (or to depress a modestly negative ROA into a catastrophically negative ROE). The ROA component of ROE can be further decomposed. Now let

$$ROE = (\text{Pretax income}/\text{Revenues}) \times (\text{Revenues}/\text{Total assets}) \times$$
$$(1 - \text{Tax rate}) \times (\text{Total assets}/\text{Owners' equity})$$

Restating with the names of the ratios,

$$ROE = \text{Pretax margin} \times \text{Total asset turnover} \times \text{Tax retention rate} \times \text{Asset}/\text{equity}$$

Thus the organization's ability to reward its shareholders (or the community that contributed its fund balance) depends on its ability to price its services so as to earn a pretax margin, its ability to use its assets to generate revenues (total asset turnover), its tax burden, and its financial leverage (asset/equity ratio).

SUMMARY

William Beaver (1991, pp. 9, 18) set forth guidelines on the analysis of financial statements for investors. His "10 commandments" are equally relevant for health care analysts. The commandments are as follows:

1. Thou shalt not use financial statements in isolation....

2. Thou shalt not use financial statements as the only source of firm-specific information....

3. Thou shalt not avoid reading footnotes, which are an integral part of financial statements....

4. Thou shalt not focus on a single number....

5. Thou shalt not overlook the *implications* of what is read....

6. Thou shalt not ignore events subsequent to the financial statements....

7. Thou shalt not overlook the limitations of financial statements....

8. Thou shalt not use financial statements without adequate knowledge....

9. Thou shalt not shun professional help....

10. Thou shalt not take unnecessary risks....

Beaver's comments are both pithy and worth remembering. Commandment 7 is especially worth heeding. Financial ratios are based on the numbers in the financial statements. Those numbers are accumulated, through the accounting cycle, via rules based on the accrual principle. Ratios are only as useful as the underlying data on which they are based. Chapter 3 discussed the ambiguity that is necessarily present in accounting numbers. Inventory valuation, depreciation expense, timing differences between revenue recognition and cash inflows, and the differences in definitions and classification between the not-for-profit sectors all affect the numbers on the financial statements (Sherman, 1986). The analyst must be forewarned.

CONTINUING CASES

As director and senior physician of a large, successful multispecialty medical group, Roger Jackson, MD, is unaccustomed to financial problems. Times, however, are changing. Two years ago, when the group's orthopedist (and leading revenue generator) threatened to leave, Jackson agreed to divide the group's annual surplus on a "percent of net revenue" basis. With his own attention devoted more and more to medical society matters (this year, he is president of the Clearwater County Medical Society) and to managing PCI, Inc., Dr. Jackson has seen his income from the practice plummet.

Now this: Henry Kirk presented PCI's financial statements to Dr. Jackson in a closed meeting this morning. "What do I know about financial statements?" was all that Dr. Jackson could say. "Melanie married that financial guy, but they live in Austin, and I don't trust him anyway." Worse, Tom Land down at CCB Bank ("Who do they think they are? CCB Bank! %#*%%#!!") says that the Jackson Group's credit has deteriorated badly (see the Continuing Cases section in Chapter 3).

Dr. Jackson is a plain-spoken man, a leader in the Jamestown civic affairs, and a successful entrepreneur. After graduation from medical school (University of Texas Medical Branch at Galveston, 1973) and completion of internship and residency (internal medicine) at Parkland Hospital in Dallas, he returned to his hometown of Jamestown to practice. By 1985 he had organized the Jackson Group and was ready to break ground for the structure that is now Physicians' Clinic. He and Mrs. Jackson live well by Jamestown standards. Their two daughters (both married and living away from Clearwater County) also enjoy the profits of PCI, Inc.

"Where's that Fowler woman? How are we doing, really? Cut the bull. Tom Land says we should have more cash. We're in business to take care of patients, not to hold a bank account. Do we need more cash? Four and a quarter million dollars in depreciation expense! What's that? We're being eaten alive! Can't we do something about that depreciation expense? Can we afford to continue to service all of that debt? What's the bottom line here?"

In another part of Jamestown, Billy Bob and Alice Ferguson are having coffee at their kitchen table. Going over the statements ("Computerized accounting is great, isn't it?"), Billy Bob is pleased with Lone Star Home Health Services' performance. "Alice, my dear, if I were still in banking, I believe I'd be willing to lend money to LSHHS," Billy Bob gloated. Things have not always been so rosy for LSHHS, and only a few years ago it needed regular cash infusions from its sponsoring churches.

Mrs. Ferguson, however, is a realist. "Would you really, Billy? Our excess is less than $4,000. We have about 2 months' expenses set aside in cash. It looks pretty precarious to me."

Mr. Ferguson learned long ago that he was lucky to have a cautious wife (how else could they have paid William and Mary's tuition at Baylor?). Thus he promised his wife that he would do a full financial analysis of LSHHS first thing tomorrow.

CASE QUESTIONS

The financial statements to which Dr. Jackson refers are in Table 4–3. In the absence of Janet Fowler, answer Dr. Jackson's questions.

Table 4–3 PCI, Inc., financial statements, 20XX

PCI, Inc. Balance Sheet 20XX (in $ thousand)	
Assets	
Current assets	
Cash and cash equivalents	$ 50
Marketable securities	5
Accounts receivable	240
Inventory	3
Prepaid expenses and other current assets	25
Total current assets	323
Long-term assets	
Property, plant, and equipment (net)	35,000
Intangible assets	15
Total long-term assets	35,015
Total assets	35,338
Liabilities	
Current liabilities	
Wages and salaries payable	135
Interest payable	90
Note payable	100
Other accounts payable	15
Current portion of long-term debt	1,000
Total current liabilities	1,340
Long-term liabilities	
Deferred income tax expense	30
Long-term debt	15,000
Total long-term liabilities	15,030
Total liabilities	16,370
Owners' equity	
Paid-in capital	1,000
Retained earnings	17,968
Total owners' equity	18,968
Liabilities + owners' equity	35,338
Revenues	
Net patient care revenue	11,750.00
Facilities rental revenue	12,500.00
Interest income	0.60
Other revenue	22.00
Total revenue	24,272.60

Table 4–3 (Continued)   PCI, Inc., financial statements, 20XX

PCI, Inc. Balance Sheet 20XX (in $ thousand)

Expenses

Wages and salaries	4,650.00
Maintenance and utilities	1,125.00
Equipment leases (operating leases only)	115.00
Insurance expense	145.00
Depreciation and amortization	4,250.00
Interest expense	12,000.00
Deferred income tax expense	16.00
Other expenses	2.50
Total expenses	22,303.50
Net income before taxes	1,969.10
Provision for income taxes	590.73
Net income	1,378.37

Lone Star's financial statements are shown in Table 4–4. What is the financial status of LSHHS?

Table 4–4   Lone Star Home Health Service, financial statements, 20XX

Statement of Revenues and Expenses

Revenues

Total revenues	$225,750
Expenses	
Wages and salaries	14,500
Payments to contract providers	122,000
Supplies and cost of goods sold	24,575
Maintenance and utilities	3,500
Equipment operation expenses	2,800
Insurance expense	15,500
Depreciation expense	3,694
Other expenses	35,250
Total expenses	221,819
Excess of revenues over expenses	3,931

Balance Sheet

Assets	
Current assets	
Cash and cash equivalents	38,900
Accounts receivable	7,500
Inventory	1,245
Other current assets	2,150
Total current assets	49,795
Long-term assets	
Property, plant, and equipment (net)	33,250
Total long-term assets	33,250
Total assets	83,045

Table 4–4 (Continued) Lone Star Home Health Service, financial statements, 20XX

Statement of Revenues and Expenses

Liabilities	
Current liabilities	
Wages and salaries payable	1,500
Contractual fees payable	3,500
Other accounts payable	2,200
Total current liabilities	7,200
Fund balance	75,845
Liabilities + fund balance	83,045

Discussion Questions

1. How is liquidity different from debt service coverage? Don't they both measure ability to pay debts?

2. In ratio analysis, an individual organization is usually compared to an appropriate industry average. How can one tell if the entire industry is doing poorly or well?

3. Which is more important, ROA or ROE? Why?

REFERENCES

Anthony, R.N. (1986). Accounting rate of return. *American Economic Review, 76*(1), 244–246.

Beaver, W.H. (1991). Ten commandments of financial statement analysis. *Financial Analysts Journal, 47*(1), 9, 18.

Cleverly, W.O. and Cameron, A.E. (2002). *Essentials of health care finance* (5th ed.). Gaithersburg, MD: Aspen.

Cleverly, W.O. & Rohleder, H. (1985). Unique dimensions of financial analysis service ratios. *Topics in Healthcare Finance, 11*(4), 81–88.

Coyne, J.S. (1985). Measuring hospital performance in multi-institutional organizations using financial ratios. *Health Care Management Review, 10*(4), 35–42.

Fisher, F.M. & McGowan, J.J. (1983). On the misuse of accounting rates of return to infer monopoly profits. *American Economic Review, 73*(1), 82–97.

Foster, G. (1978). *Financial statement analysis*. Englewood Cliffs, NJ: Prentice-Hall.

Johnsson, J. (1992, January 5). Financial performance data: HCIA, HFMA battle over methodology, market share. *Hospitals*, pp. 35–37.

Long, W.F. & Ravenscraft, D.J. (1984). The misuse of accounting rates of return: Comment. *American Economic Review, 74*(3), 494–500.

McCue, M.J. (1991). The use of cash flow to analyze financial distress in California hospitals. *Hospital and Health Service Administration, 36*(2), 223–241.

Salaman, G.L. (1985) Accounting rates of return. *American Economic Review, 75*(3) 495–504.

Sherman, H.D. (1986). Interpreting hospital performance with financial statement analysis. *Accounting Review, 61*(3), 526–550.

Standard & Poor's Corporation. (1989). *S&P's municipal finance criteria*. New York: Author.

Tenet Healthcare Corporation. (2000). *Annual report, 2000*. Los Angeles.

White, G.I., Sondhi, A.C., and Fried, D. (1997). *The analysis and use of financial statements* (2nd ed.). New York: John Wiley.

SELECTED READINGS

Cleverly, W.O. and Cameron, A.E. (2002). *Essentials of health care finance* (5th ed.). Gaithersburg, MD: Aspen.

Standard & Poor's Corporation. (1989). *S&P's municipal finance criteria*. New York: Author.

White, G.I., Sondhi, A.C., and Fried, D. (1997). *The analysis and use of financial statements* (2nd ed.). New York: John Wiley.

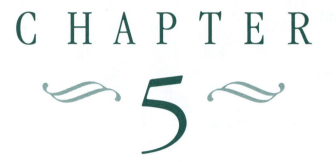

C H A P T E R

5

The Time Value of Money

Learning Objectives

After reading this chapter, the student should be able to:

1. Explain the opportunity cost basis for the time value of money.
2. Recognize situations that call for time value of money calculations.
3. Calculate future values and present values of single payments.
4. Calculate present values of annuities and other cash flow streams.
5. Perform simplified bond valuation calculations.

Key Terms

Annuity	Interest
Compound	Par value
Coupon payment	Present value
Coupon rate	Principal
Discounting	Rate of discount
End-of-period assumption	Time value of money
Future value	

Chapter 1 introduced the five pillars of finance (primacy of cash flows, recognition of maximizing behavior, risk aversion, time value of money, and recognition of opportunity cost). This chapter develops one of the pillars, that the value of money depends on when it is to be received.

In financial decision making, it is usually the case that one must evaluate a cash flow, or a stream of cash flows, that are expected in the future. In deciding whether or not to purchase a bond, one must examine the stream of interest and principal payments that the bond issuer promises to make in the future. In deciding whether or not to open a satellite clinic, one must consider the stream of cash flows that the clinic will generate in the future. In managing an organization's pension plan, the investment manager must consider the plan's obligations to make cash payments to retirees in the future.

In order to evaluate future cash flows, or streams of cash flows, one must understand the **time value of money**, the relationship between money today and money tomorrow. That relationship is neat and precise and depends on the time until the future cash flow and the interest rate that can be earned in the intervening period. Cash in the future is not the same as cash today. Because one can earn interest, it takes less than $1 in hand today to generate $1 at some future time. Many financial professionals describe this phenomenon by saying, "A dollar today is worth more than a dollar tomorrow." One might better say, "A dollar today is worth more than today's promise of a dollar tomorrow, even if that promise is without risk and there is no possibility of inflation."

It is important to recognize that money's time value exists because of money's ability to earn interest over time. A dollar in hand today is worth more than an IOU for a dollar because the dollar today can be lent at interest. The time value of money exists even if the purchasing power of the dollar will be constant over time (even if there will be no inflation) and even if the IOU carries no risk (there is an ironclad guarantee attached to the promise to pay). The forgone interest (the source of the time value of money) is an opportunity cost. Although they are distinct pillars of financial decision making, it is opportunity cost that generates the time value of money.

Expected inflation can affect the time value of money by increasing the interest rates that lenders demand. Similarly risky promises to pay may require higher interest rates than nonrisky promises and, therefore, may have lower present values. However, it is through the necessary interest rate that the effects of inflation and risk on the time value of money are manifest. The specific roles of expected inflation and of risk on interest rates are discussed further in Chapter 9. This chapter focuses on the skills necessary to study asset valuation, the selection of lines of business, and capital budgeting.

COMPOUNDING: THE CALCULATION OF FUTURE VALUE

The first Baron Rothschild, when asked what he considered the world's greatest natural wonder, is said to have replied, "Compound interest." **Interest** is a periodic payment made to induce some person (or institution) to delay consumption and to lend money to others. Interest is the price of money. It is the price one party receives for lending money and the price another party pays to borrow. Interest is always quoted as a percentage of the amount of money put aside or borrowed (a percentage of the **principal**). The determination of the level of interest rates is beyond the scope of this text but is a major topic in any textbook of macroeconomics (Mankiw, 2000).

Interest **compounds** when the interest paid in one period earns interest in the next period. It is that interest on interest that allows loans to grow from small to substantial amounts (such as the Rothschild family's fortune). Figure 5-1 shows how a dollar put aside (lent) at some rate of interest (r) accumulates over time.

Assume that one can lend money without any risk of loss of principal. At time zero ($t = 0$), \$1 is lent at interest rate r. r is expressed as a decimal, such as 0.08 (8 percent) or 0.10 (10 percent). After one period (at $t = 1$), the lender still has the \$1 lent and also has $r \times \$1$ in interest. The new principal, at $t = 1$, is $\$1 \times (1 + r)$.

If the lender allows interest to continue to compound, the full $\$1 \times (1 + r)$ will earn interest during the second period. At the end of the second period, the lender still has the $\$1 \times (1 + r)$ that she had at $t = 1$. The lender also has earned interest in the amount of $r \times \$1 \times (1 + r)$. A little algebraic manipulation shows that, at $t = 2$, the lender has a total of $\$1 \times (1 + r)^2$.

If the lender allows interest to continue to compound, the full $\$1 \times (1 + r)^2$ will earn interest during the third period. At the end of the third period the lender still has the principal she held at $t = 2$. The lender also earned interest in the amount

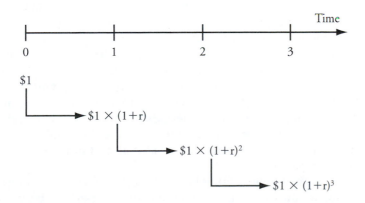

Figure 5-1 Annual compounding of \$1 deposit

$r \times \$1 \times (1 + r)^2$. Adding the old principal to the third period's interest and simplifying, one can see that the new principal is $\$1 \times (1 + r)^3$.

Following the same logic, after n periods of compounding at interest rate r, the original \$1 loan will have grown to be $\$1 \times (1 + r)^n$. The \$1 became a larger amount due to the passage of time, the earning of interest, and the compounding of interest on interest. The \$1 at $t = 0$ and the larger, future value are equivalent sums, evaluated at different points in time. They are generated by the same \$1 loan.

For convenience, the value of any amount at the end of five years ($t = 5$) is abbreviated V_5. The value in the present of a future amount at the present ($t = 0$) is abbreviated V_0. More generally, the value of a cash flow (or of a stream of cash flows) at the time t is abbreviated V_t.

Suppose that one loans \$1,000 to PCI, Inc. (the investor-owned firm in the continuing cases). PCI signs a contract agreeing to compound interest, annually, at the rate of 6 percent, on the anniversary date of the loan. At the end of 5 years, what would be the face value of the outstanding loan (V_5)? Table 5-1 provides the information necessary to solve that problem.

Table 5-1 shows the future value factors (FVFs) for various years and for various rates of compounding. For example, the future value factor for 5 percent for 5 years ($FVF_{5\%,\ 5\ yrs}$) is 1.2763. That is, if \$1 were lent at compound interest for 5 years at 5 percent interest, the outstanding loan would grow to be $\$1 \times 1.2763$, or about \$1.28. That $FVF_{5\%,\ 5\ yrs} = 1.2763$ is another way of saying that $(1 + 0.05)^5 = 1.21763$. Algebraically, $FVF_{r\%,\ n\ yrs} = (1 + r)^n$. In Table 5-1, the column labeled N shows the number of periods over which compounding takes place.

To solve for the **future value** of the principal of the \$1,000 loan to PCI, find the entry in Table 5-1 for 6 percent and 5 years. That amount ($FVF_{6\%,\ 5\ yrs}$) is 1.3382. The value of the principal, after 5 years of annual compounding at 6 percent (V_5), is the amount of the original loan (\$1,000) multiplied by the future value factor (1.3382). The solution, then is $\$1,000 \times 1.3382$, or \$1,338.20. PCI, Inc., must pay the lender \$1,338.20 at the end of 5 years to extinguish its debt obligation.

Now change the nature of the loan contract. Rather than compounding interest annually, say that PCI agrees to compound interest (to post the interest to the principal of the loan and to begin paying interest on interest) every 6 months. By convention, that problem is solved by dividing the annual interest rate by 2 and multiplying the number of payment periods by 2. Thus the loan in question is now 6 percent compounded semi-annually, or 3 percent for 10 periods.

To solve this revised problem, find $FVF_{3\%,\ 10\ periods}$ in Table 5-1. That factor is 1.3439. Multiply the $FVF_{3\%,\ 10\ periods}$ by the amount of the original loan (\$1,000) to find the principal at the end of 5 years. The new principal (V_5) will be \$1,343.90.

Mathematically sophisticated readers will note that dividing the annual interest rate in half and doubling the number of periods does not lead to a strictly correct solution to the problem. The convention of multiplying the number of periods and dividing the annual interest rate, however, is used almost universally, perhaps because it facilitates use of tables such as Table 5-1.

The two examples just given highlight an interesting fact about compounding: for any given annual rate of interest and any given total period of accumulation, the more frequently interest is compounded, the greater is the future value. For

Table 5-1   Future value of $1 after *n* periods

Rate of Compounding

N	0.01	0.02	0.03	0.04	0.05	0.06	0.07	0.08	0.09	0.10	0.11	0.12	0.15	0.20
0	1.0000	1.0000	1.0000	1.0000	1.0000	1.0000	1.0000	1.0000	1.0000	1.0000	1.0000	1.0000	1.0000	1.0000
1	1.0100	1.0200	1.0300	1.0400	1.0500	1.0600	1.0700	1.0800	1.0900	1.1000	1.1100	1.1200	1.1500	1.2000
2	1.0201	1.0404	1.0609	1.0816	1.1025	1.1236	1.1449	1.1664	1.1881	1.2100	1.2321	1.2544	1.3225	1.4400
3	1.0303	1.0612	1.0927	1.1249	1.1576	1.1910	1.2250	1.2597	1.2950	1.3310	1.3676	1.4049	1.5209	1.7280
4	1.0406	1.0824	1.1255	1.1699	1.2155	1.2625	1.3108	1.3605	1.4116	1.4641	1.5181	1.5735	1.7490	2.0736
5	1.0510	1.1041	1.193	1.2167	1.2763	1.3382	1.4026	1.4693	1.5386	1.6105	1.6851	1.7623	2.0114	2.4883
6	1.0615	1.1262	1.1941	1.2653	1.3401	1.4185	1.5007	1.5869	1.6771	1.7716	1.8704	1.9738	2.3131	2.9860
7	1.0721	1.1487	1.2299	1.3159	1.4071	1.5036	1.6058	1.7138	1.8280	1.9487	2.0762	2.2107	2.6600	3.5832
8	1.0829	1.1717	1.2668	1.3686	1.4775	1.5938	1.7182	1.8509	1.9926	2.1436	2.3045	2.4760	3.0590	4.2998
9	1.0937	1.1951	1.3048	1.4233	1.5513	1.6895	1.8385	1.9990	2.1719	2.3579	2.5580	2.7731	3.5179	5.1598
10	1.1046	1.2190	1.3439	1.4802	1.6289	1.7908	1.9672	2.1589	2.3674	2.5937	2.8394	3.1058	4.0456	6.1917
11	1.1157	1.2434	1.3842	1.5395	1.7103	1.8983	2.1049	2.3316	2.5804	2.8531	3.1518	3.4785	4.6524	7.4301
12	1.1268	1.2682	1.4258	1.6010	1.7959	2.0122	2.2522	2.5182	2.8127	3.1384	3.4985	3.8960	5.3503	8.9161
13	1.1381	1.2936	1.4685	1.6651	1.8856	2.1329	2.4098	2.7196	3.0658	3.4523	3.8833	4.3635	6.1528	10.6993
14	1.1495	1.3195	1.5126	1.7317	1.9799	2.2609	2.5785	2.9372	3.3417	3.7975	4.3104	4.8871	7.0757	12.8392
15	1.1610	1.3459	1.5580	1.8009	2.0789	2.3966	2.7590	3.1722	3.6425	4.1772	4.7846	5.4736	8.1371	15.4070
16	1.1726	1.3728	1.6047	1.8730	2.1829	2.5404	2.9522	3.4259	3.9703	4.5950	5.3109	6.1304	9.3576	18.4884
17	1.1843	1.4002	1.6528	1.9479	2.2920	2.6928	3.1588	3.7000	4.3276	5.0545	5.8951	6.8660	10.7613	22.1861
18	1.1961	1.4282	1.7024	2.0258	2.4066	2.8543	3.3799	3.9960	4.7171	5.5599	6.5436	7.6900	12.3755	26.6233
19	1.2081	1.4568	1.7535	2.1068	2.5270	3.0256	3.6165	4.3157	5.1417	6.1159	7.2633	8.6128	14.2318	31.9480
20	1.2202	1.4859	1.8061	2.1911	2.6533	3.2071	3.8697	4.6610	5.6044	6.7275	8.0623	9.6463	16.3665	38.3376
21	1.2324	1.5157	1.8603	2.2788	2.7860	3.3996	4.1406	5.0338	6.1088	7.4002	8.9492	10.8038	18.8215	46.0051
22	1.2447	1.5460	1.9161	2.3699	2.9253	3.6035	4.4304	5.4365	6.6586	8.1403	9.9336	12.1003	21.6447	55.2061
23	1.2572	1.5769	1.9736	2.4647	3.0715	3.8197	4.7405	5.8715	7.2579	8.9543	11.0263	13.5523	24.8915	66.2474
24	1.2697	1.6084	2.0328	2.5633	3.2251	4.0489	5.0724	6.3412	7.9111	9.8497	12.2392	15.1786	28.6252	79.4968
25	1.2824	1.6404	2.0938	2.6658	3.3864	4.2919	5.4274	6.8485	8.6231	10.8347	13.5855	17.0001	32.9190	95.3962

Table 5-1 *(continued)* Future value of $1 after *n* periods

						Rate of Compounding								
N	0.01	0.02	0.03	0.04	0.05	0.06	0.07	0.08	0.09	0.10	0.11	0.12	0.15	0.20
26	1.2953	1.6734	2.1566	2.7725	3.5557	4.5494	5.8074	7.3964	9.3992	11.9182	15.0799	19.0401	37.8568	114.4755
27	1.3082	1.7069	2.2213	2.8834	3.7335	4.8223	6.2139	7.9881	10.2451	13.1100	16.7386	21.3249	43.5353	137.3706
28	1.3213	1.7410	2.2879	2.9987	3.9201	5.1117	6.6488	8.6271	11.1671	14.4210	18.5799	23.8839	50.0656	164.8447
29	1.3345	1.7758	2.3566	3.1187	4.1161	5.4184	7.1143	9.3173	12.1722	15.8631	20.6237	26.7499	57.5755	197.8136
30	1.3478	1.8114	2.4273	3.2434	4.3219	5.7435	7.6123	10.0627	13.2677	17.4494	22.8923	29.9599	66.2118	237.3736
35	1.4166	1.9999	2.8139	3.9461	5.5160	7.6861	10.6766	14.7853	20.4140	28.1024	38.5749	52.7996	133.1755	590.6682
40	1.4889	2.2080	3.2620	4.8010	7.0400	10.2857	14.9745	21.7245	31.4094	45.2593	65.0009	93.0510	267.8635	1,469.7716
45	1.5648	2.4379	3.7816	5.8412	8.9850	13.7646	21.0025	31.9204	48.3273	72.8905	109.5320	163.9876	538.7693	3,657.2620
50	1.6446	2.6916	4.3839	7.1067	11.4674	18.4202	29.4570	46.9016	74.3575	117.3909	184.5648	289.0022	1,083.6574	9,100.4382

example, at 7 percent interest and a period of 5 years, semiannual compounding results in a greater future value (greater value of V_5) than does annual compounding. Similarly, all else equal, V_5 will be greater with quarterly compounding than with semiannual compounding. For any given period and annual rate of interest, the greatest achievable value of V_t is that which results from continuous compounding.

The formula for continuous compounding is

$$V_t = V_0 e^{rt}$$

where r is the annual rate of interest, t is the time over which compounding takes place (expressed in years), and e is the base of the natural logarithms (approximately 2.71828). Under continuous compounding, PCI's end-of-year-5 debt, in these examples, would be

$$V_5 = (\$1,000 \times e^{6\% \times 5}) = (\$1,000 \times 1.3499) = \$1,349.90$$

The difference between future values under annual and continuous compounding is so great that banks that offer continuously compounded savings often quote two rates: the nominal rate and the effective rate, or yield. Consider a bank account that offers an annual rate of 10 percent compounded annually. A depositor places $100 in that account on the first business day of the year (January 2) and, on the last business day of the year, realizes a value of $110. He realizes a yield of 10 percent. That is, the change in the account's value divided by the initial deposit is 10 percent [($110 - $100)/$100].

Now consider the same depositor and the same nominal rate of interest (10 percent), but say the account offers continuous compounding. At the end of the year, the balance of the account is $110.51 ($100 x $e^{0.10}$). The effective yield on the deposit is the change in the account's value divided by the initial deposit. That yield is 10.51 percent [($110.51 - $100)/$100]. Over a 1-year period, the difference is minor (about half a dollar), but for longer time periods and for greater account sizes, the dollar differences can be great.

Table 5-2 compares the future values of the PCI loan compounded at 6 percent for 5 years under annual, semiannual, quarterly, and continuous compounding. The data show that, as the compounding period grows shorter, interest is added to principal and begins to earn interest on interest more quickly. The result is that the terminal value (V_5) becomes larger.

Table 5-2 Future value of $1,000 compounded at 6 percent for 5 years

Compounding Intervals	Value at t = 0	Future Value Factor for 5 Years at 6 Percent	Value at t = 5
Annual	$1,000	1.3382	$1,338.20
Semiannual	1,000	1.3439	1,343.90
Quarterly	1,000	1.3469	1,346.86
Continuous	1,000	1.3499	1,349.86

The nature of the compounding process leads to three generalizations about the future value of any given amount held in the present (any given value of V_0):

1. All other factors held equal, the greater the rate of compounding, the greater is the future value (the value of V_t).

2. All other factors held equal, the longer is the time over which compounding occurs (the greater is t), the greater is the future value (the value of V_t).

3. All other factors held equal, the more often interest is compounded, the greater is the future value (the value of V_t).

DISCOUNTING: THE CALCULATION OF PRESENT VALUE

An amount of money in the present (V_0) can be associated with the amount to which it will grow in the future (V_t), given a specified time period, annual interest rate, and compounding period. Similarly, any amount of money to be received in the future (V_t) can be associated with the amount that, if held today, would generate the future amount under the conditions assumed (V_0). That amount needed today (V_0) is the **present value** of the future sum. The process by which a present value is computed, given some future value or values, is called **discounting**.

The present value of any future sum is the amount that, if lent today at a specified rate of interest, would generate the future sum on the specified future date. The present value, then, depends on (1) the size of the future amount, (2) the time to receipt of the future amount, (3) the assumed rate of interest, and (4) the frequency of compounding.

The derivation of future value showed that

$$V_t = V_0 \times (1 \times r)^t$$

The same relationship can be used to derive the formula for present value:

$$V_0 = V_t / (1 + r)^t,$$

$$V_0 = V_t \times [1/(1 + r)^t], \text{ or}$$

$$V_0 = V_t \times (1 + r)^{-t}$$

Table 5-3 shows the values of $1/(1+r)^t$ for various values of r (the **discount rate**) and t (the time to receipt of the future value). These figures are the present value factors at r percent for n periods ($\text{PFV}_{r\%, \, n \text{ periods}}$). Using the values in that table, one can find the present value of any future amount for the rates of discount and the numbers of periods given. For example, suppose that PCI, Inc., wishes to retire $400,000 of its long-term debt at its first possible opportunity. According to the terms under which its bonds were issued, those bonds can be "called" 3 years from today. The firm wishes to put aside enough funds today to have the $400,000 in 3 years. Assume that PCI can earn 8 percent, compounded annually, on the funds it sets aside.

PCI's problem is to compute the present value of $400,000 to be paid at the end of 3 years, assuming a discount rate of 8 percent. In Table 5-3, find the entry for the

Table 5-3   Present value of $1 to be received after *N* periods

Rate of Discount

N	0.01	0.02	0.03	0.04	0.05	0.06	0.07	0.08	0.09	0.10	0.11	0.12	0.15	0.20
0	1.0000	1.0000	1.0000	1.0000	1.0000	1.0000	1.0000	1.0000	1.0000	1.0000	1.0000	1.0000	1.0000	1.0000
1	0.9901	0.9804	0.9709	0.9615	0.9524	0.9434	0.9346	0.9259	0.9174	0.9091	0.9009	0.8929	0.8696	0.8333
2	0.9803	0.9612	0.9426	0.9246	0.9070	0.8900	0.8734	0.8573	0.8417	0.8264	0.8116	0.7972	0.7561	0.6944
3	0.9706	0.9423	0.9151	0.8890	0.8638	0.8396	0.8163	0.7938	0.7722	0.7513	0.7312	0.7118	0.6575	0.5787
4	0.9610	0.9238	0.8885	0.8548	0.8227	0.7921	0.7629	0.7350	0.7084	0.6830	0.6587	0.6255	0.5718	0.4823
5	0.9515	0.9057	0.8626	0.8219	0.7835	0.7473	0.7130	0.6806	0.6499	0.6209	0.5935	0.5674	0.4972	0.4019
6	0.9420	0.8880	0.8375	0.7903	0.7462	0.7050	0.6663	0.6302	0.5963	0.5645	0.5346	0.5066	0.4323	0.3349
7	0.9327	0.8706	0.8131	0.7599	0.7107	0.6651	0.6227	0.5835	0.5470	0.5132	0.4817	0.4523	0.3759	0.2791
8	0.9235	0.8535	0.7894	0.7307	0.6768	0.6274	0.5820	0.5403	0.5019	0.4665	0.4339	0.4039	0.3269	0.2326
9	0.9143	0.8368	0.7664	0.7026	0.6446	0.5919	0.5439	0.5002	0.4604	0.4241	0.3909	0.3606	0.2843	0.1938
10	0.9053	0.8203	0.7441	0.6756	0.6139	0.5584	0.5083	0.4632	0.4224	0.3855	0.3522	0.3220	0.2472	0.1615
11	0.8963	0.8043	0.7224	0.6496	0.5847	0.5268	0.4751	0.4289	0.3875	0.3505	0.3173	0.2875	0.2149	0.1346
12	0.8874	0.7885	0.7014	0.6246	0.5568	0.4970	0.4440	0.3971	0.3555	0.3186	0.2858	0.2567	0.1869	0.1122
13	0.8787	0.7730	0.6810	0.6006	0.5303	0.4688	0.4150	0.3677	0.3262	0.2897	0.2575	0.2292	0.1625	0.0935
14	0.8700	0.7579	0.6611	0.5775	0.5051	0.4423	0.3878	0.3405	0.2992	0.2633	0.2320	0.2046	0.1413	0.0779
15	0.8613	0.7430	0.6419	0.5553	0.4810	0.4173	0.3624	0.3152	0.2745	0.2394	0.2090	0.1827	0.1229	0.0649
16	0.8528	0.7284	0.6232	0.5339	0.4581	0.3936	0.3387	0.2919	0.2519	0.2176	0.1883	0.1631	0.1069	0.0541
17	0.8444	0.7142	0.6050	0.5134	0.4363	0.3714	0.3166	0.2703	0.2311	0.1978	0.1696	0.1456	0.0929	0.0451
18	0.8360	0.7002	0.5874	0.4936	0.4155	0.3503	0.2959	0.2502	0.2120	0.1799	0.1528	0.1300	0.0808	0.0376
19	0.8277	0.6864	0.5703	0.4746	0.3957	0.3305	0.2765	0.2317	0.1945	0.1635	0.1377	0.1161	0.0703	0.0313
20	0.8195	0.6730	0.5537	0.4564	0.3769	0.3118	0.2584	0.2145	0.1784	0.1486	0.1240	0.1037	0.0611	0.0261
21	0.8114	0.6598	0.5375	0.4388	0.3589	0.2942	0.2415	0.1987	0.1637	0.1351	0.1117	0.0926	0.0531	0.0217
22	0.8034	0.6468	0.5219	0.4220	0.3418	0.2775	0.2257	0.1839	0.1502	0.1228	0.1007	0.0826	0.0462	0.0181
23	0.7954	0.6342	0.5067	0.4057	0.3256	0.2618	0.2109	0.1703	0.1378	0.1117	0.0907	0.0738	0.0402	0.0151
24	0.7876	0.6217	0.4919	0.3901	0.3101	0.2470	0.1971	0.1577	0.1264	0.1015	0.0817	0.0659	0.0349	0.0126
25	0.7798	0.6095	0.4776	0.3751	0.2953	0.2330	0.1842	0.1460	0.1160	0.0923	0.0736	0.0588	0.0304	0.0105

Table 5-3 (continued) Present value of $1 to be received after *N* periods

					Rate of Discount									
N	0.01	0.02	0.03	0.04	0.05	0.06	0.07	0.08	0.09	0.10	0.11	0.12	0.15	0.20
26	0.7720	0.5976	0.4637	0.3607	0.2812	0.2198	0.1722	0.1352	0.1064	0.0839	0.0663	0.0525	0.0264	0.0087
27	0.7644	0.5859	0.4502	0.3468	0.2678	0.2074	0.1609	0.1252	0.0976	0.0763	0.0597	0.0469	0.0230	0.0073
28	0.7568	0.5744	0.4371	0.3335	0.2551	0.1956	0.1504	0.1159	0.0895	0.0693	0.0538	0.0419	0.0200	0.0061
29	0.7493	0.5631	0.4243	0.3207	0.2429	0.1846	0.1406	0.1073	0.0822	0.0630	0.0485	0.0372	0.0174	0.0051
30	0.7419	0.5521	0.4120	0.3083	0.2314	0.1741	0.1314	0.0994	0.0754	0.0573	0.0437	0.0334	0.0151	0.0042
35	0.7059	0.5000	0.3554	0.2534	0.1813	0.1301	0.0937	0.0676	0.0490	0.0356	0.0259	0.0189	0.0075	0.0017
40	0.6717	0.4529	0.3066	0.2083	0.1420	0.0972	0.0668	0.0460	0.0318	0.0221	0.0154	0.0107	0.0037	0.0007
45	0.6391	0.4102	0.2644	0.1712	0.1113	0.0727	0.0476	0.0313	0.0207	0.0137	0.0091	0.0061	0.0019	0.0003
50	0.6080	0.3715	0.2281	0.1407	0.0872	0.0543	0.0339	0.0213	0.0134	0.0085	0.0054	0.0035	0.0009	0.0001

PVF$_{8\%, 3 \text{ yrs}}$ (0.7938). Multiply that number by $400,000 to obtain $317,520. $317,520 is the present value, at 8 percent, of $400,000 to be received at the end of 3 years. That is, $317,520, put aside at 8 percent, compounded annually for 3 years, will become $400,000. If PCI puts aside $317,520 today at 8 percent, it will have the $400,000 it needs to call its bonds 3 years from today.

Table 5-3 was constructed using an **end-of-period assumption**. That is, the cash flows being discounted are assumed to take place at the end of the period in question. The table also assumes that discounting takes place once each period. Were PCI, in the example, to put its funds aside in an account earning and compounding interest every 6 months, the problems would be different. Then one would divide the 8 percent annual interest rate by 2 and double the number of periods. One would find the PVF for six periods at 4 percent per period (0.7903). Multiplying the PVF$_{4\%, 6 \text{ periods}}$ by $400,000, one sees that PCI would need to set aside $316,120 today in order to have $400,000 in 3 years.

Just as more frequent compounding increases the future value of any amount set aside in the present, more frequent discounting decreases the present value of any amount to be received in the future. The present value of any future amount is minimized, for any given annual rate of discount, when discounting is continuous. Working from the formula for future value, one can derive the formula for the present of a future sum when discounting is continuous:

$$V_0 = V_t \times e^{-rt}$$

where r is the annual rate of interest, t is the time until receipt of the future sum (expressed in years), and e is the base of the natural logarithms (about 2.71828).

Table 5-4 shows the present value factors for various annual rates of discount and for various time periods when discounting is continuous. For the example just given, when discounting is continuous, find the PVF for 8 percent at 3 years (0.7866). To find the present value of the $400,000 payment necessary, multiply 0.7866 by $400,000 to obtain $314,640. Under continuous discounting, PCI would need only $314,640 today to have, at 8 percent, $400,000 at the end of 3 years.

As was true of compounding, the mathematics of discounting provides some generalizations for the relationship between any given future value and its present value:

1. All other factors held equal, the longer the time until the receipt of that value, the smaller is the present value.

2. All other factors held equal, the greater the discount rate, the smaller the present value.

3. All other factors held equal, the more frequent is the discounting interval, the smaller is the present value.

SPECIAL PROBLEMS IN PRESENT VALUE

Discounting single payments is uncomplicated, given the availability of Tables 5-3 and 5-4. One usually faces more complex situations when solving time value of money problems. Rather than demanding the present value of a single payment,

Table 5-4 Present value of $1 to be received after N periods (continuous discounting)

N	Rate of Discount													
	0.01	0.02	0.03	0.04	0.05	0.06	0.07	0.08	0.09	0.10	0.11	0.12	0.15	0.20
0	1.0000	1.0000	1.0000	1.0000	1.0000	1.0000	1.0000	1.0000	1.0000	1.0000	1.0000	1.0000	1.0000	1.0000
1	0.9900	0.9802	0.9704	0.9608	0.9512	0.9418	0.9324	0.9231	0.9139	0.9048	0.8958	0.8869	0.8607	0.8187
2	0.9802	0.9608	0.9418	0.9231	0.9048	0.8869	0.8694	0.8521	0.8353	0.8187	0.8025	0.7866	0.7408	0.6703
3	0.9704	0.9418	0.9139	0.8869	0.8607	0.8353	0.8106	0.7866	0.7634	0.7408	0.7189	0.6977	0.6376	0.5488
4	0.9608	0.9231	0.8869	0.8521	0.8187	0.7866	0.7558	0.7261	0.6977	0.6703	0.6440	0.6188	0.5488	0.4493
5	0.9512	0.9048	0.8607	0.8187	0.7788	0.7408	0.7047	0.6703	0.6376	0.6065	0.5769	0.5488	0.4724	0.3679
6	0.9418	0.8869	0.8353	0.7866	0.7408	0.6977	0.6570	0.6188	0.5827	0.5488	0.5169	0.4868	0.4066	0.3012
7	0.9324	0.8694	0.8106	0.7558	0.7047	0.6570	0.6126	0.5712	0.5326	0.4966	0.4630	0.4317	0.3499	0.2466
8	0.9231	0.8521	0.7866	0.7261	0.6703	0.6188	0.5712	0.5273	0.4868	0.4493	0.4148	0.3829	0.3012	0.2019
9	0.9139	0.8353	0.7634	0.6977	0.6376	0.5827	0.5326	0.4868	0.4449	0.4066	0.3716	0.3396	0.2592	0.1653
10	0.9048	0.8187	0.7408	0.6703	0.6065	0.5488	0.4966	0.4493	0.4066	0.3679	0.3329	0.3012	0.2231	0.1353
11	0.8958	0.8025	0.7189	0.6440	0.5749	0.5169	0.4630	0.4148	0.3716	0.3329	0.2982	0.2671	0.1920	0.1108
12	0.8869	0.7866	0.6977	0.6188	0.5488	0.4868	0.4317	0.3829	0.3396	0.3012	0.2671	0.2369	0.1653	0.0907
13	0.8781	0.7711	0.6771	0.5945	0.5220	0.4584	0.4025	0.3535	0.3104	0.2725	0.2393	0.2101	0.1423	0.0743
14	0.8694	0.7558	0.6570	0.5712	0.4966	0.4317	0.3753	0.3263	0.2837	0.2466	0.2144	0.1864	0.1225	0.0608
15	0.8607	0.7408	0.6376	0.5488	0.4724	0.4066	0.3499	0.3012	0.2592	0.2231	0.1920	0.1653	0.1054	0.0498
16	0.8521	0.7261	0.6188	0.5273	0.4493	0.3829	0.3263	0.2780	0.2369	0.2019	0.1720	0.1466	0.0907	0.0408
17	0.8437	0.7118	0.6005	0.5066	0.4274	0.3606	0.3042	0.2567	0.2165	0.1827	0.1541	0.1300	0.0781	0.0334
18	0.8353	0.6977	0.5827	0.4868	0.4066	0.3396	0.2837	0.2369	0.1979	0.1653	0.1381	0.1153	0.0672	0.0273
19	0.8270	0.6839	0.5655	0.4677	0.3867	0.3198	0.2645	0.2187	0.1809	0.1496	0.1237	0.1023	0.0578	0.0224
20	0.8187	0.6703	0.5488	0.4493	0.3679	0.3012	0.2466	0.2019	0.1653	0.1353	0.1108	0.0907	0.0498	0.0183
21	0.8106	0.6570	0.5326	0.4317	0.3499	0.2837	0.2299	0.1864	0.1511	0.1225	0.0993	0.0805	0.0429	0.0150
22	0.8025	0.6440	0.5169	0.4148	0.3329	0.2671	0.2144	0.1720	0.1381	0.1108	0.0889	0.0714	0.0369	0.0123
23	0.7945	0.6313	0.5016	0.3985	0.3166	0.2516	0.1999	0.1588	0.1262	0.1003	0.0797	0.0633	0.0317	0.0101
24	0.7866	0.6188	0.4868	0.3829	0.3012	0.2369	0.1864	0.1466	0.1153	0.0907	0.0714	0.0561	0.0273	0.0082
25	0.7788	0.6065	0.4724	0.3679	0.2865	0.2231	0.1738	0.1353	0.1054	0.0821	0.0639	0.0498	0.0235	0.0067

Table 5-4 (*continued*)   Present value of $1 to be received after *N* periods (continuous discounting)

N	\multicolumn{20}{c}{Rate of Discount}

N	0.01	0.02	0.03	0.04	0.05	0.06	0.07	0.08	0.09	0.10	0.11	0.12	0.15	0.20
26	0.7711	0.5945	0.4584	0.3535	0.2725	0.2101	0.1620	0.1249	0.0963	0.0743	0.0573	0.0442	0.0202	0.0055
27	0.7634	0.5827	0.4449	0.3396	0.2592	0.1979	0.1511	0.1153	0.0880	0.0672	0.0513	0.0392	0.0174	0.0045
28	0.7558	0.5712	0.4317	0.3263	0.2466	0.1864	0.1409	0.1065	0.0805	0.0608	0.0460	0.0347	0.0150	0.0037
29	0.7483	0.5599	0.4190	0.3135	0.2346	0.1755	0.1313	0.0983	0.0735	0.0550	0.0412	0.0308	0.0129	0.0030
30	0.7408	0.5488	0.4066	0.3012	0.2231	0.1653	0.1225	0.0907	0.0672	0.0498	0.0369	0.0273	0.0111	0.0025
35	0.7047	0.4966	0.3499	0.2466	0.1738	0.1225	0.0863	0.0608	0.0429	0.0302	0.0213	0.0150	0.0052	0.0009
40	0.6703	0.4493	0.3012	0.2019	0.1353	0.0907	0.0608	0.0408	0.0273	0.0183	0.0123	0.0082	0.0025	0.0003
45	0.6376	0.4066	0.2592	0.1653	0.1054	0.0672	0.0429	0.0273	0.0174	0.0111	0.0071	0.0045	0.0012	0.0001
50	0.6065	0.3679	0.2231	0.1353	0.0821	0.0498	0.0302	0.0183	0.0111	0.0067	0.0041	0.0025	0.0006	0.0000

valuation problems usually involve calculating the present value (V_0) of a stream of cash flows (V_1, V_2, ..., V_n). Fortunately, such problems are straightforward. Figure 5-2 pictures one such problem for three future cash flows. Each of the future cash flows is discounted back to the present. The present value of the stream of cash flows is the sum of the present values of the individual cash flows.

Table 5-5 shows the calculation of the present value (V_0) of a series of three future cash flows (V_1, V_2, V_3), each discounted at 5 percent (annual discounting). To find the present value of the stream, each of these is multiplied by the present value factor, for 5 percent, for the appropriate time period. Multiply V_1 by the $\text{PVF}_{5\%, 1\,yr}$, V_2 by the $\text{PVF}_{5\%, 2\,yrs}$, and V_3 by the $\text{PVF}_{5\%, 3\,yrs}$. Having found the present values of each of the three component cash flows, one sums them to find the present value of the stream of cash flows ($5,446.50).

The interpretation of the solution shown in Table 5-5 is straightforward. If one had $5,446.50 today and put it aside at 5 percent interest (compounded annually on the anniversary of the deposit), one could withdraw $2,000 1 year from today, $2,000 2 years from today, and $2,000 3 years from today. The third withdrawal would completely exhaust the account.

Some cash flow streams are so long that calculating the present value of each cash slow in the stream is impractical. For example, when one looks at the present value of the stream of cash flows that will accrue from owning a share of common stock, one assumes that the firm issuing the stock will continue to exist for the

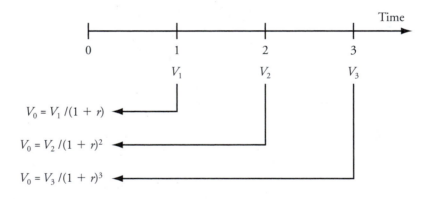

Figure 5-2 Discounting of future cash flows

Table 5-5 Present value of three future cash flows

Year	Future Cash Flow	PVF at 5%	Discounted Cash Flow
1	$2,000	0.9524	$1,904.76
2	2,000	0.9070	1,814.06
3	2,000	0.8638	1,727.68
Total			5,446.50

forseeable future. When evaluating a possible new line of service, one usually assumes that one will continue to provide the service indefinitely. Preferred stock, which promises to pay its holder a fixed annual dividend in perpetuity, can be evaluated as a perpetual stream of cash flows, as long as the issuing firm is solvent. The formula for the present value of a constant, perpetual stream (a perpetuity) is

$$V_0 = V_1 \,/\, r$$

where V_1 is the first cash flow in the stream (since the stream is constant, all of the future cash flows are equal) and r is that rate of discount.

In some cases, cash flow streams are assumed to be perpetual, but the cash flows that constitute them are not constant. If the rate of growth of the cash flows is constant, the formula for the present value of the stream is

$$V_0 = V_1 \,/\, (r - g)$$

where V_1 is the first cash flow in the stream, r is the discount rate, and g is the rate of growth of the cash flows (assumed constant).

ANNUITIES

Another special case of present value problem is that of an **annuity**. An annuity is a series of equal, evenly spaced cash flows. Many problems in finance can be solved by calculating the present value of an annuity. An individual planning for retirement might purchase an annuity contract, promising to pay a constant amount every month from retirement until death. The insurance company offering such a retirement annuity must determine the contract's price by determining the present value of the expected stream of annuity payments. That present value is the amount that, if put aside today, will generate exactly the expected stream of payments.

The insurance company, of course, cannot know in advance the number of annuity payments that it will make to any given individual (the number of months after retirement the retiree will live). Individuals' postretirement life spans cannot be known with certainty. Actuaries can, however, provide estimates of the expected life span of a representative retiree. By selling annuity contracts to a very large number of individuals, the insurance company can make a profit by pricing its contract of the basis of expected years of life. Bonds represent annuities, paying their holders an interest payment (also known as a **coupon payment**) every 6 months until maturity. Their valuation (see Chapter 6) involves finding the present value of the annuity of coupon payments.

The formula for the present value of an annuity is easily derived. Look again at Table 5-5. The cash flow stream illustrated there is a 3-year annuity of amount $2,000. The present value of that annuity is

$$V_0 = (V_1 \times \mathrm{PVF}_{5\%,\ 1\ \mathrm{yr}}) + (V_2 \times \mathrm{PVF}_{5\%,\ 2\ \mathrm{yrs}}) + (V_3 \times \mathrm{PVF}_{5\%,\ 3\ \mathrm{yrs}})$$

Because the cash flows are equal, $V_1 = V_2 = V_3$, the present value can be rewritten as

$$V_0 = (V_1 \times \text{PVF}_{5\%,\ 1\ \text{yr}}) + (V_1 \times \text{PVF}_{5\%,\ 2\ \text{yrs}}) + (V_1 \times \text{PVF}_{5\%,\ 3\ \text{yrs}})$$

One can factor V_1 from each of the expressions in parentheses to obtain

$$V_0 = V_1 \times \sum_{t=1}^{3} \text{PVF}_{5\%,\ t\ \text{yrs}}$$

The sum of the three PVFs is the present value factor for an annuity for 5 percent for 3 years ($\text{PVFA}_{5\%,\ 3\ \text{yrs}}$). Table 5-6 shows the PVFAs for a variety of interest rates and periods. Like the other tables in this chapter, Table 5-6 assumes that each annuity payment is made at the end of the period. Therefore, when using Table 5-6 to calculate the present value of an annuity, one is calculating the value of the annuity as evaluated at the point one period prior to the first payment in the annuity.

The PVFA can be derived either as the sum of the present value factors for single payments over the life of the annuity or by using the formula

$$\text{PVFA}_{r\%,\ n\ \text{yrs}} = [1 - 1 / (1 + r)^n] / r$$

That formula, or any of several that are algebraically equivalent forms, can be derived by subtracting from the present value of a perpetual annuity of $1 per period $(1/r)$ the present value of that part of the perpetuity that is to be received after the termination of the annuity in question $[1 / r \times 1 / (1 + r)^n]$ (Brealey & Myers, 2000, p. 42).

Return to the problem in Table 5-5. To use Table 5-6 to find the present value of the three-period annuity, find the PVFA for 5 percent for 3 years (2.7232). Multiply that factor by the (annual) amount of the annuity ($2,000). The result is the present value of the annuity, $5,446.40, within rounding error of the present value calculated using the three PVFs for single payments.

Consider a simplified pension planning problem. PCI, Inc. (from the continuing case), has promised its director of facilities $35,000 per year in deferred compensation for the first 10 years of his retirement (in lieu of a traditional pension plan). The first of these payments is to be made on the date of retirement, with a payment on each of the nine succeeding retirement anniversaries. How much must PCI have tucked away on the retirement date in order to have that obligation fully covered? Assume that PCI can earn 12 percent on its funds.

Table 5-7 shows the calculations involved in solving that problem. The 10 payments promised the facilities director constitute an annuity amount of $35,000 for 10 years. The relevant interest rate (rate of discount) is 12 percent. Therefore, to find the present value of the annuity stream (10 payments of $35,000 each), multiply $35,000 by $\text{PVFA}_{12\%,\ 10\ \text{years}}$ (5.6502). The product ($197,757.00) is the present value of the annuity evaluated 1 year prior to the first annuity payment.

However, that amount is not the answer to the problem. Using the table for present value factors for annuities, one calculates the present value as valued one period prior to the first cash flow. As the problem was stated, PCI needed to know how much it needed in the bank on the director's retirement date, the date of the first cash flow. Between the date 1 year prior to the first cash flow and the date of the first cash flow, the required amount would grow by exactly 12 percent (the

Table 5-6   Present value of an annuity of $1 per period for N periods

Rate of Discount

N	0.01	0.02	0.03	0.04	0.05	0.06	0.07	0.08	0.09	0.10	0.11	0.12	0.15	0.20
0	1.0000	1.0000	1.0000	1.0000	1.0000	1.0000	1.0000	1.0000	1.0000	1.0000	1.0000	1.0000	1.0000	1.0000
1	0.9901	0.9804	0.9709	0.9615	0.9524	0.9434	0.9346	0.9259	0.9174	0.9091	0.9009	0.8929	0.8696	0.8333
2	1.9704	1.9416	1.9135	1.8861	1.8594	1.8334	1.8080	1.7833	1.7591	1.7355	1.7125	1.6901	1.6257	1.5278
3	2.9410	2.8839	2.8286	2.7751	2.7232	2.6730	2.6243	2.5771	2.5313	2.4869	2.4437	2.4018	2.2832	2.1065
4	3.9020	3.8077	3.7171	3.6299	3.5460	3.4651	3.3872	3.3121	3.2397	3.1699	3.1204	3.0373	2.8550	2.5887
5	4.8534	4.7135	4.5797	4.4518	4.3295	4.2124	4.1002	3.9927	3.8897	3.7908	3.6959	3.6048	3.3522	2.9906
6	5.7955	5.6014	5.4172	5.2421	5.0757	4.9173	4.7665	4.6229	4.4859	4.3553	4.2305	4.1114	3.7845	3.3255
7	6.7282	6.4720	6.2303	6.0021	5.7864	5.5824	5.3893	5.2064	5.0330	4.8684	4.7122	4.5638	4.1604	3.6046
8	7.6517	7.3255	7.0197	6.7327	6.4632	6.2098	5.9713	5.7466	5.5348	5.3349	5.1461	4.9676	4.4873	3.8372
9	8.5660	8.1622	7.7861	7.4353	7.1078	6.8017	6.5152	6.2469	5.9952	5.7590	5.5370	5.3282	4.7716	4.0310
10	9.4713	8.9826	8.5302	8.1109	7.7217	7.3601	7.0236	6.7101	6.4177	6.1446	5.8892	5.6502	5.0188	4.1925
11	10.3676	9.7868	9.2526	8.7605	8.3064	7.8869	7.4987	7.1390	6.8052	6.4951	6.2065	5.9377	5.2337	4.3271
12	11.2551	10.5753	9.9540	9.3851	8.8633	8.3838	7.9427	7.5361	7.1607	6.8137	6.4924	6.1944	5.4206	4.4392
13	12.1337	11.3484	10.6350	9.9856	9.3936	8.8527	8.3577	7.9038	7.4869	7.1034	6.7499	6.4235	5.5831	4.5327
14	13.0037	12.1062	11.2961	10.5631	9.8986	9.2950	8.7455	8.2442	7.7862	7.3667	6.9819	6.6282	5.7245	4.6106
15	13.8651	12.8493	11.9379	11.1184	10.3797	9.7122	9.1079	8.5595	8.0607	7.6061	7.1909	6.8109	5.8474	4.6755
16	14.7179	13.5777	12.5611	11.6523	10.8378	10.1059	9.4466	8.8514	8.3126	7.8237	7.3792	6.9740	5.9542	4.7296
17	15.5623	14.2919	13.1661	12.1657	11.2741	10.4773	9.7632	9.1216	8.5436	8.0216	7.5488	7.1196	6.0472	4.7746
18	16.3983	14.9920	13.7535	12.6593	11.6896	10.8276	10.0591	9.3719	8.7556	8.2014	7.7016	7.2497	6.1280	4.8122
19	17.2260	15.6785	14.3238	13.1339	12.0853	11.1581	10.3356	9.6036	8.9501	8.3649	7.8393	7.3658	6.1982	4.8435
20	18.0456	16.3514	14.8775	13.5903	12.4622	11.4699	10.5940	9.8181	9.1285	8.5136	7.9633	7.4694	6.2593	4.8696
21	18.8570	17.0112	15.4150	14.0292	12.8212	11.7641	10.8355	10.0168	9.2922	8.6487	8.0751	7.5620	6.3125	4.8913
22	19.6604	17.6580	15.9369	14.4511	13.1630	12.0416	11.0612	10.2007	9.4424	8.7715	8.1757	7.6446	6.3587	4.9094
23	20.4558	18.2922	16.4436	14.8568	13.4886	12.3034	11.2722	10.3711	9.5802	8.8832	8.2664	7.7184	6.3988	4.9245
24	21.2434	18.9139	16.9355	15.2470	13.7986	12.5504	11.4693	10.5288	9.7066	8.8947	8.3481	7.7843	6.4338	4.9371
25	22.0232	19.5235	17.4131	15.6221	14.0939	12.7834	11.6536	10.6748	9.8226	9.0770	8.4217	7.8431	6.4641	4.9476

Table 5-6 *(continued)* Present value of an annuity of $1 per period for *N* periods

							Rate of Discount							
N	0.01	0.02	0.03	0.04	0.05	0.06	0.07	0.08	0.09	0.10	0.11	0.12	0.15	0.20
26	22.7952	20.1210	17.8768	15.9828	14.3752	13.0032	11.8258	10.8100	9.9290	9.1609	8.4881	7.8957	6.4906	4.9563
27	23.5596	20.7069	18.3270	16.3296	14.6430	13.2105	11.9867	10.9352	10.0266	9.2372	8.5478	7.9426	6.5135	4.9636
28	24.3164	21.2813	18.7641	16.6631	14.8981	13.4062	12.1371	11.0511	10.1161	9.3066	8.6016	7.9844	6.5335	4.9697
29	25.0658	21.8444	19.1885	16.9837	15.1411	13.5907	12.2777	11.1584	10.1983	9.3696	8.6501	8.0218	6.5509	4.9747
30	25.8077	22.3965	19.6004	17.2920	15.3725	13.7648	12.4090	11.2578	10.2737	9.4269	8.6938	8.0552	6.5660	4.9789
35	29.4086	24.9986	21.4872	18.6646	16.3742	14.4982	12.9477	11.6546	10.5668	9.6442	8.8552	8.1755	6.6166	4.9915
40	32.8347	27.3555	23.1148	19.7928	17.1591	15.0463	13.3317	11.9246	10.7574	9.7791	8.9511	8.2438	6.6418	4.9966
45	36.0945	29.4902	24.5187	20.7200	17.7741	15.4558	13.6055	12.1084	10.8812	9.8628	9.0079	8.2825	6.6543	4.9986
50	39.1961	31.4236	25.7298	21.4822	18.2559	15.7619	13.8007	12.2335	10.9617	9.9148	9.0417	8.3045	6.6605	4.9995

Table 5-7   Calculations for a deferred compensation retirement plan

Annual amount of deferred compensation	$ 35,000.00
Years annuity is to be paid	10
Effective interest rate	12.00%
Present value factor for an annuity (12%, 10 yrs)	5.6502
Present value of the annuity evaluated 1 year prior to the first payment	197,757.00
Present value of the annuity evaluated on the date of the first payment	221,487.84

annual rate of interest). Therefore one must multiply the present value 1 year prior to the first cash flow ($197,757.00) by 1.12 to take account of the accumulation of interest during the following year. The result is that, on the director's retirement date, PCI needs to have set aside $221,487.84 to be able to cover the promised 10-year annuity.

SOME EXAMPLES

Knowledge of the time value of money is necessary in solving a great many financial problems. One type of application, valuation of assets and securities, is the subject of Chapter 6. Another type of application of time value of money calculation is capital budgeting, the subject of Chapters 10 and 11. Present value problems are also at the heart of many financing and working capital decisions. A few examples of the application of time value of money calculations will serve both as a guide in performing those calculations and as an illustration of their importance.

Consider the problem of bidding on the purchase of a corporate bond. Such a bond is a contact promising that the borrower will pay the lender a fixed amount of interest every 6 months for some specified period (the life of the bond) and, on the maturity date, will repay the principal of the loan in full. In the United States, corporate bonds are usually issued with a face value (or **par value**) of $1,000, for terms of up to 30 years. The semiannual payments (coupon payments) are specified as a percentage of the face value (two payments whose sum, divided by $1,000, is the **coupon rate**). In most cases, the coupon payments are fixed for the life of the bond. Prevailing market rates of interest will vary over the life of the bond. The bond's price must change to bring the rate of return the bond offers into line with prevailing market interest rates. Chapter 6 will shows that a bond buyer will bid no more than the present value of all of the future cash flows that the bond promises. If there are enough bidders, the market price will settle at that present value.

Table 5-8 shows the determination of a potential buyer's bid for a $1,000 bond with a coupon rate of 8 percent when the prevailing market rate of interest is 6 percent. The bond is issued today, the first coupon is due 6 months from today, and the principal is due (the bond matures) 30 years from today.

The bond's coupon payments and its return of principal to the bondholder represent 60 future cash flows. The present value of a stream of cash flows is the sum of the present values of the individual cash flows. In Table 5-8 each of these future cash flows is discounted at the semiannual rate of 3 percent (remember that, when discounting is semiannual, one follows the convention that the annual rate of

Table 5-8 Bidding on a 30-year bond

Bond promises to pay 8% on a face value of $1,000
Coupon payments are to be made every 6 months.
Required annual interest rate is 6% (semiannual rate is 3%).

Period	Bond's Promised Cash Flow	PVF at 3%	Bond's Promised Cash Flow Discounted
1	$40	0.9709	$38.83
2	40	0.9426	37.70
3	40	0.9151	36.61
4	40	0.8885	35.54
5	40	0.8626	34.50
6	40	0.8375	33.50
7	40	0.8131	32.52
8	40	0.7894	31.58
9	40	0.7664	30.66
10	40	0.7441	29.76
11	40	0.7224	28.90
12	40	0.7014	28.06
13	40	0.6810	27.24
14	40	0.6611	26.44
15	40	0.6419	25.67
16	40	0.6232	24.93
17	40	0.6050	24.20
18	40	0.5874	23.50
19	40	0.5703	22.81
20	40	0.5537	22.15
21	40	0.5375	21.50
22	40	0.5219	20.88
23	40	0.5067	20.27
24	40	0.4919	19.68
25	40	0.4776	19.10
26	40	0.4637	18.55
27	40	0.4502	18.01
28	40	0.4371	17.48
29	40	0.4243	16.97
30	40	0.4120	16.48
31	40	0.4000	16.00
32	40	0.3883	15.53
33	40	0.3770	15.08
34	40	0.3660	14.64
35	40	0.3554	14.22
36	40	0.3450	13.80
37	40	0.3350	13.40
38	40	0.3252	13.01
39	40	0.3158	12.63
40	40	0.3066	12.26
41	40	0.2976	11.91
42	40	0.2890	11.56
43	40	0.2805	11.22
44	40	0.2724	10.89

Table 5-8 (continued) Bidding on a 30-year bond

Period	Bond's Promised Cash Flow	PVF at 3%	Bond's Promised Cash Flow Discounted
45	40	0.2644	10.58
46	40	0.2567	10.27
47	40	0.2493	9.97
48	40	0.2420	9.68
49	40	0.2350	9.40
50	40	0.2281	9.12
51	40	0.2215	8.86
52	40	0.2150	8.60
53	40	0.2088	8.35
54	40	0.2027	8.11
55	40	0.1968	7.87
56	40	0.1910	7.64
57	40	0.1855	7.42
58	40	0.1801	7.20
59	40	0.1748	6.99
60	1,040	0.1697	176.52
			Present value = 1,276.76

interest is divided in half). The final cash flow is different from the others in that it consists of both the 60th coupon payment and the return of the face value of the bond (the principal of the loan) to the bondholder. Summing the discounted cash flows shows that, under these circumstances, a potential bond buyer would bid $1,276.76 for the bond in question.

Table 5-9 looks at the same facts in a different way. The bond promises 60 equal evenly spaced payments. That flow of payments is an annuity of 60 payments. Thus multiplying $40 (the amount of each payment) by the present value factor for an annuity for 60 periods at 3 percent ($PVFA_{3\%, 60 \text{ periods}}$) will yield the present value of the annuity that the bond promises. The $PVFA_{3\%, 60 \text{ periods}}$ does not appear in Table 5-4 but can be computed using the formula for such factors

Table 5-9 Bidding on a 30-year bond

Bond promises to pay 8% on a face value of $1,000.

Coupon payments are to be made every 6 months.

Required interest rate is 6%.

Bond offers an annuity of $40 per period for 60 periods.

Annuity is followed by a single payment of $1,000 when the face value (principal) is redeemed at the end of 30 years.

Present value = $40 \times PVFA_{3\%, 60 \text{ periods}}$ + $1,000 \times PVF_{6\%, 30 \text{ yrs}}$

$PVFA_{3\%, 60 \text{ periods}}$ = 27.6756; $PVF_{6\%, 30 \text{ yrs}}$ = 0.1741

Present value = $1,281.13

$[(1 - (1 + r)^n / r]$. PVFA$_{3\%, 60 \text{ periods}}$ = 27.6756. Why is 3 percent used as the periodic discount rate? Because the effective annual interest rate is given as 6 percent. As payments are made every 6 months, the convention of dividing the annual rate in half and multiplying the number of periods by 2 is used to arrive at a periodic discount rate of 3 percent and 60 periods.

In addition to the 60-period annuity, the issuer of the bond promises to repay the principal amount at the end of the life of the bond (the maturity date). That $1,000 is to be received at the end of 30 years. It must be discounted by multiplying by the present value factor (for a single payment) for 6 percent for 30 years (PVFA$_{6\%, 30 \text{ yrs}}$) *or* by the present value factor (for a single payment) for 3 percent for 60 periods (PVFA$_{3\%, 60 \text{ periods}}$). The two present value factors will give results that differ only trivially. Most professionals prefer to use the same interest rate (3 percent in this case) for both parts of the bond's value.

The calculations shown in Table 5-9 show the present value of the bond's cash flows to be $1,281.13. This approach generates a present value less than $5 different (due to rounding error) from the approach used in Table 5-8.

Table 5-10 shows the solution to a very different type of problem. A small community hospital has installed a new computerized axial tomography (CAT) scanner and expects to be able to use it for 3 years. It wants to begin today to save for the necessary replacement device (this process is called "funding the depreciation"). The hospital's facilities planners estimate that replacement in 3 years will cost $525,000. How much money should the hospital set aside today ($t = 0$), 1 year from today ($t = 1$), and 2 years from today ($t = 2$) in order to have the necessary $525,000 in 3 years (at $t = 3$)? The hospital's funded depreciation account will earn interest at 10 percent.

The problem requires setting the future value of the sum of the 3 equal payments equal to $525,000 (it is a future value of an annuity problem). The procedure requires that, first, the future value factors (for single payments) for one, two, and

Table 5-10   Saving to replace an asset

Current CAT scanner will remain in place until 3 years from today.
Expect replacement CAT scanner to cost $525,000.
Can earn 10%, compounded annually.

Year	Amount to Set Aside	FVF$_{10\%, 3 - t + 1 \text{ yrs}}$	Future Value of Annual Savings
1	$144,191.16	1.3310	$191,918.43
2	144,191.16	1.2100	174,471.30
3	144,191.16	1.1000	158,610.27
	Sum	3.6410	525,000.00

Steps:
1. Let X be the constant annual amount to be set aside.
2. Set $X \times \text{FVF}_{10\%, 3 \text{ yrs}} + X \times \text{FVF}_{10\%, 2 \text{ yrs}} + X \times \text{FVF}_{10\%, 1 \text{ yr}}$ = $525,000.
3. Solve for X.
4. Use the matrix above to test results.

three periods at 10 percent ($FVF_{10\%, 3 \text{ yrs}}$, $FVF_{10\%, 2 \text{ yrs}}$, and $FVF_{10\%, 1 \text{ yr}}$) be found. These factors can be found in Table 5-1. Then the value of the equal annual deposit to the funded depreciation account (the unknown quantity) is multiplied by each of the FVFs and the sum is set equal to $525,000:

$$\$525,000 = (X \times FVF_{10\%, 3 \text{ yrs}}) + (X \times FVF_{10\%, 2 \text{ yrs}}) + (X \times FVF_{10\%, 1 \text{ yr}})$$

That equation implies that

$$\$525,000 = X \times \sum_{t=1}^{3} FVF_{10\%, t \text{ yrs}}$$

Solving for X, one finds the required annual deposit to be $144,191.16. That $144,191.16 is the necessary amount can be verified by substituting into a spreadsheet like that shown in Table 5-5.

Table 5-11 illustrates an important principle of financial decision making: two streams of cash flows can be compared at any common point in time. Henry Kirk of Physicians' Clinic (in the continuing case) plans to retire 5 years from today. Although his pension and deferred compensation from PCI, Inc., will give him an adequate income, he realizes that he will need additional savings to purchase one of the beach front condominiums he and Mrs. Kirk have coveted since their first visit to South Padre Island years ago. Mr. Kirk estimates that a two-bedroom model will cost $250,000 in 5 years.

Mr. Kirk wants to pay level annual payments into a savings account to accumulate the purchase price of his condominium. He will make the first payment in 1 year and the last on his retirement date. He can earn 9 percent in a long-term deposit account at CCB Bank. How large must each annual payment be?

The "trick" to the solution to this problem is to realize that the $250,000, to be paid in 5 years, and Mr. Kirk's stream of five payments can be compared at any common point in time. The most convenient point for most comparisons, including this one, is the present time ($t = 0$). To solve for Mr. Kirk's necessary annual

Table 5-11   Planning for the purchase of a beach home for retirement

Retirement will be 5 years from today.
Need $250,000 on the retirement date to purchase desired beach home.
Relevant interest rate is 9%.

Year	Needed Cash	PVF at 9%	Discounted Needed Cash
5	$250,000	0.6499	$162,475

Solving:
$162,475 = X × PVFA for 9% for 5 years
$162,475 = X × 3.8897
     X = $41,770.57

1. Five deposits constitute an annuity to be valued today.
2. Compare the present value of the needed cash flow to that of the 5-year annuity.
3. Solve for the annual amount of the annuity.

contribution, the present value, evaluated today (V_0), of the anticipated purchase price and of the stream of deposits must be calculated.

The present value of the purchase price is straightforward. The purchase will be a single payment, 5 years from today. To calculate its present value, multiply the anticipated payment ($250,000) by the present value factor for a single payment for 9 percent for 5 years ($PVF_{9\%, \, 5 \, yrs}$). Table 5-3 shows that $PVF_{9\%, \, 5 \, yrs}$ is 0.6499. The present value of the condominium's purchase price is $162,475.

For a stream of payments to be adequate to pay the purchase price, the present value of the stream of payments must equal the present value of the purchase price ($162,475). The five payments, made at $t = 1$, $t = 2$, $t = 3$, $t = 4$, and $t = 5$, represent a five-period annuity. Multiplying a fixed payment (X) by the present value factor for an annuity for 9 percent for 5 years ($PVFA_{9\%, \, 5 \, yrs}$) gives the value of that four-period annuity as measured today (V_0). Table 5-6 shows that $PVFA_{9\%, \, 5 \, yrs}$ is 3.8897.

Mr. Kirk will set the present value of his five payments equal to the present value of the anticipated price of the condominium. Algebraically,

$$\$162,475 = X \times PVFA_{9\%, \, 5 \, yrs}$$

Equivalently,

$$\$162,475 = X \times 3.8897$$

Solving for X, one finds that the required annual deposit is $41,770.57

SUMMARY

That the value of a dollar (or of a crown, a euro, a pound, or a yen) depends on when it is to be received (or paid) is one of the fundamental pillars of financial decision making. The burden that an obligation represents for an organization declines when paying that obligation can be pushed into the future. That fact is the key to solving a wide variety of financial problems in investment analysis, valuation (Chapter 6), and asset selection (Chapters 10 and 11).

The relation between money today and money in the future can be measured precisely. It depends on how far in the future a payment is to be made, what interest rate will prevail in the interim period, and how often interest is to be compounded. Understanding the simple mathematics of present value is the key to the valuation of assets and is the first step in making capital investment and financing decisions.

The present value of any future amount is greater

1. The lower is the discount rate.

2. The shorter is the time to receipt of the future value.

3. The less frequent is the period of discounting.

The lowest present value of any future cash flow (for a given discount rate and time to receipt) is that associated with continuous discounting.

QUESTIONS AND PROBLEMS

1. To what future value will $1,250 grow if it is put aside to earn 7 percent interest today and left to compound for 5 years? For 10 years? For 20 years?

2. One puts $50 into a savings account on the first business day of each month, beginning on January 2. The account earns 12 percent per year, compounded monthly. What is the balance of the account on New Year's Eve?

3. What is the present value of $250,000 to be received at the end of 15 years if the discount rate is 5 percent (discounted annually)? 10 percent? 20 percent?

4. What is the present value of $500,000 to be received 15 years from now if the annual rate of discount is 10 percent and discounting is continuous?

5. One year from today, Mr. Guenther will retire from his position as chief information officer at Presbyterian Hospital. The hospital's retirement plan guarantees Mr. Guenther $45,000 per year, payable on the retirement date and on each anniversary thereafter. The plan's actuary estimates that Mr. Guenther will live to collect 15 of those payments. The plan earns 6 percent on its investments. How much must the retirement have in place now to fund its expected obligation to Mr. Guenther?

6. What is the most that a rational investor would be willing to pay for the following bond: face value = $1,000; annual coupon rate = 9 percent; semiannual coupon payments; issued today, first coupon payment is 6 months from today; matures 10 years from today? The effective market rate of interest is 6 percent. What would a rational investor pay for the bond if the effective market rate of interest were 12 percent?

7. Explain why the future value is greater under quarterly compounding than under annual compounding, for any given present value and annual rate of interest.

8. Compare two annuity contracts. Annuity Contract A pays its holder $10,000 per year for 10 years, at the end of each year, beginning 1 year from today. Annuity Contract B pays its holder $10,000 per year for 10 years, at the beginning of each year, beginning today. The relevant rate of discount for both contracts is 8 percent. Which of the annuity contracts has the higher present value? How much higher? How can one adjust the information in Table 5-4 to calculate the present value of Contract B?

9. What annual payment (made at the end of each year) is necessary to retire a $150,000 debt in 8 years? The eight payments are to be equal and made at the end of each year. The interest rate on the loan is 12 percent. Explain how to approach this problem.

10. Consider a share of common stock whose annual dividend, 1 year from today, is expected to be $12. The annual dividend is expected to grow at a constant rate of 2 percent in perpetuity. The relevant discount rate is 8 percent. What is the present value of all of the expected future dividends from holding the share of stock?

REFERENCES

Brealey, R.A. & Myers, S.C. (2000). *Principles of corporate finance* (6th ed.). New York: McGraw-Hill.

Mankiw, N.G. (2000). *Macroeconomics* (4th ed.). New York: Worth.

SELECTED READING

Ayers, F.J. (1968). *Mathematics of finance*. New York: McGraw-Hill (Schaum's Outline Series).

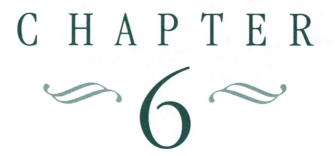

CHAPTER
6

Valuing Assets

Learning Objectives

After reading this chapter, the student should be able to:

1. Explain the differences among the major approaches to valuation.
2. Explain the conceptual origin of discounted cash flow valuation.
3. Apply discounted cash flow models to the valuation of health care organizations.
4. Apply discounted cash flow models to the valuation of securities for which no active trading is available to establish a reliable market price.

Key Terms

Adjusted book value	Goodwill
Appraisal	Market value
Discounted cash flow	Valuation
Dividend discount model	

One of the most useful applications of the time value of money is in the valuation of assets. Simply put, valuation is the estimation of "what things are worth." In the health care arena, a great many types of assets must be valued, and as demonstrated in the following sections, calculation of the present value of a stream of cash flow is the most appropriate means of doing so. After completing this chapter, the reader will be able to determine the implicit value of an asset, an organization, or a security according to accepted financial procedures.

VALUE

In health care settings, valuation was seldom important until the 1980s. Recent trends in hospitals' purchases and sales of group practices, sales of whole hospitals by not-for-profit owners to investor-owned firms (and vice versa), and leveraged buyouts of hospital firms have created the need to understand the valuation process.

Many items are traded in markets in which no well-defined price can be observed. For example, young internists are invited, upon completion of their residencies, to "buy into" established medical practices. That is, the recent resident is offered the opportunity to buy an ownership share in the practice of several established senior colleagues. What is such an ownership share worth? Unlike the price of a share of General Motors stock, there is no continuous bidding to establish a market price for a share of a practice. The young internist must determine if the price quoted, and the terms under which he or she will pay that price, is fair.

The internist is faced with the purchase of more than just some equipment and a share of an office lease (Baumann & Oxaal, 1993). The diagnostic equipment, the office supplies and machinery, and the right to occupy space have been put together into a bundle, a practice. The physicians who built the practice have devoted their care and professional skills to building a roster of loyal patients. Those patients trust the incumbent physicians to know them and their conditions, to treat them when necessary, and to refer them to other specialists when appropriate. The loyalty of those patients, and the revenues that they will provide, have value. The practice may have contracts with one or more managed care plans. The revenues that those contracts will generate also have value. The value of the practice, then, depends on the cash-generating power of patient and business relationships (**goodwill** is the accounting term) rather on the market value of the things the practice owns.

The valuation of a practice, a clinic, a hospital, or a subsidiary does not depend on the market values of its physical assets. In that sense, **valuation** is different from **appraisal**, the process in which one determines the market values of compo-

nent assets. Valuation depends on the uses to which assets are put, on name identification and customer loyalty, and on the degree of control being transferred.

As the health care sector has changed, the role of valuation has grown. Not
only are more assets involved in the delivery of health care, but their ownership changes much more frequently than was true in the past. The example
just outlined, the pricing of a share of a medical practice, illustrates a common
application of valuation. Today, not only do young physicians purchase shares
in practices (and older physicians "cash out" of them), but new applications of
valuation have emerged. When practices merge, each of them must be valued
so that ownership of the new, combined practice can be distributed appropriately among the owners of the two preexisting ones. When a medical center
purchases a group practice, the owners of the practice insist on fair compensation for their sale. When not-for-profit holding organizations sell their hospitals
to investor-owned firms, they want to know that they were properly compensated for the sale. When hospital pension funds are offered bonds for their
portfolios, they need to know that they are not giving up too much of their
beneficiaries' funds in exchange.

APPROACHES TO VALUATION

There is a substantial body of literature, both scholarly and applied, on valuation in general (Copeland, Koller, & Murrin, 1990; Damodaran, 1996; McCarthy
& Healy, 1971; Smith, 1988; Veit, 1990) and on valuation in health care (Burik
& Millar, 1987; Federa & Ketcham, 1993). Those books and articles suggest four
possible approaches to valuing firms, practices, assets, and securities. These
four methods are the use of rules of thumb, the use of adjusted book (accounting) value (Nicholas, 1990), the use of market value (Wolf, 1990), and the use
of discounted cash flows (Gilbert, 1990). This section will explain how one
might use each of the four methods. The next section will argue that the
fourth (discounted cash flows) is the best method.

People often simplify their lives by adopting rules of thumb. These are shortcuts
in decision making, rules that work in most cases. A manager might say, "Nurses
on the night shift should earn 1.25 times as much per hour as nurses on the day
shift." That manager can go through life with that rule and never need to conduct
an external wage analysis or to hire a compensation consultant. Applying that
compensation rule simplifies decision making. The rule of thumb works as long as
nothing disturbs the local labor market for nurses.

Similarly, many financial managers have adopted rules of thumb for valuing
organizations. One such rule is that an organization (whether a consulting firm, a
hospital, or a medical practice) is worth twice its annual revenues. By analogy, a
share of corporate stock would be worth twice the issuing firm's revenues per
share. Another rule of thumb, advocated in a widely read business magazine, is
that a firm is worth "equipment and fixtures (at fair market value), inventory
(valued at seller's cost), leasehold improvements (market value) and one year's
net income," ("How to Price a Small Business," 1984).

As convenient as rules of thumb may be, their use, inevitably, means making assumptions about how much one could realize from the sale of assets and about the relation between current revenues (or earnings) and market price. Those assumptions may or may not be valid in any real case at any given time.

Adjusted Book Value

The **adjusted book value** approach holds that the numbers on the balance sheet, specifically, owners' equity (or net assets), are an accurate reflection of an organization's value. This approach would have a share of corporate stock sell for owners' equity per share. Chapter 3 reviewed the ambiguities in the meaning of accounting numbers. Although sophisticated users of the adjusted book value approach attempt to value inventory and accounts receivable at market values, ambiguities remain.

Consider Herman, a fictitious consultant, who wants to publish a newsletter, "The Health Care Financial Reporter." To begin, Herman incorporates his firm, which buys a state-of-the-art desktop computer, printer, and desktop publishing software for $10,000. The would-be author also buys some used office furniture and a mailing list of the area's hospitals. He leases his office space. Over time, Herman's newsletter grows in popularity. The firm's net income grows, all of which Herman withdraws from his corporate accounts each month as his personal income.

After 5 years, Herman's newsletter is a national bestseller. Herman, now accustomed to a six-figure income, has grown bored with the regular grind of publishing and wants to work the lecture circuit. He looks for a buyer for his newsletter publishing firm.

Herman's books show his equipment, fully depreciated, as having zero value. Even on a market-value basis, a 5-year-old computer system has minimal worth. Office furniture that was used 5 years ago is now worthless. Herman has no cash in his business accounts, having withdrawn all cash each month. The book value of Herman's firm is zero.

A major commercial publisher of newsletters approaches Herman and wants to purchase "The Health Care Financial Reporter." Would Herman agree to sell for the book value of his private publishing organization? Not on a bet. His corporation, and the right to market his popular newsletter, is worth much more than the book value of the assets that produce it. After all, Herman has drawn a nice check for his work each month for the last 5 years. Accounting book values do not necessarily reflect market values.

Market Value

The **market value** approach takes another tack. Users of this approach seek to value one practice by identifying several comparable practices whose market values are known. Thus one might begin to value the ABC Clinic by finding out the recent sale price of comparable XYZ Clinic. XYZ's recent sale price can be divided by its previous year's net income to determine its price/earnings ratio. That ratio can then be multiplied by ABC's previous annual income to determine a market value for ABC. Again, sophisticated users of this approach will compare ABC's market area (demographics, income, insurance coverage) to that of XYZ and adjust the price/earnings ratio accordingly (Wolf, 1990).

The market value approach is very similar to the most commonly used methods of real estate valuation (or appraisal). In real estate appraisal, one values parcel A by identifying comparable parcels (B, C, and D) whose prices have recently been determined in the open market. A's market value is then estimated by its relationship, in size and improvements, to the values of its "comparables."

The market value approach to valuation yields reasonable results *if* comparables can be identified. If one is negotiating the first sale of a cardiology practice in the state, the method will not work. Moreover, the market value approach assumes that the same price/earnings ratio will apply to the organization being valued as to the comparable organization(s). When the market value approach works, it is because its use of an appropriate price/earnings ratio mimics the fourth approach: discounted cash flows.

THE LOGIC OF DISCOUNTED CASH FLOW VALUATION

The method of valuing a financial asset or a going business concern (whether not for profit or investor owned) that is best justified by financial theory is the **discounted cash flow** method. The discounted cash flow approach is based on the assertion that any asset is worth the present value of all of the cash flows that the asset will generate for its owner. Thus advocates of this approach hold that a bond's market value should be equal to the present value of the cash flows that its issuers promise to pay to its buyers. The value of a medical practice is the present value of the cash flows that the practice will generate for its owners.

What is the logic that underlies the use of the discounted cash flow method? First, consider the issue of cash flows. Why is it the present value of cash flows that matter? It is for the expectation of cash flows, now or in the future, that one purchases financial assets. Financial and business assets are different from the collection of great art, bottle caps, or old road signs; they are purchased to generate cash. One might purchase an asset because one expects its value to rise (one expects it to generate a capital gain), but the hoped-for capital gain will materialize only if other investors, in the future, bid a higher price for the asset in the expectation of cash flows. History is replete with examples of people (or whole nations) who believed assets would rise in value for no obvious reason. The Dutch tulip craze, with the price of a single tulip bulb reaching an entire year's wages, is a famous example. Such "bubbles," with asset values based on something (often imagined) other than future cash flows, always end in crashes.

Remember Herman the consultant from a few pages back, however. Herman will take his newsletter publishing firm to the auction block with something to offer a potential buyer: the cash flows that the buyer can realize from publishing and selling the newsletter. It is the cash flows that the newsletter offers, not the few, paltry assets in place, that make the purchase of the firm attractive.

Consider a simple case, a zero-coupon bond. A zero-coupon bond represents a loan from the buyer of the bond to the issuer of the bond. The issuer promises to pay the face (or par) value of the bond to the buyer on the date the loan is due (maturity date). In the meantime, the issuer will make no interest payments to the buyer (the issuer makes no coupon payments, hence it is a zero-coupon bond).

Consider a zero-coupon bond with a par value of $1,000, maturing 10 years from today. The prospective bond buyer's best alternative financial investment pays 8 percent compounded annually. What is that bond worth? The problem is shown in Table 6–1. The zero-coupon bond's value, its market price, will gravitate toward $463.19.

If the potential bond buyer were to pay more than $463.19, he would be incurring opportunity costs. That is because were he to loan, for example, $475 today at 8 percent, compounded annually, at the end of 10 years he would have $1,025.49. Therefore $475 is too much to bid for a $1,000 bond maturing 10 years from now, when the relevant interest rate is 8 percent. Invested in an alternative asset, the $475 could, become an amount ($1,025.49) greater than the promised $1,000. The bond buyer who bids $475 for the bond today incurs an opportunity cost of $25.49 at the end of 10 years.

Similarly, the seller of the bond will not accept any amount less than $463.19 for her $1,000 bond. Were the seller to accept a bid of, say, $400 for a $1,000 bond maturing in 10 years, she would be offering to pay more than the required 8 percent. In fact, to accept $400 for the $1,000 10-year bond would be to pay 9.6 percent ($[1000/400]^{1/10} - 1 = 0.096$). Thus for the seller to accept less than $463.19 would be to incur an unnecessary interest rate on her debt. The seller, then, will accept no less than the present value of the promised cash flows to avoid unnecessary interest rate costs. The buyer, on the other hand, will offer no more than the present value of the promised cash flows to avoid incurring opportunity cost. The market price of the bond must be equal to the present value of the cash flows that its seller promises to pay to its buyer.

The greater the competition in bidding for the bond, the more rapidly its price will approach the present value of its cash flows. If the seller of the bond acts as an auctioneer, competitive bidding will force the price of the bond to the maximum that any buyer is willing to pay. If 8 percent is the rate of interest on the next best alternative, then a price of, say, $450 represents a bargain for the buyer. In the next best alternative, at 8 percent, $450 would become only $971.52, $1,000 × $(1.08)^{10}$, in 10 years. If the bond buyer could pay only $450 for the bond, he would reap a windfall gain of $28.48 at the end of 10 years. So long as the market price of the bond implies such a windfall gain, other potential bond buyers will bid more. The bidding will stop when the price of the bond reaches the present value of the promised cash flows, $463.19.

Table 6-1 Value of a zero-coupon bond maturing in 10 years

Value in 10 years	$1,000.00
PVF for 10 years for 8%	0.4632
Present value of the bond's par value	463.19

SOME APPLICATIONS

Applications of valuation abound in finance. Whenever the value of an asset must be determined but cannot be observed in a competitive market, one is faced with a valuation problem. Any market price, such as the price of a share of corporate stock, will settle at the present value of its expected cash flows, with or without anyone's actually performing the calculations.

Corporate Bond

Consider a typical corporate bond, promising to pay its holder interest (the coupon payment) every 6 months (beginning 6 months from today) for 10 years and to repay its principal at the end of the 10-year period. Assume that the par value of the bond is $1,000 and that the coupon rate is 6 percent. The coupon payments form an annuity of 20 periods and with periodic payments of $30 ($1,000 × 0.06/2). The return of principal is a single payment at the end of 10 years. Assume that the interest rate now prevailing on the next best investment is 8 percent.

To value the bond, one needs to find the present value, at 8 percent, of all of the cash flows (principal and interest) that the bond's issuer promises to pay. First, consider the annuity formed by the coupon payments. The present value of an annuity of 20 $30 payments, at 4 percent per period (8 percent per year implies 4 percent per 6-month period), is equal to

$$V_0 \text{ (annuity)} = \$30 \times \text{PVFA}_{4\%, \, 20 \text{ periods}}$$

or

$$V_0 \text{ (annuity)} = \$30 \times 13.5903$$

or

$$V_0 \text{ (annuity)} = \$407.71$$

The present value of the return of the bond's principal is also straightforward. The present value of $1,000 to be received at the end of 10 years at 8 percent is

$$V_0 \text{ (principal)} = \$1,000 \times \text{PVF}_{8\%, \, 10 \text{ yrs}}$$

or

$$V_0 \text{ (principal)} = \$1,000 \times 0.4632$$

or

$$V_0 \text{ (principal)} = \$463.19$$

Alternately, one can use the PVF for 20 periods at 4 percent. The result will differ but little.

The present value of all of the cash flows that the bond's issuer promises to pay is the sum of the present value of the annuity component and the present value of the principal component:

$$V_0 \text{ (total)} = \$407.71 + \$463.19$$

or

$$V_0 \text{ (total)} = \$870.90.$$

The bidding for the bond will stop when the market price equals that number.

Preferred Stock

Preferred stock is an interesting application. Corporations that issue preferred stock promise to pay a fixed dollar dividend in perpetuity. As long as the corporation exists, the holder of the share of preferred stock is entitled to a fixed annual payment. Unless the stock carries some atypical legal right (such as convertibility), the corporation has no obligation to repurchase, or otherwise "cash in," the stock. The price of a share of preferred stock will be the present value of an annuity of amount equal to the stock's promised annual payment. Consider a share of preferred stock promising to pay $50 per year in perpetuity. If the interest rate on the next best alternative investment is 4 percent, the price of the share of stock will be

$$V_0 = \text{Annual amount/interest rate}$$

or

$$V_0 = \frac{\$50}{0.04}$$

or

$$V_0 = \$1{,}250.$$

Common Stock

Common stock is one of the most difficult assets to value, because the corporation issuing the stock has no legal obligation to pay anything to its common stock holders. Financial analysts frequently use **dividend discount models**, based on the rule that the stock is worth the present value of the future dividends it will pay, to value corporate shares (Ferrell, 1985; Sorenson & Williamson, 1985). The simplest dividend discount model assumes that dividends will be constant forever. In that case, the valuation of the common shares is just like the valuation of preferred shares, shown earlier.

In real life, dividends are seldom constant over time. Some boards of directors form implicit covenants with their shareholders to increase dividends each period. One form that such an implicit covenant might take is that dividends will increase by some fixed annual percentage. Consider again a corporation that promises to pay $50 dividends beginning 1 year from today and that now promises to increase that dividend by 1 percent per year. The formula for the present value of that dividend stream is

$$V_0 = \frac{D_1}{(r-g)}$$

where D_1 is the dividend to be paid 1 year hence, r is the required rate of interest, and g is the annual rate of growth of the dividend. If the opportunity cost of capital is 4 percent, the value of the stock would be

$$V_0 = \frac{\$50}{0.04 - 0.01}$$

or

$$V_0 = \frac{\$50}{0.03}$$

or

$$V_0 = \$1,666.67$$

In the case just cited, $1,666.67 is the equilibrium market value of the share of stock in question, assuming no market frictions (such as transactions costs) and assuming that all market participants accept the promise of the growing dividend. Why is that the market value? If a potential stockholder were to take $1,666.67 and put it away at 4 percent interest, she could withdraw $50 in 1 year, $50 × (1.01) in 2 years, $50 × (1.01)^2 in 3 years, and so on. The $1,666.67, at 4 percent, could duplicate the stock's promised cash flows. To sell the stock for less than $1,666.67, the seller would be giving the buyer some future cash flows for free. To buy the share for more than $1,666.67, the buyer is surrendering some future cash flows that she could have earned in an alternative security.

In practice, one often projects more complex cash flows than the constant growth dividend discount model can handle. The rule is still the same, the organization is worth the present value of its expected future cash flows, but the calculations become substantially more complex. Consider the case of a corporation that owns and operates free-standing imaging centers, and is expected to pay a $5 per share dividend one year from today. The Corporation is now experiencing high growth in dividends (12 percent per year), expected to continue for 2 more years. At the end of that period, 3 years from today, analysts project that dividend growth will decline to 4 percent per year, and remain at that level in perpetuity. The current required rate of return is 8 percent.

Although tedious, the calculations are straightforward. One cannot use the constant growth rate model, since the current growth rate (12 percent) is greater than the required rate of return (8 percent). As the growth rate approaches the required rate of return in the simple model, the value of the organization approaches infinity. Thus, for the first three years, the analyst must calculate the present value of each dividend.

For dividends after the period of explosive growth, one can use the constant growth model ($D_4/(r - g)$, D_4 because that is the first dividend after the high growth period), but must discount that value back to the present from $t = 3$.

The calculation, then, is

$$V_0 = [\$5 \times PVF_{8\%, \, 1 \, year}] = [\$5(1.12) \times PVF_{8\%, \, 2 \, years}] + [\$5(1.12)^2 \times PVF_{8\%, \, 3 \, years}] + [\$5(1.12)^2(1.04) \, / \, (0.08 - .04] \times PVF_{8\%, \, 3 \, years};$$

or

$$V_0 = [\$5 \times 0.9259] + [\$5.60 \times 0.8573] + [\$6.27 \times 0.7938] +$$
$$[\$6.52 / (.04)] \times 0.7938;$$

or

$$V_0 = \$143.80.$$

A CASE STUDY

Figure 6–1 shows the 1992 financial statements for the Mayo Foundation. It is interesting to contemplate exactly what the Mayo Foundation was worth at that time. That value cannot be observed, as the Mayo Foundation has no common stock outstanding (it is a not-for-profit entity) and the assets of the foundation (the Mayo Clinic, its affiliated facilities, and some financial assets) have not been traded in open markets (where their prices could be observed) in recent memory.

If one uses the rule of thumb that an organization is worth 2 years' net revenues, the Mayo Foundation (and all of its holdings) is worth $3,141,244,000, or about $3 billion. To find that value, add up the foundation's sources of revenue, operating and other. Operating revenue for 1992 was $1,491,740,000. Other revenues (listed separately, below the operating expenses category) were $78,882. In this case, it is important to recognize nonoperating revenues, as investment income and the ability to raise donations are important aspects of the value of the foundation. Doubling the total of operating and nonoperating revenue gives the $3 billion figure.

The second valuation method discussed earlier was the adjusted book value method. The book value of owner's equity (fund balance in this case) is the difference between the book value of assets and the book value of liabilities. The Mayo Foundation's book value of assets at the end of 1992 was $2,592,120,000. Refer to Chapter 3 to review the accounting rules that produce that value. Land is booked at its historical cost. Other physical assets are booked at cost less depreciation. That these assets are joined with a high level of medical expertise is ignored in computing book value, as is the name recognition of the Mayo Clinic.

The foundation's book value of liabilities was $924,530,000 at the end of 1992. Thus the book value of the foundation's fund balance at year-end 1992 was $1,667,590,000. That figure can be calculated either by subtracting the book value of liabilities from the book value of assets or by adding the two classes of fund balance (restricted and unrestricted) shown in the statements. The book value method, then, gives a value for the Mayo Foundation of about $1.7 billion, much lower than the "2 years' revenue" rule of thumb.

One cannot use the market value approach to value the Mayo Foundation. There simply are no comparable organizations whose price earnings multiple one can apply to Mayo's bottom line.

The fourth approach to valuation, the one best justified by financial theory, is the discounted cash flow approach. Mayo reports its cash flows at the bottom of its one-page financial statements. The relevant figure among the cash flow items is cash flow from operating activities, $226,774,000 for 1992. That cash was expended

MAYO FOUNDATION

Comparative Financial Statement Summary
Unrestricted and Restricted Funds Combined — 1992 and 1991
(In thousands of dollars)

Balance Sheets — December 31	1992	1991	Change
Assets			
Cash	$ 2,687	$ 11,451	$ (8,764)
Receivables for medical services — net	271,204	269,771	1,433
Investments — at market	1,155,764	956,271	199,493
Other assets	114,305	102,191	12,114
Land and facilities — cost less depreciation	1,048,160	942,156	106,004
TOTAL	**$2,592,120**	$ 2,281,840	$ 310,280
Liabilities and Fund Balances			
Accounts payable and other liabilities	$ 343,291	$ 312,959	$ 30,332
Long-term debt	581,239	425,109	156,130
Fund balance — restricted	261,299	238,824	22,475
Fund balance — unrestricted	1,406,291	1,304,948	101,343
TOTAL	**$2,592,120**	$ 2,281,840	$ 310,280

Statements of Revenues and Expenses — For the Year			
Operating Revenues			
Medical services — net	$1,312,405	$ 1,204,229	$ 108,176
Grants and contracts	61,807	54,571	7,236
Auxiliary and other	84,972	77,666	7,306
Allocated investment return	32,556	34,301	(1,745)
	$1,491,740	$ 1,370,767	$ 120,973
Operating Expenses			
Compensation	$ 916,060	$ 843,366	$ 72,694
Other	530,744	487,679	43,065
	1,446,804	1,331,045	115,759
Net Operating Income*	$ 44,936	$ 39,722	$ 5,214
Other Revenue/Expense			
Contributions net of expense	$ 51,974	$ 53,843	$ (1,869)
Unallocated investment return	4,816	135,347	(130,531)
Other	22,092	(108,556)	130,648
TOTAL	$ 78,882	$ 80,634	$ (1,752)
Excess of Revenues Over Expenses*	$ 123,818	$ 120,356	$ 3,462

Statements of Funds Flow — For the Year	1992	1991	Change
Operating activities (adjusted for non-cash items)	$ 226,774	$ 214,361	$ 12,413
Facilities and equipment	(190,375)	(178,623)	(11,752)
Net increase in investments	(192,984)	(20,211)	(172,773)
Net long-term debt changes and other	147,821	(9,928)	157,749
(Decrease) Increase in Cash	$ (8,764)	$ 5,599	$ (14,363)

* Used for working capital, research and education endowments and facilities and equipment.

The above summary is intended to present a brief review of Mayo's financial condition and activities for 1992 compared with 1991. The financial statements of Mayo Foundation for the years ended December 31, 1992 and 1991 were examined by Deloitte & Touche. A copy of their report and financial statements can be obtained by writing to the Treasurer, Mayo Foundation, Rochester, Minnesota 55905.

Figure 6-1 Mayo Foundation financial statements, 1992.

for facilities and equipment and for investments, and that cash was raised by issuing long-term debt is irrelevant for the valuation of the organization as a going concern.

The discounted cash flow value of the Mayo Foundation, then, can be calculated as

$$V_0 = \frac{\$226,774,000}{r}$$

where r is some rate of discount (or rate of capitalization). What rate should one use? As developed in Chapter 10, the appropriate rate of discount is the cost of capital for the organization doing the valuing. It is in the choice of capitalization rate that ambiguity enters the valuation process. Asset values vary inversely with capitalization rates, and the effect of a change in the capitalization rate can be large. Table 6–2 shows the discounted cash flow values for the Mayo Clinic for five rates, varying from 4 to 12 percent.

The various values shown in Table 6–2 represent what a purchaser might bid for the foundation were his cost of capital from 4 to 12 percent and could he capture the same cash flows that Mayo now enjoys. The values range from about $1.9 billion (only a little above the adjusted book value) to almost $5.7 billion (well above the "2 years' revenue" rule of thumb value).

A FEW COMPLICATIONS

Valuing assets is not always as straightforward as the preceding pages make it seem. Negotiations over the prices of business, legal actions brought by the beneficiaries of trusts, and the settlement of wills and estates would be much simpler if a few complications did not exist. The value of any asset or business is, ultimately, what a buyer will pay for it. When there are no transactions to observe (when no one has made a viable bid for the assets), value is notoriously difficult to establish.

Often, when firms are up for sale, the price bid by a potential buyer is substantially lower than that asked by the seller. Sometimes such a spread (securities dealers would call it a negative *bid-ask spread*) is merely a bargaining ploy by the buyer. Often, however, such spreads are the result of the value to the seller's being greater than the value to the buyer. The seller may have a lower cost of capital. The

Table 6–2 Discounted cash flow values for the Mayo Foundation, 1992

Cash flow = $226,774,000

Rate of Capitalization	Value
4%	$5,669,350,000
6%	3,779,566,667
8%	2,834,675,000
10%	2,267,740,000
12%	1,889,783,333

seller may, perhaps by virtue of not-for-profit status, be able to generate greater cash flows than some would-be buyer. Whichever is the case, the value of the asset or business is the value as determined by the potential buyer willing to pay the highest price.

An especially difficult (and common) complication in valuing health care assets is that potential buyers and sellers may face very different tax regimes. A not-for-profit organization (if qualified under Section 501(c)(3) of the Internal Revenue Code) pays no income tax on its net income. In most places, such an organization pays no property tax on its land and improvements. A shift to (or away from) not-for-profit status, then, involves a change in after-tax cash flows. Further, as discussed in Chapter 13, not-for-profit health care organizations can benefit from tax-exempt municipal debt, providing a substantially higher cost of capital (and higher asset values) than would be the case for investor-owned organizations. To complicate things even further, investor-owned organizations, although paying higher pretax interest rates on debt, can deduct their interest payments from their tax liabilities, lowering their own true, after-tax cost of capital. The result is that a clinic may have a very different value to a not-for-profit hospital than it has for a partnership of physicians.

Yet another complication in valuation involves the passage of control. Ownership of majority interest in a clinic involves control over the business decisions of that organization. Ownership of a minority share of a clinic entitles one to a share of cash flows but leaves the minority owner at the mercy of the decisions of those in control. In effect, the majority owner(s) become agents in making decisions for the minority owners. As discussed in Chapter 2, such agents can enrich themselves at the expense of the principals. Valuation of such an organization, then, involves the estimation of premiums for control and discounts for minority status (Pratt, 1990).

SUMMARY

Often a value must be determined for assets that have no directly observable market price. These assets include bonds offered for sale, inactively traded shares of stock, and whole business units. The approach to valuation that is best justified by economic and financial theory is that value is the present value of all of the future cash flows that would accrue to the asset's owner. It is to gain those cash flows, not to gain control of individual assets, that individuals and organizations purchase health care organizations.

In financial markets, asset values (the prices of stocks and bonds, for example) approach the present values of the cash flows that those assets promise to their owners. To value organizations and securities, one must learn the methods of discounted cash flow analysis presented in Chapter 5. Valuation calculations in health care, however, are complicated by several questions. Will the purchaser, acting as a provider, be able to generate the same cash flows as the seller? Will the purchaser's cash be subject to different tax treatment (and therefore different "take-home amounts") than the seller? Is the value of one party's share of the organization affected by subjugation to a majority owner? Let the valuer beware!

Discussion Questions

1. List the strengths and weaknesses of each of the four approaches to valuation (rules of thumb, adjusted book value, market value, and discounted cash flow).

2. For medical practices, hospitals, and other health care organizations, the value of the whole is usually much more than the sum of the values of the organizations' assets. Explain why this is so.

3. ABC Corporation (investor owned) is considering the purchase of Charity Hospital (not-for-profit). Why would the cash flows realized by the facility under ABC's ownership be different from those realized under its current status? How should ABC adjust its cash flow calculations in arriving at a fair price for the hospital?

4. A young physician, fresh out of surgical residency, has sought your advice. She has been offered a share of an established practice but is unsure if the price required (to be deducted from her share of earnings over a 10-year period) is fair or not. Explain to her how she should proceed in making her decision.

CONTINUING CASE

Dr. Roger Jackson's mood was a mixture of anger, frustration, and confusion. He was angry at Tom Land, his loan officer at CCB Bank, for restricting the credit of PCI, Inc., and of the Jackson Group (see the Continuing Case for Chapter 4). He was also angry at Henry Kirk and Janet Fowler because he believes they are responsible for the hard times on which PCI has fallen. He is frustrated by his inability to correct the financial situation at PCI, and he is confused as to exactly what the financial situation of PCI is.

Thursday morning, Dr. Jackson kept an appointment with Tom Land. Tom had requested a meeting with Dr. Jackson to discuss PCI's relationship with CCB. Dr. Jackson had, at first, thought nothing of Tom's request that Henry Kirk and Janet Fowler not be told of the meeting. "Just you and me this time, like the old days," was all that Tom had said.

"In the old days," Dr. Jackson thought, "it was Clearwater County State Bank, and Tom Land was a benchwarmer for the Jamestown High School Lobos."

When he arrived at Tom Land's office, Dr. Jackson was introduced to R.J. McFarland ("just R.J."), an agent of Medical Corporation of the Southwest (MCS). Mr. McFarland has visited Jamestown several times in the past few weeks and has asked Tom to set up this morning's meeting. Until today, the only information about PCI to which Mr. McFarland had access was the corporation's financial statements (introduced in Chapter 4 and reproduced in Table 6–3).

Table 6–3 PCI, Inc., financial statements

PCI, Inc. Balance Sheet 20XX (in $ thousand)

Assets	
Current assets	
Cash and cash equivalents	$50
Marketable securities	5
Accounts receivable	240
Inventory	3
Prepaid expenses and other current assets	25
Total current assets	323
Long-term assets	
Property, plant, and equipment (net)	35,000
Intangible assets	15
Total long-term assets	35,015
Total assets	35,338
Liabilities	
Current liabilities	
Wages and salaries payable	135
Interest payable	90
Note payable	100
Other accounts payable	15
Current portion of long-term debt	1,000
Total current liabilities	1,340
Long-term liabilities	
Deferred income tax expense	30
Long-term debt	15,000
Total long-term liabilities	15,030
Total liabilities	16,370
Owners' equity	
Paid-in capital	1,000
Retained earnings	17,968
Total owners' equity	18,968
Liabilities + owners' equity	35,338

(continues)

MCS has a proposal. For $40,000,000 it will purchase all of the shares of PCI, Inc. Thus they would own Physicians' Clinic, all of the assets of the inpatient facility ("fat lot of good that will do them"), and the few other assets that PCI holds. A little detective work has shown Mr. McFarland that if Jackson, as the largest single shareholder, approves the sale, it is "a done deal." The number Mr. McFarland offers was developed at headquarters and is not negotiable.

MCS offers its standard purchase agreement. The transaction is to be done in cash on the date of closing. All existing office lease arrangements and purchase contracts will continue in force. The existing level of uncompensated care will be continued for at least 3 years (a meaningless provision in this case, as Physicians' Clinic has never admitted a

Table 6–3 (continued)   PCI, Inc., financial statements

PCI, Inc. Income Statement, 20XX (in $ thousand)	
Revenues	
Net patient care revenue	11,750.00
Facilities rental revenue	12,500.00
Interest income	0.60
Other revenue	22.00
Total revenue	24,272.60
Expenses	
Wages and salaries	$4,650.00
Maintenance and utilities	1,125.00
Equipment leases (operating leases only)	115.00
Insurance expense	145.00
Depreciation and amortization	4,250.00
Interest expense	12,000.00
Deferred income tax expense	16.00
Other expenses	2.50
Total expenses	22,303.50
Net income before taxes	1,969.10
Provision for income taxes	590.73
Net income	1,378.37

nonpaying in-patient). Of course, MCS would assume all of PCI's outstanding liabilities. Dr. Jackson would vacate his PCI office but would, of course, be welcome to remain upstairs with the Jackson Group. All current PCI corporate staff and all clinic administrative staff would be paid 2 months' salary and terminated ("that would show that Fowler woman!"). Clinical, ancillary, and maintenance staff of the clinic would be retained.

MCS is a fledgling firm, headquartered in Tyler (expenses are much lower than in Dallas or Houston). Owned by its founders, none more than 40 years old, it has grown rapidly by purchasing medical practices, clinics, medical laboratories, and specialty hospitals in intermediate-size cities in Central and East Texas. It standardizes operations, takes advantage of volume purchasing discounts, and (some say) plays fast and loose with regulations on self-referrals. MCS does not overpay for the facilities it purchases.

Dr. Jackson left the meeting more confused than ever. His share of the sale price would pay for that condominium on South Padre Island and an appropriate lifestyle. But is the price fair? Can't really ask Janet Fowler for advice on this one. Would MCS try to recapture its purchase price by milking the Jackson Group for exorbitant rent when the current lease comes due? "What it boils down to, I guess, is whether or not $40,000,000 is really what the corporation is worth," Dr. Jackson told his wife over coffee after dinner.

CASE QUESTIONS

1. What is PCI, Inc.'s current level of cash flow?

2. Assuming that level of cash flow to be fixed for all time, and assuming an 8 percent rate of discount, what is PCI really worth on a discounted cash flow basis? What is PCI worth on a book value basis?

3. Holding the rate of discount fixed and assuming fixed cash flows, what does MCS expect to be able to realize as a net annual cash flow, beginning next year?

4. Although MCS will not negotiate its purchase price, it might make adjustments in other aspects of the purchase agreement. What safeguards should Dr. Jackson seek to protect himself legally (from future action by vendors, employees, and others) and economically (in his role as lead partner of the Jackson Group).

5. Does Dr. Jackson have any ethical responsibilities that he is neglecting in focusing only on the price that MCS offers? Consider his responsibilities to other shareholders in PCI, Inc., to employees (corporate and clinic), to patients, to lenders, and to those with whom PCI has made contracts.

REFERENCES

Baumann, Barbara H. & Oxaal, M.R. (1993). Estimating the value of group medical practices: A primer. *Healthcare Financial Management, 47*(12), 58–65.

Burik, D. & Millar, J. (1987, October/November). How to evaluate a physician group practice. *Price Waterhouse Health Industry Update*, 8–10.

Copeland, T., Koller, T., & Murrin, J. (1990). *Valuation*. New York: J. Wiley.

Damodaran, Aswath. (1996). *Investment valuation*. New York: J. Wiley.

Federa, R.D. & Ketcham, J.S. (1993). The valuation of medical practices. *Topics in Health Care Financing, 19*(3), 67–75.

Ferrell, J.L., Jr. (1985). The dividend discount model: A primer. *Financial Analysts Journal, 41*(6), 16–25.

Gilbert, G.A. (1990). Discounted-cash-flow approach to valuation. In E.T. Veit (Ed.), *Valuation of closely held companies and inactively traded securities* (pp. 23–27). Charlottesville, VA: Institute of Chartered Financial Analysts.

How to price a small business. (1984, August 13). *Forbes*, p. 112.

McCarthy, G.D. & Healy, R.E. (1971). *Valuing a company*. New York: Wiley (Ronald Press).

Nicholas, D.W. (1990). Adjusted-book-value approach to valuation. In E.T. Veit (Ed.), *Valuation of closely held companies and inactively traded securities* (pp. 31–35). Charlottesville, VA: Institute of Chartered Financial Analysts.

Pratt, S.P. (1990). Discounts and premia. In E.T. Veit (Ed.), *Valuation of closely held companies and inactively traded securities* (pp. 38–50). Charlottesville, VA: Institute of Chartered Financial Analysts.

Smith, G.V. (1988). *Corporate valuation*. New York: Wiley.

Sorenson, E.H. & Williamson, D.A. (1985). Some evidence on the value of dividend discount models. *Financial Analysts Journal, 41*(6), 60–69.

Veit, E.T. (Ed.). (1990). V*aluation of closely held companies and inactively traded securitie*s. Charlottesville, VA: Institute of Chartered Financial Analysts.

Wolf, J.G. (1990). Market approach to valuation. In E.T. Veit (Ed.), *Valuation of closely held companies and inactively traded securities* (pp. 13–21). Charlottesville, VA: Institute of Chartered Financial Analysts.

SELECTED READINGS

Copeland, T., Koller, T., & Murrin, J. (1990). *Valuation*. New York: Wiley.

Damodaran, Aswath. (1996). *Investment valuation*. New York: J. Wiley.

Veit, E.T. (Ed.). (1990). *Valuation of closely held companies and inactively traded securities*. Charlottesville, VA: Institute of Chartered Financial Analysts.

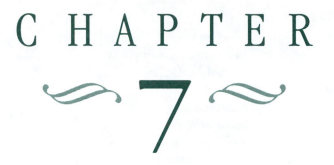

CHAPTER 7

Cost Behavior

Learning Objectives

After reading this chapter, the student should be able to:

1. Define *cost*.
2. Distinguish variable from fixed cost for a service or process.
3. Distinguish direct from indirect cost for a responsibility center or service.
4. Allocate indirect costs to revenue centers using appropriate techniques.
5. Perform simple statistical cost analyses.
6. Perform simple cost/volume/profit analyses.

Key Terms

Activity-based costing	Indirect cost
	Per-unit contribution margin
Cost	Reciprocal cost allocation
Cost allocation	method
Cost center	Responsibility center
Cost drivers	Revenue center
Cost/volume/profit analysis	Shadow cost center
Direct allocation method	Step-down allocation method
Direct cost	Step-fixed cost
Double distribution method	Variable cost
Fixed cost	

Controlling costs is not, strictly speaking, a financial function. Controlling costs involves attention to internal controls (rules for making purchases and for using assets), parsimony in spending, and the elimination of waste of materials and repetition of service. Process improvement staff, operating personnel, and purchasing authorities all play roles in cost control.

Most health care professionals, however, view cost control as being in the realm of financial management. The financial management staff certainly have a role in educating their colleagues as to the nature and level of cost. Managerial accountants, part of the financial team, are charged with measuring and analyzing costs. In addition, understanding the behavior of costs as volume changes (the subject of this chapter) is essential to carrying out the critical financial function of budgeting (the subject of Chapter 8).

After completing this chapter, the reader should be able to (1) allocate costs from cost centers to revenue centers, (2) perform simple statistical cost analyses, and (3) predict the level of service volume at which a health care organization can break even, equating its revenue to its costs.

COSTS

There may be no word more widely used, but more misunderstood, than **costs**. Consumers speak of what a service "costs" when they mean the price of the service. Policy analysts speak of national health care costs when they mean total national spending on health care. All of this verbal sloppiness is very confusing and obscures the meaning of costs as accountants, economists, and managers use it.

In accounting, economics, and managerial decision making, the cost of a good or service is its cost of production. That is, the cost of a home health visit is the market value of all of the resources that are employed in the delivery of that visit (Burik & Duval, 1985). The cost of an appendectomy and of a day's inpatient stay is the market value of *all* of the resources that are involved in delivering that appendectomy and overnight stay. The costs of producing a service are not necessarily the same as the price that the consumer (or his insurance carrier) pays for the service. In fact, good managers work hard to keep cost well below price. Consumers pay a price; providers bear the cost.

Thus the costs of minor surgery and an overnight stay include the obvious items: the wholesale price (not the price charged to the patient) of the patient's food, the wholesale price of the surgical packs used, the wholesale price of all of the pharmaceuticals consumed, the wholesale price of laundry products, and the patient's share of the labor costs involved in delivering care. The cost of care also involves some indirect costs that are as real and as important as the obvious items. These include a share of the cost of construction and maintenance of the hospital building, a share of the cost of running the hospital's administrative units (administration, human resources, finance, marketing, patient accounts, information systems), and a share of the organization's financing costs. For society, the costs of care are greater than they are for the hospital. These nonhospital costs include the market value of physicians' services, the costs of home care after discharge, and any earnings the patient loses during illness and recovery.

For any organization, including health care providers, knowledge of costs is critical to sound management decision making. One can't control costs without knowing what they are. Without knowledge of what costs were in September, one cannot determine whether or not one is successful in controlling costs in October. For an organization to survive, the prices it charges must be at least as great as its costs. Pricing, then, depends on knowledge of costs. One cannot budget (plan) resource use for the next year without knowing what costs one is likely to incur during that period (the subject of Chapter 8).

Costs in Health Care

As important as knowledge of costs is to any organization, it is still rare among health care providers. As hospitals evolved during the late 19th and early 20th centuries (Stevens, 1999), they were either small adjuncts to physicians' practices or charitable organizations. Management expertise was in short supply. Overt concern with cost flew in the face of the ethos of charity. Hospital costs were simply ignored. Medical practices often kept track of their expenses but seldom had the resources or the inclination to determine the cost of any one service. Public health departments, often the most financially strapped health care organizations, were required to prepare financial reports for their governments, but were loathe to do any more involved analysis.

With the passage of the Social Security Amendments of 1965, particularly with the original structuring of Medicare payment, cost determination took on new meaning, at least in the hospital sector. Medicare Part A promised to "reimburse" hospitals for 80 percent of their "allowable costs" and required hospitals to file Medicare Cost Reports on which those reimbursements would be based. Parenthetically, it was this payment structure that introduced the myth that all payments to providers were merely "reimbursement" for costs incurred.

After 1965 hospitals not only were required to file cost data with the U.S. Health Care Financing Administration (administrators of the Medicare system, now the

Centers for Medicare and Medicaid Services) but also had incentives to treat their costs in a very special way. As discussed in the following section, the costs of facilities and administration can be allocated in any of several different ways. Medicare's cost-based payment system, and the adoption of similar systems by other third-party payors, provided hospitals with the incentive to allocate the most costs possible to the most generous payer. Cost finding was not intended to support managerial decision making but to maximize reimbursement. The cost accounting systems marketed and serviced by public accounting firms were not designed to support either cost control or budgeting but were "revenue maximization" systems (Balachandran & Dittman, 1978). Although investor-owned hospitals (and a few aggressive not-for-profit hospitals) had decision support systems for cost analysis, they represented only a very small share of hospitals and of hospital beds.

With the passage of the Social Security Amendments of 1983, Medicare "reimbursement" entered a new era, that of prospectively determined payment. The new payment system promised hospitals a fixed payment for each admission, based on diagnosis (Koch, 1999). Cost-based reimbursement was to become a thing of the past. Now cost analysis had a new function. The cost of caring for an angina patient, for example, was important, not because those costs would be reimbursed, but because the hospital needed to keep average angina care costs below their (fixed) Medicare payment level. It is in this prospective payment era that, slowly, cost analysis systems to support managerial decisions have been introduced into the hospital sector (Burik & Duval, 1985).

COSTS CLASSIFICATION

The cost of producing an item (a bandage, for example) or of providing a service (a bed-day in the medical unit) is the market value of all of the resources employed in producing the item or providing the service. Cost includes the market value of administrative inputs, outlays to repay financiers, and the periodic expenses associated with running an organization that are not tied to any single product or service (rent, utilities, and professional license fees, for example).

Costs can be classified in several ways. First, costs are either **direct** or **indirect**. Direct costs are those incurred directly as a result of providing a specific good or service. Thus, the direct cost of a bed day in the adult medicine unit of a hospital includes all resources tied directly to that bed day: nursing care, food consumed, drugs administered, and others. Indirect costs are those that, although very real, cannot be tied directly to the patient's stay in the bed. These include shares of depreciation, the cost of the administrative division, and the fixed costs (see below) of laundry and food service.

The direct/indirect distinction above is the one preferred by most accountants, as it focuses on the unit of service as the cost object. An older way of making the distinction focuses on the budget unit (or responsibility center, see below). In that view, costs incurred within the budget unit are direct, and costs incurred in other budget units are indirect to the unit in question.

Second, costs are **fixed**, **variable**, or **step-fixed**. Fixed costs are those that do not vary as service volume varies. Those include rent and utilities, which are set for each month regardless of whether or not any patients appear. Costs need not be immutable, forever unchanging, in order to be fixed. The definition of a fixed cost is only that it does not change as volume changes. Variable costs do change as volume changes.

Step-fixed (or semivariable) costs behave in complex ways. These are costs that are fixed over some range of service volume but rise to a new level for a higher range of service volumes. For example, three nurses may be needed if there are 5 or fewer patients on a floor. For 6 to 10 patients, however, one might need to call in a fourth nurse. Nursing costs, then, would be step-fixed: fixed over ranges, but changing in discrete increments as patient volume rises from range to range.

Figure 7–1 shows the classification of costs, for a hospital nursing unit, along two dimensions, direct/indirect and fixed/variable, and provides some examples. The salaries of the unit managers and the depreciation of the equipment specifically assigned to the unit are both direct (they can be tied directly to the care of specific patients) and fixed (they would be incurred even if the patient census were zero). Note that they are fixed with respect to patient census only, the managers' salaries could be increased by hiring more management.

The nursing unit will usually be assigned costs from other responsibility centers (discussed later). These are indirect from the standpoint of the unit's patients.

Variable costs change with patient volume. The purchase price of the syringes used within the nursing unit (and of other supplies) varies with patient volume, as do the wages paid to nurses on call by the unit. These are both variable and direct.

Algebraically, total costs (TC) equals fixed costs (FC) plus variable cost per unit (VC_u) times the quantity of units delivered (Q):

$$TC = FC + (VC_u \times Q)$$

	Direct	Indirect
Fixed	- Salaries of unit managers - Depreciation of unit equipment	- Allocated depreciation of facility - Allocated salaries from administration
Variable	- Supplies - Wages of nurses on call	

Figure 7-1   Classification of costs for a nursing unit.

RESPONSIBILITY CENTERS

Costs occur somewhere. The places where costs occur, and which have budgets, are called **responsibility centers**. A responsibility center is a subunit of the larger organization that is responsible for some type of budget. Responsibility center accounting, the assignment of costs to responsibility centers and the evaluation of the budgetary and cost-control performance of those centers, is an important component of internal control and good budget practice.

Some responsibility centers, **cost centers**, are charged with managing their costs only. Cost centers have no revenue budgets (see Chapter 8 for definitions of the various types of budgets) and no obligation to earn revenues for the organization. *Administration* is always a cost center, as are *human resources* and *housekeeping*. Being a cost center does not make a unit any less important than any other unit in the organization. For example, in many hospitals, nursing (to the great chagrin of many nurses) is a cost center. Although it is true that a hospital cannot function without nursing service, nursing's being a cost center merely means that, in those hospitals, "nursing service" does not bill for its services. Managers who starve cost centers in order to control organizational costs are not practicing good management.

Some cost centers, **shadow cost centers**, exist as budgets on paper only. For example, *rent and utilities* and *depreciation of plant and equipment* are large-budget items for any organization. These are cost centers even though there is no one in the center. For cost allocation purposes, however, rent, utilities, and depreciation need to be treated as cost centers.

Those centers that are charged with controlling costs and with generating revenue for the organization are **revenue centers**. A revenue center is charged with both an expense budget and a revenue budget. It is evaluated on its ability to meet the goals embedded in its revenue budget. An organization's revenue centers, collectively, have the obligation to meet, through their production of revenues, the costs of all cost centers and of all revenue centers.

COST ALLOCATION: MANAGERIAL DECISIONS UNDER AMBIGUITY

Revenue centers, collectively, must meet the total costs of their organizations. In order to determine how effectively any one revenue center is doing its share in meeting costs, one must allocate to that revenue center its proper share of cost centers' costs. This section and the one that follows present simplified models of **cost allocation** and discuss their effects on managerial decisions. Readers wishing to study these methods in greater detail should consult a textbook on managerial accounting (Finkler & Ward, 1999).

In the cost allocation process, one assigns to every responsibility center benefiting from the services of cost center X some share of the costs generated in center X. Thus, as every responsibility center in the organization "benefits" from the services of the chief executive's office, every center is assigned a share of the costs of that office. Any cost allocation is based on (1) an allocation method and (2) a set of allocation criteria.

Suver, Neumann, and Boles (1992) describe four cost allocation methods: direct, step-down, double distribution, and reciprocal. Figures 7–2 through 7–6 show how costs would be allocated in a simple organization, Sample Clinic, using the direct and step-down methods, respectively. Sample Clinic has two revenue centers, pediatrics and adult medicine. These are served by six cost centers: rent and utilities (a shadow center), the executive office, financial affairs, imaging, nursing, and the laboratory. The cost allocation problem for Sample Clinic is to allocate the costs generated in the six cost centers to the two revenue centers.

Direct Allocation Method

The **direct allocation method** is the easiest to implement, but it ignores intermediate cost flows. Figure 7–2 shows that, under direct allocation, all costs incurred in each of the cost centers are allocated, through some set of allocation criteria, directly to the revenue centers, with no intermediate allocations. That the financial affairs office enjoys the services of rent and utilities is ignored in this allocation method.

Step-Down Allocation Method

The **step-down allocation method**, although somewhat more difficult to implement, improves on the direct allocation method by recognizing intermediate cost flows. Figure 7–3 illustrates the first steps in that method. In the first step, responsibility centers are arrayed in a hierarchy. At the top of that hierarchy is the center that provides resources to the most other centers, in this case, rent and utilities. The costs of that "top" center are then allocated, according to the appropriate allocation criterion, to all other centers. After all of the costs of the "top" center are allocated, it is "closed." Once the top responsibility center is closed, no costs are allocated to it.

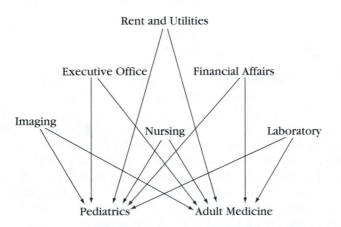

Figure 7–2 Direct cost allocation, Sample Clinic (adapted from Balachandran & Dittman, 1978).

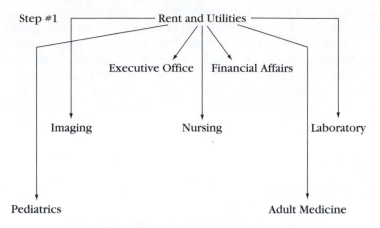

Figure 7–3 Step-down cost allocation, Sample Clinic (adapted from Balachandran & Dittman, 1978).

Figure 7–4 shows the second step in the step-down process. Rent and utilities has been closed. Now all of the costs (including those that were allocated from rent and utilities) of the next center (or centers) in the hierarchy are allocated to the remaining responsibility centers. In this case, all of the costs of the executive office (including the costs that were allocated to the executive office from rent and utilities) are allocated, via application of the appropriate allocation criterion, to the remaining responsibility centers. The executive office is then closed and no costs are allocated to it.

Figures 7–5 and 7–6 show the remainder of the step-down process, with all of the costs (including those allocated from above) being allocated down from each succeeding layer of responsibility centers. The process ends when all cost centers have been closed and all of the organization's costs are allocated to the revenue centers.

Double or Multiple Distribution Method

The **double (or multiple) distribution method** of cost allocation improves on the step-down method by recognizing that resources flow in more than one direction. For example, in Sample Clinic, financial affairs enjoys the supervision and direction of the executive office, but also may provide services (analysis, counseling) to the executive office. In the double distribution method, centers are not closed on the first pass of costs through the hierarchy of responsibility centers. Rather, during the first pass through the hierarchy, costs are allocated "upward" as appropriate. Only in the second pass through the hierarchy (double distribution) or in some later pass (multiple distribution) are centers closed. The process ends when all of the organization's costs are allocated to the revenue centers.

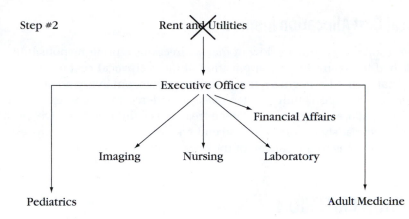

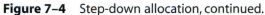

Figure 7–4   Step-down allocation, continued.

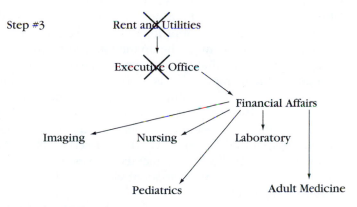

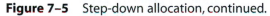

Figure 7–5   Step-down allocation, continued.

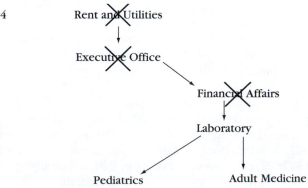

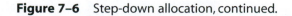

Figure 7–6   Step-down allocation, continued.

Reciprocal Cost Allocation Method

The recognition that resources flow in many directions among responsibility centers is pushed to the limit in the application of the **reciprocal cost allocation method**. That method recognizes that resources flow from every responsibility center to every other responsibility center. Once considered too complex to manage, reciprocal cost allocation problems can be treated as solutions to matrix problems with modern spreadsheet software. The end result of this allocation process, like that of every other, is to allocate all of the organization's costs to its revenue centers.

ALLOCATION CRITERION

The allocation of costs from any one center to other centers, whichever allocation method is used, depends on an allocation criterion. The allocation criterion is the rule for how to divide the costs of Center A among the centers it serves. For example, the costs of rent and utilities might reasonably be divided among the other centers on the basis of each center's proportion of net allocatable square feet of space. The costs of financial affairs might be divided according to each center's percentage of budget (taking care that it is the percentage of the budget of centers below financial affairs in the hierarchy that is used). The cost of the human resources office might be divided according to each center's percent of payroll (again, payroll of centers below human resources in the hierarchy). There is no one correct criterion for allocating the cost of any responsibility center. One must, however, take care to ensure that the allocation criteria for fixed costs used are not functions of service volume. To allocate indirect fixed costs on the basis of service volume (percent of bed-days, percent of inpatient visits) would be to treat fixed costs as if they were variable costs.

Table 7–1 shows the step-down allocation of monthly costs for fictitious Sample Clinic. The hierarchy of responsibility centers shown is the same as that in Figures 7–3 through 7–6. The allocation criteria are given next to the name of each center. Rent and utilities is to be allocated on a percentage-of-square-feet basis (the square feet for the responsibility centers, including public spaces, are also shown). Thus, because the executive office occupies 17 percent of total square feet, it is allocated 17 percent ($2,482.76) of total monthly rent and utilities. After the $15,000 in rent and utility costs are allocated to the other seven responsibility centers, rent and utilities is closed.

In the second step, the executive office has its own $12,000 of direct cost to allocate to other responsibility centers, *plus* the $2,482.76 that it was allocated from rent and utilities. These costs are allocated on the basis of percentage of direct cost. Of the total $14,482.76 to be allocated from the executive office, the financial office will be allocated $428.77, because direct costs in that responsibility center constitute 2.96 percent of total direct costs for those responsibility centers below the executive office in the hierarchy. After the executive office's $14,482,76 in total costs are allocated, it is closed.

Table 7–1 Step-down cost allocation, Sample Clinic

From	Direct Cost	Executive Office	Financial Affairs	Imaging	Nursing	Laboratory	Pediatrics	Adult Medicine
				To				
Rent and utilities (percentage of square feet)	$15,000	$2,482.76	$517.24	$1,241.38	$413.79	$1,241.38	$4,137.93	$4,965.52
Executive office (direct cost as percentage of total)	12,000		428.77	1,191.02	1,524.50	2,096.19	4,287.66	4,954.63
Financial affairs (direct cost as percentage of total)	4,500			461.53	590.75	812.29	1,661.49	1,919.95
Imaging (direct cost as percentage of total)	12,500						7,141.51	8,252.41
Nursing (direct cost as percentage of total)	16,000						8,595.95	9,933.10
Laboratory (direct cost as percentage of total)	22,000						12,131.38	14,018.48
Pediatrics	45,000							
Adult medicine	52,000							
Total	179,000						82,955.92	96,044.08

	Square Feet	Percentage of Total
Executive office	1,200	0.17
Financial affairs	250	0.03
Imaging	600	0.08
Nursing	200	0.03
Laboratory	600	0.08
Pediatrics	2,000	0.28
Adult medicine	2,400	0.33
Total	7,250	1.00

In the third step, financial affairs' costs are allocated. These include the $4,500 in direct costs *plus* the $517.24 that it was allocated from rent and utilities *plus* the $428.77 that it was allocated from the executive office. The total costs of financial affairs are then allocated on a percentage-of-direct-cost basis, where the percent of direct cost is based on the direct costs of the responsibility centers below financial affairs in the allocation hierarchy. After all of the costs of the financial office have been allocated, it is closed.

At the end of the process, all of the organization's costs ($179,000) have been allocated to the two revenue centers ($82,955.92 + $96,044.08 = $179,000). Remember that different allocation criteria lead to different final cost allocations. Use of another allocation method, such as reciprocal allocation, would also change the final allocation. Decisions based on the cost of operating the pediatric product line in Sample Clinic, then, are based on ambiguous information. There is no one correct measure of the monthly cost of operating that revenue center.

THE ABCS OF ABC

One of the most important recent innovations in cost analysis has been the development of **activity-based costing (ABC)** (Baker, 1998; Chan, 1993). ABC has helped to identify the costs of particular services better than was previously possible, and has been a valuable tool in the performance evaluation approach known as the "Balanced Scorecard" (Kaplan and Norton, 1992).

In a traditional (pre-ABC) approach, costs are allocated to revenue centers (as above, and the allocation process stops). If a revenue center has more than one service line (as is usually the case), costs are simply divided among those service lines, often on a "per visit" or "per bed day" basis. The similarity to spreading peanut butter evenly on a slice of bread has given this process the derogatory name "peanut butter costing." Peanut butter costing can lead to overestimation of the costs of some services and underestimation of the costs of others.

ABC seeks to improve on the shortcomings of peanut butter costing by identifying the **cost drivers** that use resources within a revenue center. Consider a clinical laboratory. A hemoglobin A1-c test uses more resources than a simple serum glucose measurement (both are used in the assessment of diabetic control). Peanut butter costing allocates the same cost to each. ABC costing identifies the drivers that move cost, such as set-up time, and allocates the laboratory's cost based on each test's use of those drivers. The result is that the cost object, or cost pool, is the service, not the center. In a system in which the costs of specific diagnoses, and, therefore, specific product lines, are important inputs into decisions, ABC has become an important tool, indeed.

SEPARATING FIXED AND VARIABLE COSTS

Just as finding the total (direct plus indirect) cost of a service or of a revenue center is essential to good budgeting and decision making, so is separating fixed from variable cost. A service that at least meets its variable cost of production makes a contribution to meeting the organization's fixed cost and ought, at least in the short-run, to be continued. Decisions as to which services to keep, which to terminate, and which to subject to flexible budgeting (discussed in Chapter 8) require that one be able to separate the fixed and variable components of costs.

Unfortunately, costs rarely come with their fixed and variable components broken down. Rather, one is usually faced with data on the total costs of operating a responsibility center, if one has cost data at all. Also, whereas some costs are clearly fixed (depreciation, for example) and others are clearly variable (vials of vaccine for a public health clinic), others cannot be identified as fixed or variable before the fact. The fixed/variable distinction is, ultimately, an empirical question.

Two methods are widely used for separating fixed and variable costs: the high-low method and least squares regression analysis. The latter has become, with advances in spreadsheet software, so easily applied that it has largely replaced the former. Table 7–2 extends the cost analysis of fictitious Sample Clinic's pediatric revenue center. The allocated overhead cost column reflects the amount of indirect costs that are allocated to pediatrics each month. *Overhead* is only another way of expressing *fixed costs*. Various numbers of visits are recorded for each month in a sample year. Figure 7–7 shows the cost data graphically. The figure reveals data on direct fixed and variable costs that would not be available to a decision maker without detailed analysis. The reader can easily verify that variable costs per unit are $30. The director of the pediatric center does not yet know that. What the clinic director knows is revealed in Table 7–3.

High-Low Method

The *high-low method* is very simple, easy to apply, and accurate over small ranges of output. The method is shown in Table 7–4. In the high-low method, one selects one high-volume month (it need not be the month with the highest volume) and one low-volume month (it need not be the month with the lowest volume).

Table 7–2   Sample Clinic, monthly costs for pediatrics

Month	Visits	Allocated Overhead Costs	Direct Fixed Costs	Variable Costs	Total Costs
January	600	$83,000	$45,000	$18,000	$146,000
February	660	83,000	45,000	19,800	147,800
March	630	83,000	45,000	18,900	146,900
April	570	83,000	45,000	17,100	145,100
May	525	83,000	45,000	15,750	143,750
June	480	83,000	45,000	14,400	142,400
July	390	83,000	45,000	11,700	139,700
August	460	83,000	45,000	13,800	141,800
September	660	83,000	45,000	19,800	147,800
October	700	83,000	45,000	21,000	149,000
November	715	83,000	45,000	21,450	149,450
December	680	83,000	45,000	20,400	148,400

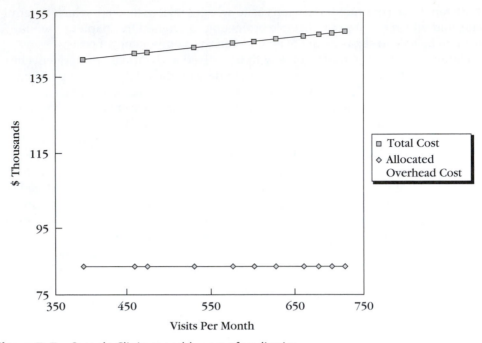

Figure 7–7 Sample Clinic, monthly cost of pediatrics

Table 7–3 Sample Clinic monthly costs for pediatrics: what the clinic director knows

Visits	Allocated Overhead Costs	Total Costs
390	$83,000	$139,700
460	83,000	141,800
480	83,000	142,400
525	83,000	143,750
570	83,000	145,100
600	83,000	146,000
630	83,000	146,900
660	83,000	147,800
660	83,000	147,800
680	83,000	148,400
700	83,000	149,000
715	83,000	149,450

Subtracting the low volume from the high volume and the associated low cost from the associated high cost, one determines how much total costs will change for a given change in volume. In Table 7–4 a change of 325 visits per month causes a change of $9,750 in total cost.

All of the change in total cost associated with the change in total volume must be variable cost. Fixed costs, by definition, don't change as volume changes.

Table 7–4   Sample Clinic: pediatrics breakdown of fixed and variable costs, high-low method

	Visits	Total Costs
High month	715	$149,450
Low month	390	139,700
Difference	325	9,750

Variable cost/Unit = $9750/325 = $30

High-month fixed cost = TC − (VC$_u$ × Q)
$$= \$149{,}450 - (\$30 \times 715)$$
$$= \$128{,}000$$

Dividing the total change in cost by the change in volume, then, yields variable cost per unit ($9750/325 = $30).

Remember that total cost is equal to fixed cost plus the product of variable cost per unit and quantity of units. In equation form:

$$TC = FC + (VC_u \times Q)$$

Using the high-volume month, one knows that fixed cost is equal to total cost minus variable cost per unit times the number of units (quantity). Subtracting variable cost per unit ($30) times quantity (715) from total cost, one finds that monthly fixed cost is $128,000. Because $83,000 of that fixed cost is allocated overhead, it follows that $45,000 must be the monthly direct fixed cost of the pediatric clinic. These results are consistent with the data in Table 7–2.

The high-low method works well when variable cost per unit is constant and when fixed costs do not change over the time period used. When fixed costs vary widely (for example, when utility bills are very different in the summer and winter months, or when a new facility has been opened between the high-volume and low-volume months), the high-low method is less reliable.

Least Squares Regression Analysis

An alternative to the high-low method is the use of ordinary least squares regression analysis to separate fixed and variable costs. Regression analysis, properly employed, is a powerful, flexible tool. Contemporary students and financial analysts are fortunate in that regression analysis is now a standard feature of spreadsheet software. Readers unfamiliar with the method should consult a textbook on econometrics (Lardaro, 1993, especially chapters 4 and 5; Maddala, 1992, especially chapter 3).

To use the linear regression model to separate fixed and variable costs, one specifies a model of the form

$$Y = a + \beta X$$

or

$$\text{Total cost} = \text{Fixed cost} + (\text{Variable cost per unit} \times \text{Quantity})$$

That is, total cost is specified as determined by a causal relationship in the form of a straight line. Total cost is the dependent variable, fixed cost is the estimated intercept term (what total cost would equal were volume equal to zero), and variable cost per unit is the estimated coefficient (β) of quantity (the independent variable). In the language of spreadsheets, the column labeled Total Cost in Table 7–3 is the Y-range (the dependent variable) and the column labeled Visits is the X-range (the independent variables).

Table 7–5 shows the Output Range from a spreadsheet regression, estimating the fixed and variable cost components from Table 7–3. The "constant" ($128,000) is the estimated value for fixed cost. The estimated X coefficient shows variable cost per unit, how much the dependent variable (total cost) changes with a one unit change in the independent variable (service volume or quantity). That estimated variable cost per unit is $30. As was the case for the high-low method, the regression model yields an estimated fixed cost per month of $128,000.

R-squared indicates the proportion of the total variation in the dependent variable that is explained by the model. In this case, but seldom in real life, the relationship is exact and R squared is at its maximum value, 1.00. Because the relationship estimated is exact, the test for the statistical significance of the estimated coefficient is trivial, the standard error of the coefficient is 0.00. In most cases, one would need to divide the estimated coefficient by its standard error. The resulting t-statistic should then be subjected to a significance test to determine whether variable cost per unit is, in fact, significantly different from zero.

What is the advantage of using statistical cost analysis rather than the high-low method? Regression is a more "robust" method. It works even if fixed costs are nonconstant (so long as the analyst can model the causes of the change in fixed cost). Linear regression is also, in the age of desktop computing, easy. With only a spreadsheet, one can run regressions instantly, at the touch of a button

Finally, the use of linear regressing allows the development of richer models of more complex cost behavior. For example, a clinic offering both vaccinations (X_1) and well-baby visits (X_2) might specify and estimate a cost function of the form:

$$TC = \alpha + \beta_1 X_1 + \beta_2 X_2,$$

Table 7–5   Sample Clinic: Pediatrics breakdown of fixed and variable costs, linear regression method

Regression Output	
Constant	$128,000.00
Std. err. of Y est	0.00
R squared	1
No. of observations	12
Degrees of freedom	10
X coefficient(s)	30.00
Std err of coef.	0.00

where α is estimated fixed cost, β_1 is estimated variable cost per unit for vaccinations, and β_2 is estimated variable cost per unit for well-baby visits.

Sometimes, fixed costs change within a data collection period. Consider the case of moving to a new facility and wanting to know the effect of the move on costs. Our clinic could model:

$$TC = \alpha + \beta_1 X_1 + \beta_2 X_2 + \beta_3 X_3,$$

where the initial variables are interpreted as above, and $X_3 = 1$ for months in the new facility and $X_3 = 0$ otherwise. β_3, then, is the estimated effect of the new facility on fixed costs.

COST-VOLUME-PROFIT ANALYSIS, TRADITIONAL

The previous sections showed how costs will behave as volume changes and how to separate fixed from variable costs. The **cost-volume-profit (CVP) analysis** model is a useful framework for analyzing that information (Cleverly, 1979).

Consider Sample Clinic's pediatric unit once again. No matter what its monthly volume, it generates $45,000 in direct fixed cost and is assigned $83,000 in overhead costs. Each visit generates $30 in variable cost (variable cost per unit, VC_u). Suppose the pediatric clinic charges $50 per visit. The $50 is the price of a visit, or revenue per unit (R_u). Each visit, then, contributes $50—$30 toward meeting Sample Clinic's fixed cost. That amount is the **per-unit contribution margin** of a pediatric visit. It represents what each pediatric visit contributes toward meeting the clinic's fixed costs.

To find how many visits would be necessary for the pediatric unit to break even, begin with the formula:

$$\text{Total cost} = \text{Fixed cost} + (VC_u \times Q)$$

The formula for total revenue is

$$\text{Total revenue} = (R_u \times Q)$$

At the breakeven quantity (Q^*), total revenue equals total cost, so

$$(R_u \times Q^*) = \text{Fixed cost} + (VC_u \times Q^*)$$

To solve for Q^*, breakeven quantity,

$$(R_u \times Q^*) - (VC_u \times Q^*) = \text{Fixed cost}$$

$$(R_u - VC_u) \times Q^* = \text{Fixed cost}$$

$$Q^* = \frac{\text{Fixed cost}}{(R_u - VC_u)}$$

$$\text{Breakeven quantity} = \text{Fixed cost/per-unit contribution margin}$$

For the case at hand, breakeven quantity in the pediatric unit is $128,000/$20, or 6,400 visits per month. Does that mean that the pediatric unit should be shut down? Not necessarily. Note that $83,000 of Pediatrics' fixed cost is allocated overhead, costs that Sample Clinic would incur even if there were no pediatric unit. If the unit covers its direct costs (fixed and variable) and makes *any* contribution to overhead, it is worth keeping, even in the long run. Further, in the short run, Pediatrics cannot eliminate its own fixed cost ($45,000). In the short run, if the unit has a positive contribution margin (as it does), it should continue to operate to make a contribution to its own fixed costs. In the long run, if the unit cannot meet its own (direct) total costs, it should be eliminated, unless some outside entity or another revenue center is to subsidize it.

COST-VOLUME-PROFIT ANALYSIS, CAPITATION

The discussion above assumed that the provider is paid for each unit of service provided. Many health care providers face the situation in which total revenue per period is fixed, based on the receipt of per-member-per-month (PMPM) payments for an enrolled population. The fixed total revenue model is familiar in many settings: veterans' medical centers, Indian health service hospitals, primary care physicians' practices in the British National Health Service, hospitals and polyclinics in the countries of the former Soviet Union, as well as in pure health maintenance organizations in the U.S.

Let toal revenue be fixed: $\overline{TR}$. Total cost is still given by

$$TC = FC + (VC_u \times Q).$$

Setting the two equal and solving yields a breakeven quantity of

$$Q^* = (\overline{TR} - FC) / VC_u.$$

If we call $(\overline{TR} - FC)$ our "monthly cushion," then each unit of service eats away VC_u of that cushion. At service levels *above* Q^*, the provider suffers a loss. Boles and Fleming (1996) provide an interesting discussion of capitated providers' incentives to control enrollees' utilization of services.

SUMMARY

The cost of a health care service is the market value of the real resources used to produce that service. Knowledge of costs is important for budgeting, planning, and evaluating the adequacy of pricing structures.

Young and Pearlman (1993) have proposed that every health care organization implement a four-step process that integrates cost finding with managerial decision making. In the first stage, the organization would improve its systems for collecting cost data (its cost accounting systems). In the second stage, the organization would separate fixed from variable costs (determine its cost behavior patterns). In the third stage, the organization would identify its "cost drivers" and look for ways to control its costs (engage in feedback and managerial cost control). In the fourth stage, cost information is used as input into redesigning the organization and its tasks. That process, and the four stages that it incorporates, provides a way to use cost information to enhance organizational performance.

Modern computing equipment and relatively elementary statistical analysis make identification of costs possible for every health care organization. When costs are known, they can be controlled. With knowledge of costs, one can employ other models, such as cost/volume/profit analysis, that enable one to make better decisions.

Discussion Questions

1. "All allocations of indirect costs to revenue centers are purely arbitrary." Do you agree? Discuss.

2. In deciding to continue (or to discontinue) a service whose revenues do not cover total cost, which is more important in the short run, variable cost or fixed cost? In the long run? Why?

3. Many providers have both fee-for-service and capitated patients. How do their incentives differ with respect tot he two?

CONTINUING CASE

"We don't have a lot of money to go around. The State is pressing us to add two new sanitarians and we have a mandate to do some new budgeting of our own (see the Continuing Case for Chapter 8). You know that our tax base isn't growing. We don't expect you to lose money, but I have to be able to justify your charge per visit to the Board of Health."

Joleen Garza, Health Director of Clearwater County, explained her request to Billy Bob Ferguson. She needed a breakdown of what it actually cost Lone Star Home Health Services to send a visiting nurse to a client's home. The county was LSHHS's biggest client, with county payments amounting to about 35 percent (37.74 percent, to be exact) of total revenue.

"This is impossible, Joleen. No two visits are the same; some are in town, some are in rural areas; some take 20 minutes, some take an hour. I'm not an accountant. It would take me weeks to get you a number. Even if I could find out what a visit costs, your board wouldn't understand it any more than mine would."

"It just doesn't matter, Billy, I have to have a number for the Board. If you can't do it, I know somebody who can." She meant Central Texas Home Health, a for-profit provider based in Ft. Worth. Ferguson knew she meant business; she had hinted for over a year that she was ready to switch providers. He would have to produce some sort of cost figure before the Board of Health met at the end of the month.

Later that evening, Billy Bob sat with pencil, paper, and calculator at the Ferguson kitchen table. "Let's see what we know," Billy Bob said to himself. "For each home visit, we pay the nurse $50. She has to use her own car and gets no extra compensation. That's about all I know."

Billy Bob pulled annual expense records from the income statement (see Chapter 4) and began to look at monthly expenses (Table 7–6). "Let's think about 'visiting nurses' as a revenue center. Depreciation is charged on the vehicles used by 'meals-on-wheels,' our other revenue center. Now we're getting somewhere."

Mr. Ferguson still has some questions to answer.

Table 7–6 Lone Star Home Health Services expense analysis

Item	Last Full Year	Average per Month
Wages and salaries	$14,500.00	$1,208.33
Payments to contract providers	122,000.00	10,166.67
Supplies and cost of goods sold	24,575.00	2,047.92
Maintenance and utilities	3,500.00	291.67
Equipment operation expenses	2,800.00	233.33
Insurance expense	15,500.00	1,291.67
Depreciation expense	3,694.00	307.83
Other expense	35,250.00	2,937.50
Total	221,819.00	18,484.92

CASE QUESTIONS

1. What are reasonable bases for allocating the fixed costs of LSHHS?

2. What fixed costs should be allocated across LSHHS's revenue centers? Which fixed costs should be assigned to individual revenue centers?

3. Without data for individual months, what expenses seem likely to represent fixed costs?

4. What is the total cost of a visit? The variable cost only? The total direct cost?

5. Suppose that the Clearwater County Board of Health refuses to pay the total cost per home health visit? What is the minimum payment that LSHHS should be willing to accept to keep their contract with the county?

REFERENCES

Baker, J. (1998). *Acitivty-based costing and activity-based management for health care*. Gaithersburg, MD: Aspen.

Balachandran, V. & Dittman, D.A. (1978). Cost allocation for maximizing hospital reimbursement under third party cost contracts. *Health Care Management Review, 3*(2), 61–70.

Boles, K.E. and Fleming, S.T. (1996). Breakeven under capitation: Pure and simple? *Health Care management Review, 21*(1), 38–47

Burik, D. & Duval, T.J. (1985). Hospital cost accounting: Strategic considerations. *Healthcare Financial Management, 39*(2), 19–28.

Chan, Y.C.L. (1993). Improving hospital cost accounting with activity-based costing. *Health Care Management Review, 18*(1), 71–77.

Cleverly, W.O. (1979). Cost/volume/profit analysis in the hospital industry. *Health Care Management Review, 4*(3), 29–36.

Finkler, S.A. and Ward, D.M. (1999). *Essentials of cost accounting for health care organizations* (2nd ed.). Gaithersburg, MD: Aspen.

Kaplan, R.S. and Norton, D.P. (1992). The balanced scorecard--Measures that drive performance. *Harvard Business Review, 70*(1), 71–79.

Koch, A.L. (1999). Financing health services. In S.J. Williams & P.R. Torrens (Eds.), *Introduction to health services* (5th ed., pp. 113–148). Clifton Park, NY: Delmar.

Lardaro, L. (1993). *Applied econometrics*. New York: Harper Collins.

Maddala, G.S. (1992). *Introduction to econometrics* (2nd ed.). New York: Macmillan.

Stevens, R. (1999). *In sickness and in wealth*. (revised) New York: Basic Book.

Suver, J.D., Neumann, B.R., & Boles, K.E. (1992). *Management accounting for healthcare organizations* (3rd ed.). Chicago: Pluribus Press for the Healthcare Financial Management Association.

Young, D.W. & Pearlman, L.K. (1993). Managing the stages of hospital cost accounting. *Healthcare Financial Management, 48*(4), 58–80.

SELECTED READINGS

Finkler, S.A. and Ward, D.M. (1999). *Essentials of cost accounting for health care organizations* (2nd ed.). Gaithersburg, MD: Aspen.

Suver, J.D., Neumann, B.R., & Boles, K.E. (1992). *Management accounting for healthcare organizations*, (3rd ed.). Chicago: Pluribus Press for the Healthcare Financial Management Association.

CHAPTER

8

Budgeting and Variance Analysis

Learning Objectives

After reading this chapter, the student should be able to:

1. Explain the purpose of the budgeting process and the role of the organization's budget.
2. Make important choices about the nature of the budgeting process (fixed or flexible, top down or bottom up, incremental or zero base).
3. Prepare a statistics budget for a small health care organization.
4. Explain the relationships among the components of an organization's budget.
5. Perform a variance analysis from data on a monthly budget report.

Key Terms

Bottom-up budgeting

Budget

Budget period

Capital budget

Cash budget

Expense budget

Fixed expense budget

Flexible budget

Incremental
   budgeting

Price variance

Quantity variance

Revenue budget

Sensitivity analysis

Statistics budget

Top-down budgeting

Variance

Zero-base budgeting

Budgeting, in most administrators' minds, is the essence of financial management. Developing the budget and adhering to it during the year are what most managers consider to be their basic financial tasks (Welsch, Hilton, & Gordon, 1988). Ironically, most health care organizations do their budgeting very badly. Most misunderstand what a budget is and therefore fail to realize the power of the budget as a planning and analytical tool.

This chapter will introduce the role of the budget, its components, and its role in evaluating operating performance. After completing this chapter, the reader should be able to make informed decisions about the budgeting process and will be able to formulate a comprehensive budget.

A TOOL, NOT A TROPHY

The term **budget** means different things to different people. To some, it means an allocation of funds, as in "The State has given us our budget for the year." To others, it means an account, as in "There's not enough money in the supply budget to make that purchase." Properly understood, a budget is a *plan*. The Czech word for budget, *rozpočet* (pronounced *rosé-po-chet*), is a compound of *roz* (year) and *počet* (plan). That word conveys a meaning, to Czech speakers, about the role of the budget, that is absent in its English equivalent. A budget turns an operating plan into a program for the expenditure of funds (Seawell, 1992, pp. 473–502). Preparing the budget is an important step in planning. Spending the budget is how one turns a plan into reality.

As a plan, a budget is also a tool for ex post evaluation. Comparing budgeted amounts to actual amounts (of service volume, spending, revenue, or cash flow) provides a means of evaluating how well the organization met its operating and financial performance goals during the **budget period**, usually the fiscal year. Finally, a budget is not a document to be filed away on a shelf and forgotten. It should be a working document, important to every manager in the organization.

SOME BUDGET FABLES

Budgeting experience is an excellent teacher. As one watches and participates in budgeting, one gathers anecdotes, fables, that illustrate the process and its pitfalls. Three such fables follow.

"But We Have a Budget."

The Cutbrush County Health Department submits a funding request, through the Board of Health, to the County Commission each spring. The Commission then allots funds to the various county departments, including the Health Department, in the late summer, for the fiscal year that begins October 1. Federal funds for a few programs also become available each October.

The Cutbrush County Health Director knows his personnel budget requirements and has a few programmatic constraints on his spending. Otherwise, he allocates funds to programs and activities "as appropriate" over the course of the year. For example, when several staff members requested funds to attend the meeting of the state's Public Health Association, the Director approved the expenditure as being appropriate.

At the end of the fiscal year, a staff accountant requested funds to attend a training session in the state capital. She was told that she could not, as that would deplete funds badly needed for clinic supplies. "But what is left in the training budget?" she asked. The associate director for administration explained that the budget was not organized in categories, and that, at this time of the year, training, supplies, and miscellaneous expenses competed for what little was left over.

"So we don't actually have a budget?!?" the accountant asked, shocked.

"Sure we do," the associate director responded. "We get it from the County Commission every summer."

"Take It From the Telephone Budget."

The Rosebury Clinic has a well-defined, well-planned budget. The medical director, the board, the administrator, and the staff all take it very seriously. Toward the end of the last fiscal year, the administrator discovered that the clinic had spent 120 percent of its supply budget. He was quite concerned about this situation, and when the clinic needed $1,500 of miscellaneous supplies, he was reluctant to approve the order. After careful analysis of the situation, he arrived at a solution: the order would be placed, but charged against the telephone budget, 20 percent of which remained unspent. At the end of the year, then, $1,500 of supply expenditures were hidden in the telephone budget. The result was that all of the telephone budget had been spent, and the supply budget didn't look "as bad as it might have."

"Sit Down and Copy the Numbers from Last Year's Budget."

At Charity Hospital, the department heads are always puzzled by the budget process. Several years ago, the level of anxiety among first-level administrators was so great that the financial office staff came up with a plan. Each department director would be called to the financial office to "do" his or her budget. The budget manager would hand the director his or her budget for the current year and a worksheet for the coming year. Some items, such as salaries, had already been entered on the worksheet. These items, and those that had been decided in advance by the division director, were already filled in on the worksheet. Every other item was to be taken from the current year's sheet, multiplied by 1.045 (to take account of rising prices), and filled in on the next year's sheet. The process not only relieved staff anxiety but also guaranteed that department-level managers had direct input into the budget process.

Each of these fables is based on fact, and together they illustrate the ways that many, perhaps most, health care organizations develop and use their annual budgets. The first organization has no budget. Although it has an allocation, an overall spending constraint, it has not used the opportunity to develop an operating plan and to translate that plan into anticipated expenses. It also has no category-by-category expenditure plan against which to compare its actual spending at the end of the budget period.

The second organization confuses a budget, a planning and evaluation tool, with a set of bank accounts. When spending against the supply budget equaled the budgeted amount, the clinic administrator believed that the budget had been exhausted. As a result, further supply spending was "taken from" the telephone budget. By doing so, the clinic hid much of its spending on supplies. It created the fiction that it spent only the budgeted amount on supplies and that it spent more than it actually did on telephone calls. It prevented the budget's being a useful evaluation tool at the end of the year.

The third organization has created the impression that it is seeking input from its department directors. Actually, no information is flowing from lower levels of management to higher, and no changes in operating plans at the departmental level are being incorporated into the overall budget.

COMPONENTS OF THE BUDGET

The budget is a planning and evaluation tool. Its various components reflect those roles. The components are linked, beginning with operating plans (the statistics budget) and progressing forward to document that can be evaluated after the fact (the expense, revenue, and cash budgets).

Figure 8–1 shows the components of a full budget and the relationships among them. One begins with the **statistics budget** (or operating plan). The statistics budget includes a forecast of utilization by service type (obstetrics, pediatrics, ophthalmology, etc.), by payor mix (how many self-pay patients, how many commercial insurance, etc.), and by acuity level. It also includes items that are not forecast but are decided as matters of policy. For example, the statistics budget includes

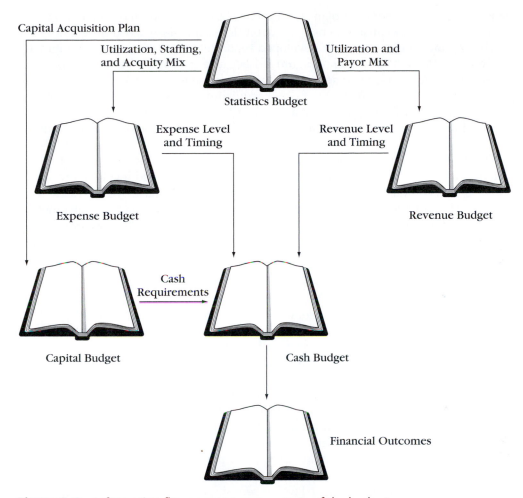

Capital Acquisition Plan

Utilization, Staffing,
and Acquity Mix

Utilization and
Payor Mix

Statistics Budget

Expense Level
and Timing

Revenue Level
and Timing

Expense Budget

Revenue Budget

Cash
Requirements

Capital Budget

Cash Budget

Financial Outcomes

Figure 8–1   Information flows among components of the budget.

employment data (how many department heads, how many maintenance personnel) and, for some items, the policy on utilization or employment per occupied bed (how many licensed professional nurses per occupied bed, how many syringes per bed-day). Many organizations have only the simplest statistics budgets, although others prepare this component in exhaustive detail.

Data on anticipated utilization by service and on payor mix go into the **revenue budget**. The revenue budget is shown on the right-hand side of Figure 8–1 because revenues are credit (right-hand side) accounting entries. The revenue budget is a prediction, a plan, for how much revenue anticipated operations will generate during the budget period.

Data on anticipated utilization, acuity levels, and staffing and supply policies go into the **expense budget**. The expense budget, what most organizations call simply "the budget," is a prediction of the total expense level that the organization will generate, given its operating plan. The expense budget is shown on the left-hand side of Figure 8–1 because expenses are debit (left-hand side) accounting entries.

The **capital budget** is usually developed separately from the expense budget. It is shown on the left-hand side of Figure 8–1 because the capital budget is the plan for acquiring new long-lived assets, which are represented by debit entries in the organization's accounts. Although capital acquisition decisions have their own processes (discussed in Chapters 10 and 11) and do not involve expense in the current period, they do require cash and therefore are a part of the overall budgeting process.

The **cash budget** (discussed in greater detail in Chapter 17) shows the anticipated flow of cash into and out of the organization. Anticipated levels of revenue, expense, and capital acquisition, and their timing, form the basis for the cash budget. All of the budget components together imply certain financial outcomes: levels of net income (or excess of revenue over expenses), net cash flow, and owners' equity (or fund balance) that one expects to be reflected in the budget period's financial statements.

PEOPLE BEHIND THE BUDGET

Budgets do not fall from the sky; someone has to prepare them. The larger the organization, the more hands that may touch the budget during its preparation. Ultimately, senior management is responsible for the budgeting process. Preparation is, typically, delegated to the chief financial officer. In large organizations (a community hospital, for example), the CFO's staff may include a budget manager, for whom preparation and review of the budget is a year-round task. In smaller organizations, the CFO herself will fill that role.

Every responsibility center director has a role in budget preparation. Questions about programmatic needs are answered at the operating level. Each responsibility center manager also receives (or should receive) periodic budget reports (prepared by the budget manager).

Most health care organizations take their semi-final budgets to their boards of directors (or trustees) for approval. In part, this is to obtain "buy-in" and legitimiacy (and, perhaps, to meet a requirement of organizational by-laws). It is also, in part, a way for senior management to protect itself during the course of the budget cycle.

BUDGETING CHOICES

Budget processes are not all alike. Some take longer than others. Some involve more feedback loops than others. Some demand more highly evolved information systems than others. There are a few basic choices that one must make about one's budget process before one can begin to make choices about the budget itself.

Fixed or Flexible?

A **fixed expense budget** is one that is specified, in advance, in dollar terms. For example, the expense budget for a clinic's laboratory might be fixed at a total of $145,000 for the year. A hospital's housekeeping department might have a fixed budget for supplies of $1,200 per month. Under a **flexible budget**, a responsibility center recognizes that some of its expenses vary with its patient load. A hospital's laundry might have a supply budget of $120 plus $12 per occupied bed-day. A unit's budget might have some fixed components (salaries, depreciation) and some flexible components (supplies, transportation).

Flexible budgeting is not an excuse to spend whatever one wants. Extraordinary spending and lack of internal cost control are the results of sloppy management practice, not of flexible budgeting. Rather, flexible expense budgets are a means of recognizing that variable costs change with volume. Without flexible budgets, units that have higher-than-expected service volumes appear to have performed badly (in the budgetary sense) due to their higher-than-budgeted levels of variable costs.

What sorts of responsibility centers are good candidates for flexible budgets? The most obvious criterion is a high proportion of variable costs. Units such as psychiatry, that have little variable costs ought to remain on fixed expense budgets. Units such as food service, in which variable costs dominate, are good candidates for flexible budgeting.

Whether an individual responsibility center's fixed or variable costs dominate, no unit within an organization is a candidate for flexible budgeting unless the organization as a whole has revenue that rises with service volume. A staff model HMO, whose monthly income is limited to its premium collections, has no business putting any responsibility center on a flexible budget. Neither does a county health department if it provides all of its services free of charge, subsisting only on its appropriations through the county. The resource limits of the county are too narrow to permit flexible budgeting. Flexible expense budgeting also generates an incentive for the unit manager to increase her level of service. Such an incentive is out of place in an organization with fixed periodic revenues. Flexible expense budgets must be matched with flexible revenue budgets.

Zero-Base, Incremental, or Something in Between?

Most organizations engage in **incremental budgeting**, in which next period's budget is justified, in part, by last period's budget. That is, this period's operating plan guides next period's operating plan, and this period's expense and revenue budgets guide next period's expense and revenue budgets. Over the past 25 years, some organizations have adopted an alternative, **zero-base budgeting** (Phyrr, 1973; Suver & Neumann, 1979). Under zero-base budgeting, each proposed item in the expense budget must be justified, without reference to any previous year, each time it is proposed. The process requires complete review of the operating plan annually, through completion of a large number of "budget packages," each justifying a specific request.

Zero-base budgeting's popularity was enhanced when then-governor Jimmy Carter mandated its use in the State of Georgia. It is intended to promote efficiency by requiring that activities and expenditures be justified by some programmatic need. It is also a lot of work. The number of budget packages that the senior management of even a small health care organization would have to review annually under zero-base budgeting is quite large.

Taking zero-base budgeting as one extreme (everything "up for grabs" every year) and incremental budgeting as the other (eveything just like it was last year), one observes two other types of processes along the continuum (Finkler and Ward, 1999, pp. 164–165). Negotiative budgeting requires each responsibility center director to make a presentation and to negotiate for increments in resources alotted. Evaluative budgeting requires some senior management group to evaluate center performance and to base changes in resources allocation on that performance.

Top-Down or Bottom-Up?

Any organization's budget, to be an effective planning tool, must be informed by information that flows up the organization chart from those who actually carry out the operating plan. To the extent that information flows from operating personnel to senior management, the organization follows a **bottom-up budget** process. Bottom-up budgeting, with responsibility centers' proposed budgets used as the starting points for the process, facilitate good planning and help to make expense and revenue budgets valid evaluation tools.

Bottom-up budgeting, however, does not promote cost control by senior management and can lead to an organization's failure to live within its overall means. Thus expense budgets must ultimately flow down from senior management. The more strongly senior management influences and controls the budget process, the more the organization has followed **top-down budgeting**.

To strike an effective balance between the informational advantages of bottom-up budgeting and the control advantages of top-down budgeting, many organizations employ an iterative process. Initial budget requests are reviewed at budget hearings, in which central budget officials provide feedback to responsibility center managers. Negotiations and adjustments can be made at that point, prior to final budget allocations being made by senior management.

AN EXAMPLE

Tables 8–1, 8–2, and 8–3 show the budget for a simple, fictitious home health service organization, Basic HomeCare, Inc. This example has been deliberately kept simple to highlight the steps in the process. Table 8–1 is a list of assumptions and a statistics budget. The firm will accept only 45 clients and has strong assurance of

Table 8–1 Basic HomeCare, Inc.: Budget for 20XX, assumptions and statistics budget

Assumptions:
1. 45 enrollees are expected for the fiscal year (maximum set at 45, current waiting list of 15).
2. Enrollees average 16 visits per month.
3. Each enrollee pays $45 per visit.
4. Contract staff receive $35 per visit.
5. Supplies per visit average $3.25.
6. No new services or expansions are anticipated in the coming year.

Table 8–2 Basic HomeCare, Inc.: Expense budget, 20XX

Item	Annual Amount
Advertising and promotion	$4,000.00
Depreciation	2,500.00
Home care supplies	28,080.00
Insurance	32,000.00
Interest on note outstanding	4,000.00
License, professional fees	3,200.00
Mailing	2,000.00
Miscellaneous	4,500.00
Office supplies	2,500.00
Payments to contract providers	302,400.00
Rent and utilities	10,800.00
Salaries and benefits	70,000.00
Telephone	4,200.00
Total	470,180.00

Table 8–3 Basic HomeCare, Inc.: Revenue budget, 20XX

	Anticipated Revenue	Anticipated Net Income
@ $45 per visit	$388,800.00	($81,380.00)
@ $50 per visit	432,000.00	(38,180.00)
@ $55 per visit	475,200.00	5,020.00
@ $60 per visit	518,400.00	48,220.00

having that many throughout the coming budget period (year). Each client will require, on average, 16 visits per month, for which he will pay $45 per visit. All visits are made by contract providers, who are paid $35 per visit. Additional variable costs per visit are $3.25. Variable cost per visit, then, is $38.25, and the contribution margin, revenue per visit minus variable cost per visit, is $6.75.

Table 8–2 takes the operating plan and assumptions from Tables 8–1, couples them with some items that are given (such as annual insurance premiums of $32,000), and provides an expense budget. By far, the largest expense item is the payments to contract providers, $302,400 (45 clients at 16 visits per month at $35 per visit for 12 months). For convenience, the expense items have been arranged in alphabetical order. Note that one item, depreciation, does not involve any cash outflow.

Table 8–3 presents Basic HomeCare's revenue budget and estimated financial results. At $45 per visit, the firm cannot break even. Remember from Chapter 7 that the formula for breakeven quantity is

$$Q^* = FC/(R_u - VC_u)$$

or breakeven quantity is fixed cost divided by the contribution margin (revenue per unit minus variable cost per unit). With a price (revenue per unit) of $45 and variable cost per unit of $38.25, Basic HomeCare's contribution margin is $6.75. With fixed costs of $139,700, their breakeven quantity is 20,696.3 visits per year, or 108 clients.

In their search for acceptable results, Basic's staff has examined results at several price levels. Holding enrollment at 45 clients, a price of $55 per visit would be adequate to cover expenses and to generate a surplus. The process of testing results under different price and quantity assumptions is known as **sensitivity analysis**.

The example of Basic HomeCare points out several of the important roles of budgeting. First, although the first round of the budget is based on an operating plan, it yields information that is useful in revising the operating plan. Among the elements of the plan for which budget feedback is important are pricing and volume decisions. Second, the amounts shown in the expense categories in Table 8–2 are projections. They are not associated with bank accounts that "run dry" at some point during the year. If Basic HomeCare needs to spend $5,000 on telephone calls, then it should spend the money and not worry about taking the excess $800 out of the supply budget. Evaluating *why* it needed to spend the additional money is an important part of cost control.

THE BUDGET CYCLE

Often managers speak of "budget season" or of "the time when we 'do' the budget." Actually, the budget cycle is a year-round process, filling the work life of the budget manager. Consider an organization whose fiscal year is the same as the calendar year. January and February are the months for preparing the annual review of the previous year's budget. January, April, July, and October are the months for preparing quarterly reports and variance analyses (see below) for the previous quarters.

As early as March, the budget manager will ask responsibility center directors for their initial input for the next year's budget. They may be asked to submit information on programmatic needs, new staffing requirements, and changing input prices. At the same time, the budget manager is preparing a new statistics budget for review by senior management. By May, this information is received and the budget manager can assemble a draft of an operating budget for review. Capital expenditure requests, reviewed separately, are due by June 1.

After thorough review, negotiation with operating directors, and balancing of projected revenues and expenses, a semi-final budget is ready in August, prior to a Labor Day weekend retreat of senior managers and trustees. A final version is printed and distributed by October 1, to take effect January 1.

VARIANCE ANALYSIS

The budget is an evaluation tool as well as a planning tool. By comparing actual amounts of quantity, expense, and revenue to budgeted (or "standard') amounts, one can get a handle on both organizational performance and the adequacy of the budget process.

In budgeting jargon, a **variance** is an actual (or realized) amount minus some budgeted (or standard) amount. It answers the question, "How much did the actual vary from the standard?" Note that this concept of variance is quite different from a statistical variance (average squared deviation from the mean). Calculating and analyzing budget variances is at the heart of ex post analysis of budgetary performance.

As a starting point, consider total revenue variance. That variance is defined as

$$\text{Total revenue variance} = \text{Actual revenue} - \text{Standard revenue}$$

or

$$\text{Total revenue variance} = (AQ \times AP) - (SQ \times SP)$$

where AQ is actual quantity (units of service sold), AP is actual price (actually recorded as revenue), SQ is standard quantity, and SP is standard price (the formulas used here are derived from Suver, Neumann, & Boles, 1992, p. 187).

The total revenue variance can be decomposed into two components. Quantity of service delivered can vary from that which was forecast in the statistics budget. That difference will be captured in the **quantity variance**, the part of the total variance due to quantity purchased or sold's being different from what was forecast. Also, the price collected for services can vary from that assumed, resulting in a **price variance**. Pricing differences may arise from loss of pricing power (causing management to lower its prices), from-higher-than expected uncollectible accounts, or from the need to grant unanticipated contractual allowances.

The formula for a price variance is

$$\text{Price variance} = (AP - SP) \times AQ$$

where AP is actual price, SP is standard price, and AQ is actual quantity.

The formula for a quantity variance is

$$\text{Quantity variance} = (AQ - SQ) \times SP$$

where AQ is actual quantity, SQ is standard quantity, and SP is standard price. The reader can verify, with a few steps of algebra, that price variance plus quantity variance equals total variance.

For revenue-related variances, positive values are desirable. That is, it is in a revenue-dependent organization's interest to have higher prices and larger quantities of services purchased than anticipated. Positive revenue-related variances represent pleasant surprises.

For expense-related variances (total expense variance, price [paid for an expense item] variance, and quantity [of some expense item] variance), negative values are desirable. Lower-than-expected supply prices and smaller-than-expected usage of materials and labor are improvements.

Where do standard costs, prices, and quantities come from? They may represent only past experience. Alternatively, they may be norms generally accepted within the industry (for example, "We need 3.0 full-time equivalent employees per occupied bed"). Whatever their sources, they are the values that go into the statistics budget and form the bases for the operating plan.

SUMMARY

An effective budget is a powerful tool for management control. Effective budgets, however, are not just statements of total allowed spending for the coming year. A budget should include a statistics budget, an expense budget, a revenue budget, a cash budget, and a capital budget. Together, those components provide a guide to expected financial outcomes for the budget period. The budget is a plan, a plan that converts organizational goals and objectives into revenue and spending forecasts.

The essence of the budget process is resource allocation. Budgeting is making choices. The manager must make some initial choices about the nature of the process itself. He must then make choices as to how to allocate resources (financial, human, technological). Well-defined financial expectations allow managers to adjust their plans (increasing prices or enrollment, cutting overhead) and, after the budget period, to compare their actual performance to their earlier expectations.

Discussion Questions

1. "There is really never pure top-down budgeting." Do you agree or disagree? Explain.

2. Explain the relationships and information flows between the components of a well-prepared budget.

3. The use of zero-base budgeting enhances rational, thoughtful resource allocation. Why have so few organizations adopted its use?

4. Is a positive price variance on an expense item good or bad? Explain. A positive quantity variance on a revenue item?

5. "If a flexible budget is properly done, there should never be a quantity variance." Explain.

CONTINUING CASES

"We've never had a budget! Until last week we didn't even know what it cost us to make a home visit," Billy Bob Ferguson complained to his wife Alice over breakfast. "Now Joleen Garza, Health Director of Clearwater County, has us jumping through hoops allocating costs. Jason [the Reverend Jason Cooper, chairman of Lone Star Home Health Services' board of directors] says that, since we know our costs now, we can budget our expenses and cut down what the churches have to give us."

"Oh, stop complaining, Billy!" Alice had little patience this morning. "I'd love to know what I can and can't spend on nursing visits (Alice is an RN and supervises LSHHS's staff, both employees and contract providers). With a budget, I'd have an answer when somebody asks why she can't get reimbursed for mileage (a constant source of complaint for the nurses who visit LSHHS's rural clients)."

Billy Bob arrived at LSHHS's office at 8:30 and set to work. "We won't have any more visits next year than this year or last year. Meals-on-wheels and visiting nurses are both holding their own, but not growing." He wondered why he couldn't just be retired, like all of his old friends from the bank. "We're not going to be able to raise our prices. Jason wouldn't approve and Joleen would just say no. I guess we can keep office expenses constant, but operating expenses on the wagons will go up." The two station wagons were aging, and repair bills and rising gasoline prices would add 4 or 5 percent to that item. Price increases for supplies and frozen prepared meals would push that item up by 10 percent. "I know Alice's and my salaries won't be going anywhere." He reasoned that the part-time employees would have to make do with what they had as well.

CASE QUESTIONS

Using last year's data (repeated below) and Billy Bob's assumptions, prepare a statistics budget and an expense budget for LSHHS.

In her storefront office, Joleen Garza was exploring new territory of her own. For years, the CHIP (Children's Health Insurance Program) Clinic had operated ("quite well, thank you very much") on a fixed budget. Planning was easy, and the clinic's director, Mary Turner, always knew exactly how much she had to spend. But times, it seems, have changed.

Table 8–4   Lone Star Home Health Service, financial statements, 20XX

Statement of Revenues and Expenses

Revenues	
Total revenues	$225,750
Wages and salaries	14,500
Payments to contract providers	122,000
Supplies and cost of goods sold	24,575
Maintenance and utilities	3,500
Equipment operation expenses	2,800
Insurance expense	15,500
Depreciation expense	3,694
Other expenses	35,250
Total expenses	221,819
Excess of revenues over expenses	3,931

Table 8–4 Lone Star Home Health Service, financial statements, 20XX (Continued)

Balance Sheet

Assets	
Current assets	
Cash and cash equivalents	38,900
Accounts receivable	7,500
Inventory	1,245
Other current assets	2,150
Total current assets	49,795
Long-term assets	
Property, plant, and equipment (net)	33,250
Total long-term assets	33,250
Total assets	83,045
Liabilities	
Current liabilities	
Wages and salaries payable	1,500
Contractual fees payable	3,500
Other accounts payable	2,200
Total current liabilities	7,200
Fund balance	75,845
Liabilities + fund balance	83,045

The Board of Health's desire for management efficiency did not stop with their demands on Lone Star Home Health Services (see the Continuing Case for Chapter 7). They had also ordered that all units of the Department of Health having variable units of service per month (that would be the CHIP Clinic) be placed on flexible budgets. Dr. Garza's graduate training in public health included only rudimentary coverage of financial management, and she had spent several hours with Tom Carter learning what flexible budgeting was all about.

"This shouldn't be too difficult," she told Tom, "except that the Board wants the new budget format in place for the next fiscal year." Joleen and Tom both knew that the next fiscal year was only 6 months away.

"Joleen, have you ever considered the information requirements of a good flexible budget?"

CASE QUESTIONS

1. What are the information requirements of a good flexible budget?

2. Plan a data collection strategy for the CHIP Clinic.

3. With only 6 months until the next fiscal year, and a budget cycle that requires that a budget be approved well in advance of October, is the development of a flexible budget a reasonable expectation for this year?

4. Is the CHIP Clinic a good candidate for a flexible budget, or should it continue to operate its budgeting process as it always has?

REFERENCES

Finkler, S.A. and Ward, D.M. (1999). *Essentials of cost accounting for health care organizations* (6th ed.). Gaithersburg, MD: Aspen Publishers.

Phyrr, P.A. (1973). *Zero-base budgeting*. New York: Wiley.

Seawell, L.V. (1992). *Introduction to hospital accounting* (3rd ed.). Dubuque, IA: Kendall/Hunt Publishing Company for the Healthcare Financial Management Association.

Suver, J.D. & Neumann, B. (1979). Zero-base budgeting. *Hospital and health services administration, 24*(1), 42–62.

Welsch, G.A., Hilton, R.W., & Gordon, P.N. (1988). *Budgeting* (5th ed.). Englewood Cliffs, NJ: Prentice-Hall.

SUGGESTED READINGS

Finkler, S.A. and Ward, D.M. (1999). *Essentials of cost accounting for health care organizations* (6th ed.). Gaithersburg, MD: Aspen.

Welsch, G.A., Hilton, R.W., & Gordon, P.N. (1988). *Budgeting* (5th ed.). Englewood Cliffs, NJ: Prentice-Hall.

PART

3

The Financial Market Environment

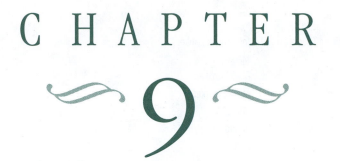

CHAPTER

9

Financial Markets: Institutions, Risk, and Return

Learning Objectives

After reading this chapter, the student should be able to:

1. Explain how external financial markets constrain health care organizations.
2. Explain the basic functions of financial markets.
3. Explain the origin (in risk aversion) and nature of the trade-off between risk and expected return.
4. Explain the role of diversification in portfolio management.
5. Show graphically and explain the capital asset pricing model.

Key Terms

Arbitrage Pricing Theory (APT)

Beta

Bond

Bond covenant

Broker

Capital Asset Pricing Model
    (CAPM)

Capital market

Capital market line

Correlation

Covariance

Dealer

Efficiency

Efficient frontier

Equilibrium

Financial market

Geometric mean

Investment banker

Market

Market maker

Money market

Portfolio

Rating agency

Return on
    investment

Risk

Risk aversion

Secondary market

Security

Security market line

Stock

Systematic risk

Unsystematic risk

External environments are important to the survival of any organization. For health care organizations, the technological environment (the talent, techniques, and pharmaceuticals available), the legal and regulatory environment, and the service market environment (the levels of income, wealth, and insurance coverage that exist in the market area) are all crucial to success. These environments are also completely external: the organization must take them as given. Similarly, conditions prevailing in financial markets form an external environment that enables health care organizations to gain external funding, constrains the actions that they can take, and serves as a barometer of general economic conditions.

After completing this chapter, the reader should understand how financial markets operate, who the major participants in those markets are, and how those markets establish prices for securities and for risk.

FINANCIAL MARKETS

A **market** is an institutional arrangement that facilitates the exchange of goods or services. It can be a place (like the New York Stock Exchange), but more often it is not. Rather, a market consists of the rules, norms, information flows, and arrangements through which goods and services are bought and sold. The market for health care in an urban area and the international market for wheat are not single places, but they are markets nevertheless.

Financial markets are arrangements for the purchase and sale of short-term (**money market**) and long-term (**capital market**) financial resources (cash). How does one purchase cash? By issuing, to the provider of funds, some type of statement of obligation, such as a bank loan, a **bond**, or a **stock** certificate. The general name for these statements of obligation is **security**. In issuing a security one promises to pay the holder some return. The rate of return one must promise to pay is the price of the cash. Financial markets are remarkably dispersed, with suppliers of funds often residing thousands of miles from those to whom they sell their cash. Financial markets are also highly competitive and impersonal. Millions of institutions and individuals trade securities. Usually, the buyer of a security (the provider of funds) will never see the issuer of the security (the user of funds). Further, the provider of funds can, in most cases, sell the securities he holds, transferring the future benefit to the new holder of the security.

FINANCIAL MARKETS: WHO AND WHAT?

Financial markets are arrangements to bring together the users of funds (issuers of securities) and the suppliers of funds (providers of funds). Figure 9–1 shows the major participants in a financial market and the relationships among them. Note that most of the major players in these markets are institutions, not individuals.

Suppliers of Funds

On the right-hand side of Figure 9–1 are the suppliers of funds. These are the bank trust departments, corporations with excess cash, endowment funds, foundations, individuals, insurance companies, mortgage investors, mutual funds, and pension funds that have cash to invest in financial assets. These individuals and organizations have cash now but need cash flows in the future. For example, a pension fund collects cash on each payday and, through the management of those cash assets, accumulates substantial wealth. The fund is obligated, however, to make streams of payments to its beneficiaries in the future. It needs to trade its current cash assets for promises of future cash flows (which is the legal definition of a security).

Providers of funds separate their charitable giving from their investment activities. In financial markets, providers seek the highest yields or returns (defined below) on their investments that are consistent with the levels of investment risk (also defined below) that they have chosen to accept. In other words, they participate in financial markets for the money that is to be made. Providers of funds don't purchase securities from one issuer only. Rather, investors form **portfolios**, assemblies of investments that are planned and purchased to meet the investors' unique needs (Markowitz, 1952).

Users of Funds

The left-hand side of Figure 9–1 shows the role of the users of funds. These are the corporations, federal government, health care organizations, households, mortgage borrowers, school districts, and specialized government agencies that need additional cash in the present. In the case of health care organizations and other corporate borrowers, cash in the present can be used to purchase fixed assets or to begin new product lines that will yield enhanced cash flows in the future. A hospital that wishes to enhance its neurosurgery service may need to borrow several million

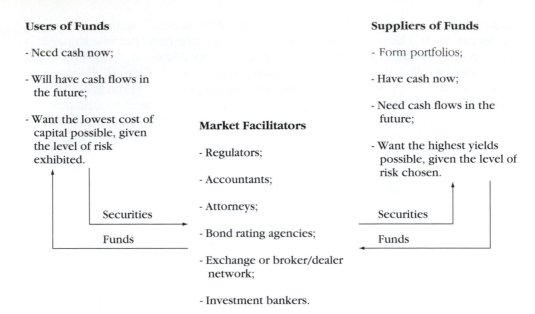

Figure 9-1 Parties in a financial market.

dollars to purchase a gamma knife. It does not have the necessary cash in the present. Operating the service in the future, however, will provide cash flows that can repay the providers of the initial cash.

The financial market structure, then, brings together those with excess cash and those who need additional cash. The match is especially good in that the providers of funds need cash flows in the future, and the users of funds will engage in activities that will generate enhanced cash flows in the future.

The users of funds both receive funds from their financial market transactions and issue obligations (securities). Those securities are a special form of contract, binding the issuer (the borrower of funds) to meet certain obligations (such as to make interest and principal payments on time) and to maintain certain conditions (such as not to allow its asset/equity ratio to exceed some specified number). These conditions, when specified in the terms under which bonds (one type of security) are issued, are known as **bond covenants**. Some observers have argued that participation in financial markets, and accepting the discipline that is required to meet bond covenants, has reduced health care organizations' abilities to pursue their missions (Wilson, Sheps, & Oliver, 1982). Participation in financial markets enables, but it also constrains.

What the providers of funds receive as payment for their money is what the users of capital must pay to secure those funds. Whereas providers seek the highest yields available at the risk levels they have chosen to accept, users seek the lowest costs of capital available at the risk levels that they display. To reconcile those conflicting desires, financial markets must perform the basic task of any market; they must bring the price of funds into **equilibrium**. The process of reaching equilibrium in financial markets involves setting a yield for risk-free debt, and of determining yield premiums for risk and length of obligation. That equilibrium is achieved through competitive bidding for securities, and its outcome is discussed below.

ROLES IN FINANCIAL MARKETS

Several market facilitator roles have emerged in modern financial markets. Securities markets are highly regulated by state and federal authorities (Pointer & Schroeder, 1986). In part as a response to the demands of regulators and in part in response to the demands of investors for information, accountants play an important role in presenting information about potential users of funds to investors. Recent corporate scandals, in which the financial health of certain corporations was misrepresented to the suppliers of funds, only underscores the importance of the accountants' role. Wherever there are regulators, and wherever legal obligations are created, attorneys are important participants. Because there are many securities issued each year, and very many securities traded in the **secondary market** (the market for resale of securities after they are issued), monitoring the riskiness of bonds available for purchase can be a full-time job. Specialized organizations, **rating agencies**, have emerged to provide credit risk analysis for the investors who subscribe to their services. Among the best known of the rating agencies are Standard and Poor's, Moody's, and Fitch's.

Securities are issued either on organized exchanges, such as the New York and American Stock Exchanges, or through negotiated markets, such as the National Association of Securities Dealers Automated Quotation (NASDAQ) system. It is important to note that, although the security may be issued *on* the New York Stock Exchange, it is not issued *by* the New York Stock Exchange. The issuer is the corporation to which funds will flow. On an organized exchange, trades are made and prices are set "by public outcry," and the process is literally an auction. In negotiated markets, one or more dealers act as **market makers** for a security, both at its issue and over its legal life. The auction process is implicit, based on the dealers' posting prices and adjusting them to market conditions. A **broker** is an institution that acts as an agent for investors, making its profit from commissions; a **dealer** is an institution that holds an inventory of securities, making its profit by trading "on its own account." Most investment corporations act as both brokers and dealers.

A special type of broker/dealer, active in both the organized exchanges and the negotiated markets, is the **investment banker** (Bloch, 1986). Investment bankers are specialists in bringing newly issued securities to market. They are the institutions most directly involved in issuing new securities and, therefore, the gatekeepers to external financial resources. Most investment bankers also serve as market makers for the securities they help to create after those securities have been issued.

RATES OF RETURN

A concept that is important to every financial market participant is that of **return on investment**. For the providers of funds, return is the rate of profitability that an investment provides. For the users of funds, return, with slight modification, is the cost of capital. For investment bankers, estimating the equilibrium return that investors require for a given level of risk is necessary to be able to market an issue of securities. One of the central roles of any well-functioning financial market is to establish equilibrium rates of return for securities that are traded in it. Determination of an equilibrium rate of return is how markets set security prices.

The rate of return to any security for any time period is

$$R_t = [(P_t - P_{t-1}) + CF_t]/P_{t-1}$$

or, after rearranging,

$$R_t = [(P_t + CF_t)/P_{t-1}] - 1$$

That is, the return in period t is equal to the change in the security's price during the period $(P_t - P_{t-1})$ plus any cash flows (interest or dividends) received during the period (CF_t), all divided by the price of the security at the beginning of the period (P_{t-1}). The rate of return to a security need not be constant over its life. Note that one way for expected future returns to rise is for the current price of the security to fall. Expected future returns can also rise if expected future price or expected future cash flow rises.

Suppose one holds a share of HealthLife Corporation (a fictitious firm) in one's portfolio. Assume that, at the end of 2000, HealthLife shares sold for $100. By the end of 2001 those shares sold for $105. During the year, HealthLife paid a $5-per-share dividend. The rate of return to HealthLife in 2001, then, was

$$R_{2001} = [(\$105 + \$5)/100] - 1$$

or

$$R_{2001} = (\$110/\$100) - 1$$

or

$$R_{2001} = (1.10) - 1 = 0.10$$

The return to holding HealthLife in 2001 was 10 percent.

The relationship between average annual returns and realized returns over time is puzzling at first. From time 0 to time T, the realized return on any investment is

$$R_{0-T} = [(P_T + CF_{0-T})/P_0] - 1$$

(purists will notice that this formula ignores any reinvestment of periodic cash flows). That price at time T is also the product of a series of annual returns and the initial price, as discussed in the section on compound interest in Chapter 5. Therefore

$$P_T = P_0 (1 + R_1) \times (1 + R_2) + (1 + R_3) \times \cdots \times (1 + R_T).$$

Because of the way annual returns compound over any holding period, the average annual return is not the familiar arithmetic average of the annual returns. Rather, the annualized return (the value that, if used in the preceding formula as a constant annual value, would yield the realized value of PT) is the **geometric mean** of "1 plus each annual return," minus one:

$$R_{\text{annualized}} = [(1 + R_1) \times (1 + R_2) \times (1 + R_3) \times \cdots \times (1 + R_T)]^{1/T} - 1$$

The return to any security over any time period is determined, in part, by how much risk the holder of that security has accepted (by how much danger there is that the provider of funds will not receive his contractual payments as promised).

RISK IN FINANCIAL MARKETS

One faces **risk** when the outcome that one expects cannot be known with certainty. Originally, economists defined risk and uncertainty differently (Knight, 1921), but in common usage, even among financial professionals, they are now interchangeable. If the outcome of a business venture is not known with absolute certainty, the venture is risky. If an investment will pay $100 in 6 months, unless the borrowing firm goes bankrupt (which it might, with a probability of .10), then the investment is risky. Risk is present when there is a probability distribution over multiple possible outcomes (whether or not that distribution is known) for some endeavor. In financial markets, risk is a fact of life.

There are, however, degrees of risk. Purchasing the bonds of highly stable, liquid corporations is risky, but less so than purchasing bonds issued by companies that are reorganizing under the protection of the federal bankruptcy laws. A common measure for risk is the standard deviation (or its square, the variance) of the distribution of potential outcomes.

Risk Aversion

Participants in financial markets are, almost universally, risk averse. In fact, one faces so few providers of funds who are not risk averse that one must treat the provider side of the market as being risk averse. Many of the agency problems discussed in Chapter 2 are the result of managers trying to shift risk to the providers of funds or of equity holders trying to shift risk to lenders. Financial markets recognize situations in which risk (risk of business failure, for example) can be shifted to lenders and treat the bonds issued by those organizations as being riskier than they would otherwise be.

The formal definition of **risk aversion** is that one is strictly risk averse if one is unwilling to participate in an actuarially fair lottery. An actuarially fair lottery is one in which one must pay the expected winnings to participate. Intuitively, one is risk averse if one won't pay $5 to participate in a lottery whose expected outcome is $5. If, faced with that choice, one would keep the $5 rather than participate in the lottery, one is risk averse.

Risk aversion makes market participants behave in particular ways. One consequence of the ubiquity of risk aversion is that providers of funds must be paid to induce them to accept risk. The determination of an equilibrium price of risk is one of the major functions of financial markets.

Risk-averse investors can moderate their exposures to risk by *diversifying* their holdings, by forming portfolios of securities and real assets (real estate, tangible property). Figure 9–2 illustrates how an investor can substantially reduce her risk by selecting two securities for her portfolio (Markowitz, 1952). Security A displays, over time, a great deal of variation in its periodic return. Sometimes its return is positive, sometimes it is negative, and in between it varies widely. The variance in return over time (the risk inherent in holding the security) for security A is substantial. Security B is also a risky security, but security B's return pattern is quite different from that of security A. In particular, the statistical **correlation** of returns between A and B is negative (correlation is a measure of the extent to which two series of measures move in the same direction over time). A and B have a negative covariance, where the **covariance** of return between security A and security B is defined as

$$\text{cov}_{A,B} = \sigma_A \sigma_B \rho_A$$

where σ is the standard deviation of security A's return, and $\rho_{a,b}$ is the correlation between the returns of securities A and B.

As an example, the dotted line in Figure 9–2 shows the returns, over time, to a portfolio that consists of equal parts of security A and security B. Its return profile is formed by adding, vertically, the returns to A and the returns to B at every point in time. Because of A and B's negative correlation (and therefore negative covariance), Portfolio A+B exhibits much less risk than either of its two components. When A's returns are up, they offset the low or negative returns to B. When B's returns are high, they counterbalance A's poor performance. Thus A+B's returns have a very low standard deviation over time, and A+B is a low-risk portfolio.

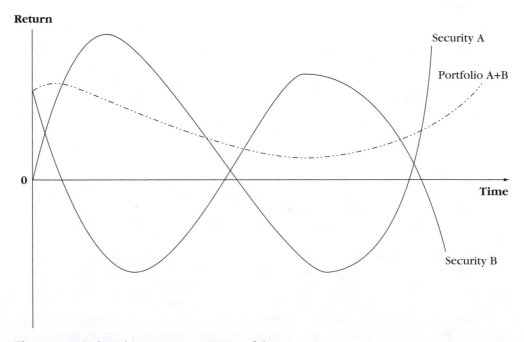

Figure 9-2 Risk within a two-security portfolio.

The variance (σ_{A+B}^2), the square of the standard deviation, of the returns to a portfolio consisting of equal parts of portfolios A and B is

$$\sigma_{A+B}^2 = \sigma_A^2 + \sigma_B^2 + 2\text{cov}_{A,B}$$

When the weights (W_A and W_B) of A and B in the combined portfolio can vary, the variance of the combined portfolio is

$$\sigma_{A+B}^2 = W_A^2\sigma_A^2 + W_B^2\sigma_B^2 + 2W_A W_B\text{cov}_{A,B}$$

More generally:

$$\tau_{\text{portfolio}}^2 = \sum_{i=1}^{N} \sum_{i=1}^{N} W_i W_j \, \tau_i \tau_j \text{cov}_{i,j}$$

As either W_A or W_B declines, the importance of σ_A or σ_B in the variance (and hence of the standard deviation) of the combined portfolio declines as well. The covariance term in the variance of the combined portfolio does not decline as rapidly, as it is multiplied by 2. Ultimately, as the number of components of a combined portfolio rises, the only significant contribution each makes to the riskiness of the portfolio is through its covariance with the portfolio as a whole.

Generally, as the number of securities in a portfolio rises, the riskiness of that portfolio declines, as shown in Figure 9–3. That declining risk is due to the effects of diversification and to the decrease in the weights of each security in the portfolio. The risk that is eliminated through diversification is that which is unique to individual securities, known as **unsystematic risk**. Not all of the risk in any portfolio of risky securities can be eliminated through diversification. There will remain a level of risk that is inherent in investing in the market, known as **systematic risk** or market risk; it is represented by the dotted line in Figure 9–3. No matter how many securities are added to a portfolio of risky securities, systematic risk remains.

Investors, the providers of funds in any financial market, form portfolios of securities. They seek to control the risk to which they are exposed, and can do so by holding diversified portfolios. Figure 9–4 depicts an investor's portfolio selection problem. The two axes represent expected return (vertical axis) and risk (horizontal axis). The vertical axis is *expected*, rather than realized, return because of the

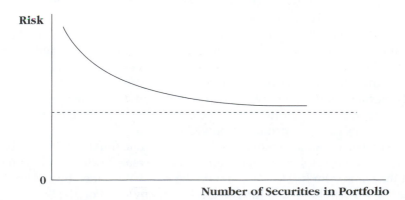

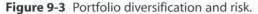

Figure 9-3 Portfolio diversification and risk.

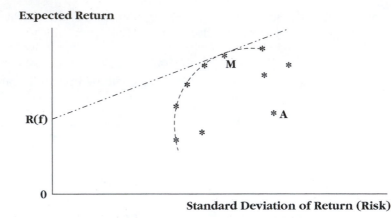

Figure 9-4 The efficient frontier.

presence of risk. When facing risky investments, one cannot know what the level of future realized return will be.

Portfolios available for investment are represented as asterisks (*) in risk-expected return space. Each portfolio is located according to its expected return and the level of risk that it displays. Only a few of the infinite number of possible portfolios are shown. If any two portfolios are available, like those labeled A and M, by investing in various combinations of the two, any portfolio on the straight line connecting them is also available (assuming that portfolios are infinitely divisible).

There is a portfolio that displays no risk at all. That is the "risk-free" portfolio, offering the risk-free rate of interest R(*f*). In practice, the risk-free portfolio consists of 90-day U.S. Treasury bills (T-bills). These mature so quickly that their values are influenced only by the approach of the maturity date (and the promise of payment of their face value) and are unaffected by any but the most extreme fluctuations in interest rates. Ninety-day T-bills are also free of any risk of default; the U.S. government will not default on its debt obligations within the next 90 days.

The curved, dashed line in Figure 9–4 is the **efficient frontier**. It shows, for any level of risk, the highest expected return available. Also, it shows the lowest level of risk at which any given level of expected return can be had. Informed, rational investors will only hold risky portfolios that lie on the efficient frontier. For example, no investor would want to hold portfolio A, because A's expected return can be obtained by assuming much less risk. Because investors love high returns and loathe risk, the efficient frontier shows the set of portfolios that are "best" for investors. Because one can invest in any combination of any two portfolios on the efficient frontier, the frontier itself must be continuous (there are no holes in it) and it must be convex (its ends cannot be bowed upward).

Because investors can loan money at the risk-free rate (buying 90-day T-bills is the equivalent of lending at the risk-free rate), they can create portfolios along the line segment that runs from R(*f*) to any point on the efficient frontier. By holding some combination of portfolio M and the risk-free asset, any point on the line segment between them can be an obtainable portfolio. In fact, if investors can borrow at the risk-free rate and use the proceeds to purchase M, the entire ray emanating from R(*f*) and tangent to the efficient frontier becomes the set of obtainable portfolios.

The portfolios that can be created along the ray from R(*f*) dominate the efficient frontier (they offer higher expected yields at any level of risk than does the efficient frontier alone). M is also the "best" risky portfolio to combine with R(*f*) in building those portfolios. Using any risky portfolio other than M will produce lower expected returns at any level of risk. M, then, takes on special importance; it is the only risky portfolio that any informed, rational investor would hold. The ray emanating from R(*f*) and tangent to the efficient frontier at M is known as the **capital market line**, the line on which all investors seek to establish portfolio positions.

EQUILIBRIUM PRICING AND RETURNS

Where on the capital market line an individual investor will establish his portfolio position depends on the investor's degree of risk aversion. Very risk-averse investors will take positions like C (for cautious) in Figure 9–5. This portfolio will "behave" much like a risk-free asset. Its returns will vary little over time, and the expected return will be about R(*f*). Less risk-averse investors will take positions like G (for gambler), which displays higher expected returns and higher risk than C. Both of those portfolios, and any other portfolio on the capital market line, involves only a combination of 90-day T-bills and M. It must follow, then, that investors will hold no risky portfolio other than M. What must M contain? It must contain the entire market. The price of any security not included in M will rise or fall, to adjust its expected return, in value until it is contained in M. M is the market portfolio.

By holding only a combination of the market portfolio and the risk-free asset, investors can eliminate all of the nonsystematic risk from their portfolios. The ease of eliminating nonsystematic risk from the portfolio implies that, in equilibrium, no investor is rewarded for assuming nonsystematic risk. The degree of risk that any portfolio contributes to a portfolio is that security's covariance with the portfo-

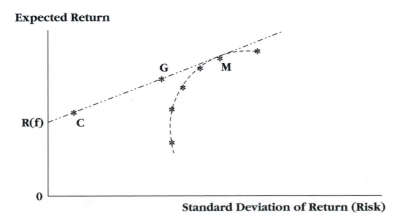

Figure 9-5 Investor preferences and portfolio position.

lio. Thus the degree of systematic risk that a security contributes to the market portfolio is the security's covariance with the market.

Is there really a market portfolio? That question has been a matter of controversy among financial economists for some time (controversies about the model developed here and in the next section are discussed in Harrington, 1987, especially Chapter 2). The theory suggests that there must be a portfolio consisting of *all* risky assets (stocks, bonds, notes, bills, certificates of deposit, bankers' acceptances, derivative securities, commercial paper, repurchase agreements, mortgage-backed securities, real estate, collectibles, jewelry). In practice, one cannot observe that portfolio. In applying models of portfolio selection and asset pricing, some market index, often the Standard and Poor's 500, is used as a proxy for the market portfolio.

Market risk can be represented as the variance in returns to the market portfolio (σ_M^2) and the reward for accepting market risk is the difference between the expected return to the market as a whole and the risk-free rate, $E[R(M)] - R(f)$. The price of a unit of market risk, then, is $\{E[R(M)] - R(f)\}/\sigma_M^2$. That is, the price of a unit of market risk is the reward for accepting market risk, divided by the amount of risk accepted.

Capital Asset Pricing Model (CAPM)

The **Capital Asset Pricing Model (CAPM)** ties the pieces just outlined into a model of market equilibrium prices, returns, and, therefore, cost of capital (Harrington, 1987; Sharpe, 1964). Figure 9–6 depicts the CAPM (pronounced "cap-m") graphically.

Every investor, for deferring current consumption is rewarded with at least the risk-free rate of interest R(*f*). In addition, those who invest in risky securities are entitled to the *expected* price of a unit of market risk, $[E[R(M)]2R(f)]/\sigma_M^2$, multi-

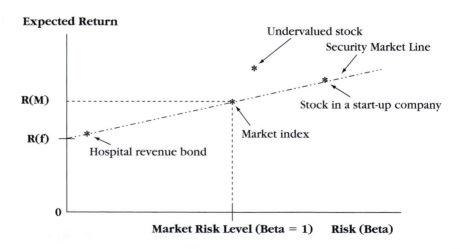

Figure 9-6 The capital asset pricing model.

plied by the amount of market risk they accept. The amount of market risk accepted by selecting any security (A) is indicated by the covariance of that security's returns with the returns to the market as a whole ($cov_{A,M}$). Therefore the expected return to security A should be

$$E[R(A)] = R(f) + ([E[R(M)] - R(f)]/\sigma_M^2)^* \ cov_{A,M}$$

or the risk-free rate plus the expected return to a unit of market risk multiplied by the amount of market risk inherent in A. Note, again, that this is an expected return, accepting risk means that expectations may not materialize.

Rewriting the previous equation,

$$E[R(A)] - R(f) = \{E[R(M)] - R(f)\} \times [cov_{A,M}/\sigma_M^2]$$

The left-hand side of the equation is the expected risk premium for investing in A. The right-hand side is especially interesting. It is the market's expected risk premium multiplied by the covariance between A and M divided by the variance of M. Covariance divided by variance is also, by happy coincidence, the coefficient of the expected price of risk, obtained by estimating an ordinary least squares regression equation, usually known as **beta (ß)**. Therefore a measure of the extent to which security A should, in equilibrium, compensate an investor for risk bearing is the ordinary least squares coefficient obtained by regressing A's expected excess return (excess over the risk-free rate) against the market's expected excess return, with the constant term suppressed (Maddala, 1992). The equation for the equilibrium expected excess return for A can thus be rewritten as

$$E[R(A)] - R(f) = \{E[R(M)] - R(f)\} \times \beta_A$$

If one were to use a spreadsheet to estimate β_A, the y-range would be $E[R(A)] - R(f)$ for a series of time periods, and the x-range would be $E[R(M)] - R(f)$ for the same series of time periods. One would need to be careful, when specifying such a regression model, to suppress the constant term.

The contribution of CAPM is that it predicts a security's equilibrium return for any given risk-free rate and expected return to the market. Once a security's beta is known, so long as it is stable, its equilibrium expected return is known (unfortunately, betas are remarkably unstable; see Blume, 1975). The beta of a portfolio is the weighted average of the betas of the securities in it. The beta of the market as a whole is always 1.00.

Figure 9–6 shows some features of the CAPM. The theory asserts that all assets' risk/return behavior should place them on a straight line, the ray emanating from the risk-free rate and passing through a point with beta equal to 1.00 and with expected return equal to R(M). That ray is known as the security market line. An overvalued security may temporarily lie below the security market line, and an undervalued security, like the one pictured, may temporarily lie above the **security market line**. A security is undervalued if its market price is less than the present value of all of the cash flows that will accrue to its holders (see Chapter 6). When a security is undervalued, investors will rush to purchase it, driving up its price. As its price rises, the expected return to the security will fall; remember that the periodic return is

$$R_t = [(P_t + CF_t)/P_{t-1}] - 1$$

As original price (P_{t-1}) goes up, expected return must fall. As investors bid for the security, its price will continue to rise, and its expected return continue to fall, until the security has returned to the security market line.

On the security market line, securities with very low risk (such as insured hospital revenue bonds) will lie close to the risk-free rate. Securities that are very risky (such as equity shares in startup companies) will lie to the right of the market index. Investors can select portfolios of assets on the bases of their own degrees of risk aversion. A very risk-averse investor will wish to form a portfolio of assets with a low beta. A less risk-averse investor will wish to form a portfolio of assets with a higher beta.

Knowing and applying security betas is not an exercise for investors and portfolio managers only. As discussed earlier, one party's return (yield) is another party's cost of capital. Therefore the CAPM yields information about providers' costs of capital as well as about portfolio managers' returns. Sloan, Valvona, and Hassan (1988) used the CAPM to estimate the cost of capital for the various components of the hospital sector. Wheeler and Smith (1988) demonstrate how to apply the CAPM to determine the proper discount rate in capital budgeting (see Chapter 10).

The CAPM is not the last word on asset pricing. For the model to represent asset pricing accurately, a number of assumptions must hold, several of them quite unrealistic (Harrington, 1987). In the CAPM, systematic (or market) risk is the only factor to which prices respond. Several alternative models have been proposed, most of which recognize that asset prices and returns can respond to more than one factor. One of the most widely used such models is the **Arbitrage Pricing Theory (APT)** (Harrington, 1987; Roll & Ross, 1984; Ross, 1976).

According to the APT, asset prices respond to several factors. These may be inflation, real economic growth, or growth in the money stock, but in practice they are not easily identified by name. Because APT hypothesizes a response term for each factor identified, it does not yield a simple summary statistic like the beta of the CAPM. APT has been used successfully, however, to estimate the cost of capital in the hospital sector (Sloan, Valvona, & Hassan, 1988).

HOW WELL DO FINANCIAL MARKETS WORK?

Undervalued stocks, like the one shown in Figure 9–6, cannot stay undervalued very long. Competitive bidding, as investors seek the stock's above-market returns, will quickly raise the stock's price, depressing its return down to the level indicated, at that level of risk, on the security market line. How quickly market participants realize that a security is undervalued (mispriced) and how quickly the price changes as a result is the degree of informational **efficiency** of the market.

If a market is inefficient, one can find mispriced securities often. Such a market does not process information quickly. Because modern financial markets have many participants, each striving to maximize his or her own position (see Chapter 1), they are not inefficient.

A market is efficient in the weak sense if all current security prices incorporate all past security prices. That is, in a market that is efficient in the weak sense, one cannot identify undervalued securities merely by knowing last week's prices. A large body of empirical research shows that price information is so widely disseminated that modern financial markets are at least efficient in the weak sense.

A market is efficient in the semistrong sense if current security prices reflect all publicly available information. In such a market, one cannot, except by accident, identify undervalued securities, unless one has special access to private information. Most modern financial markets are efficient in this sense.

A market is efficient in the strong sense if current security prices reflect all information, public and private. In such a market, even corporate insiders cannot use their information to know when a security's price will rise or fall. In real markets, there are individuals who have access to special, nonpublic information. The collapse of Enron Corporation in 2001-2002 is but an example of insiders' access to valuable information. Efficiency in the strong sense is only an ideal.

A BRIEF NOTE ON OWNERS' EQUITY

The CAPM and the APT are most often applied to the determination of the required return to (the cost of capital for) equity (common stock) financing rather than to the required returns to debt financing. Those who hold the debt securities of investor-owned corporations are entitled, by legally enforceable contract, to periodic interest payments and to repayment of principal at maturity. Those who hold the preferred stock of investor-owned corporations are entitled to a fixed annual dividend but not to any repayment of principal. Holders of common stock have no legal guarantee of any type of periodic payment. Dividends to common stock holders are payable at the discretion of the board of directors.

Many managers, directors, and trustees, therefore, believe that "equity is free." That is not the case. Providers of funds demand a required rate of return for their equity investments. In fact, because equity imposes greater risk on the investor than does debt (holders of debt securities are paid before the holders of equity securities), the required returns to equity for any individual organization are greater than the required returns to debt for that organization.

Returns to equity securities take two forms, increases in the market values of the securities and periodic dividend payments. When investor-owned organizations forget that they must pay the required return to their equity investors, a chain of events begins. Equity holders begin to sell their stock, driving its price down. The price of the stock falls until the dollar returns offered equal the required return on the now-lower market price. At the lower stock price, the firm may represent a bargain purchase for a "corporate raider." Some lessons have to be learned the hard way.

The required returns to the equity of not-for-profit organizations can take several forms. Federal tax law forbids not-for-profit firms from distributing profits to any individual, on pain of losing not-for-profit status. Not-for-profit organizations may pay returns to the communities or organizations that sponsor them through offering charity care, through reducing prices, or through offering services (burn units, neonatal intensive care) that do not generate revenues sufficient to cover their variable costs. Even in the not-for-profit sector, equity is not free (Sloan, Valvona, & Hassan, 1988).

MORE ON YIELDS

CAPM takes the general level of interest rates as given. That is, it portrays the return to holding any security as depending on the risk-free rate of interest, the expected yield to the market as a whole, and the security's degree of systematic risk. It is instructive to take a step back and to ask how the risk-free rate and the expected return to the market are determined.

To induce consumers to delay consumption, they must be compensated by a rate of interest. That "pure" rate of interest compensates savers (investors) only for delaying consumption. The determination of the pure rate of interest (r_p) is beyond the scope of this book but is a topic in macroeconomics (Mankiw, 1990).

Investors also demand compensation for the deterioration of the purchasing power of their assets, due to inflation, over time. The rate of inflation is the average rate at which prices changes. If the risk-free rate of interest does not include a premium for inflation (r_i), then investors will lose purchasing power in each year in which they hold their assets. The observed risk-free rate of interest must include a pure rate of interest plus the expected rate of inflation over the period for which the risk-free securities are issued (Fisher, 1930, pp. 493). Thus, if r_p and r_i are small, approximately,

$$R(f) = r_p + r_i$$

As expected inflation rises, the risk-free rate of interest will rise.

It is sometimes useful, especially in examining the yields on bonds, to think of the yields as being composed, like the risk-free rate of interest, of the pure rate of interest and a series of premiums. Thus the yield on some bond B might be decomposed as

$$R(B) = r_p + r_i + r_r + r_l + r_m$$

where r_p is the pure rate of interest, r_i is the premium for expected inflation, r_r is a premium for the riskiness of the bond (perhaps best defined as the probability that the bond's issuers will default on their obligations), r_l is a premium for the relative lack of liquidity (ability to sell) of the bond, and r_m is a premium for the term to maturity of the bond (the length of time until the issuer must repay the bond's principal). The relationship just shown will hold only approximately (unless compounding is continuous, in which it holds exactly).

SUMMARY

This chapter is concerned with the external financial environment in which health care organizations obtain funds. That environment *enables* health care providers to acquire and upgrade facilities and equipment. It also *constrains* them to acquire that equipment and to engage in those activities that external investors believe will produce adequate returns, at sufficiently low risk, in the future.

Financial markets are impersonal, competitive, and efficient in the semistrong sense. However, that is not to say that people do not play important roles in them. Accountants, attorneys, bond rating analysts, broker/dealers, and regulators all perform facilitating roles in financial markets, roles for which some are richly rewarded.

Financial markets reward the providers of funds with returns and charge the users of funds their costs of capital. Those returns and costs are determined, in part, by the overall level of interest rates (through the risk-free rate) and, in part, through markets' determination of the price of systematic (or market) risk. One useful approach to the pricing of systematic risk is the Capital Asset Pricing Model (CAPM). This approach suggests that the return that investors require from holding any individual security depends on the risk-free rate, the expected return to the market as a whole, and the security's own beta (the security's returns' covariance with the returns to the market as a whole, divided by the variance in return to the market as a whole). Unfortunately, CAPM may not tell the whole story on the pricing of risk (the model may not be complete), and the beta of any individual security may vary widely over time.

Discussion Questions

1. Over a lifetime, a household can play several roles in financial markets. List them and explain each.

2. Whence comes the trade-off between risk and expected return for securities?

3. What is the lowest level of risk achievable, even in the most thoroughly diversified portfolio?

4. Can anyone actually hold the market portfolio? Explain.

5. Can one really observe a risk-free rate of interest? Explain.

CONTINUING CASE

Roger Jackson, Henry Kirk, and Janet Fowler were sitting in Kirk's office, contemplating the situation of Physicians' Clinic and its parent, PCI, Inc. Kirk, the president of both corporations, spoke first: "We rely on inpatient revenues to cover our costs. Plus, if we don't have inpatient beds, we're just a medical office building. Our whole mission depends on having some occupied beds." He did not mention that his own stature as an administrator and the jobs of his many friends within PCI depended on inpatient care.

"So what's the big deal?" Dr. Jackson was characteristically blunt.

"We've got beds; we've got nurses. Heaven knows we're paying all of these people enough."

"The problem is that we're behind the technology curve. Dr. DeForest has stopped admitting any patients to the clinic. He says he needs the lab services and the imaging equipment at Memorial." Kirk's comments about Todd DeForest got Dr. Jackson's attention; DeForest, a well-liked internist, was one of the senior members, and leading revenue producers, of the Jackson Group.

Turning to Fowler, Jackson asked, "Do we have enough cash to buy some equipment?" Jackson already knew the answer (see the Continuing Case in Chapter 4).

"We don't have the cash. We would need about $22 million to revamp the lab, add a full-body CT scanner, equip an ultrasound lab, and install an MRI set-up. We just don't have it."

The three considered several options before deciding to explore ("just explore, mind you; no commitments!") the possibility of raising the necessary funds through a securities offering. But how to proceed? PCI, Inc., had never issued securities to the public. To justify diluting the ownership shares of the current shareholders, some substantial gains should be forthcoming.

Janet Fowler took the task of preparing a preliminary report and presenting it to a special meeting of the board of directors. What she found did not look promising. A call to Phil Connor, the local representative of a national investment house, put her in touch with some people in the firm's "corporate finance" office in Dallas. Their analysis was that (1) the current rate on 90-day T-bills is 4.25 percent, (2) the chief of investment strategy at the home office in New York says that his expectation for market returns over the next 12 months is 8.15 percent, and (3) PCI, Inc., looks just like a client that has a beta of 1.4 ("but we'd have to do a full work up on that"). They also explained that at least 6 months would transpire between a decision to sell securities and their actual sale. The risk premium, above the T-bill rate, on long-term corporate bonds for highly leveraged, small firms is now 5 percent.

CASE QUESTIONS

1. What external financing options are available to PCI, Inc.?

2. What are the pros and cons of a sale of equity securities as a means of financing their equipment purchases? Of a sale of debt securities?

3. If PCI decides to issue additional common stock, what is likely to be its approximate cost of capital?

4. If PCI decides to issue additional long-term debt, what is likely to be its approximate cost of capital?

REFERENCES

Bloch, E. (1986). *Inside investment banking*. Homewood, IL: Dow Jones-Irwin.

Blume, M.E. (1975). Betas and their regression tendencies. *Journal of Finance 30*(3), 785–796.

Fisher, I. (1930). *The theory of interest*. New York: Macmillan.

Harrington, D.R. (1987). *Modern portfolio theory, the capital asset pricing model and arbitrage pricing theory: A user's guide* (2nd ed.). Englewood Cliffs, NJ: Prentice-Hall.

Knight, F.H. (1921). *Risk, uncertainty, and profit*. Boston, MA: Houghton Mifflin.

Maddala, G.S. (1992). *Introduction to econometrics* (2nd ed.). New York: Macmillan.

Mankiw, N.G. (1990). A quick refresher course in macroeconomics. *Journal of Economic Literature, 28*(4), 1645–1660.

Markowitz, H.M. (1952). Portfolio selection. *Journal of Finance, 12*(1), 77–91.

Pointer, L.G. & Schroeder R.G. (1986). *Introduction to the securities and exchange commission*. Plano, TX: Business Publications, Inc.

Roll, R. & Ross, S.A. (1984). The arbitrage pricing theory approach to strategic portfolio planning. *Financial Analysts Journal, 40*(3), 14–29.

Ross, S.A. (1976). The arbitrage theory of capital asset pricing. *Journal of Economic Theory, 13*(3), 341–360.

Sharpe, W.F. (1964). Capital asset prices: A theory of market equilibrium under conditions of risk. *Journal of Finance, 19*(3), 425–442.

Sloan, F.A., Valvona, J., & Hassan, M. (1988). Cost of capital to the hospital sector. *Journal of Health Economics, 7*(1), 25–45.

Wheeler, J.R.C. & Smith, D.G. (1988). The discount rate for capital expenditure analysis in health care. *Health Care Management Review, 13*(2), 43–52.

Wilson, G., Sheps, C.G. & Oliver, T.R. (1982). Effects of hospital revenue bonds on hospital planning and operations. *New England Journal of Medicine, 307*(23), 1426–1430.

SELECTED READINGS

Bodie, Z., Kane, A., & Marcus, A.J. (2002). *Investments* (5th ed.). Chicago, IL: Irwin.

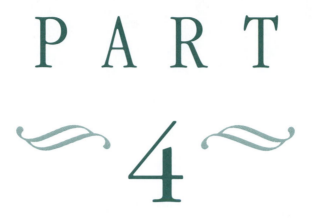

PART

4

Selecting Long-Term Assets and Programs

CHAPTER

10

The Basics of Capital Budgeting

Learning Objectives

After reading this chapter, the student should be able to:

1. Calculate cash flows after taxes for proposed capital investments.
2. Explain the appropriate decision rules for analyzing proposed investments and apply them in appropriate circumstances.
3. Calculate net present value, internal rate of return, and profitability index, given assumed cash flows and discount rates.
4. Explain the differences between the applications of the net present value and the internal rate of return rules in making mutually exclusive choice decisions.

Key Terms

Accept/reject

Capital budgeting

Capital rationing

Financing cash flow

Initial cash outflow

Internal rate of
return

Mutually exclusive choice

Net present value

Net working capital commitment

Operating cash flow

Profitability index

Tax shield

Terminating cash flow

Weighted average cost of capital (WACC)

Many assets, projects, and programs fit the model of the user of funds shown in Figure 9–1. That is, those projects require the commitment of large amounts of money in the present and offer the promise of a stream of cash flows in the future. Budgeting for these projects is complex. Should one include the entire (often very large) current outlay in the current period's expense budget? Should one expect to fund that outlay from budgeted, current revenues? Most organizations answer both of those questions with a resounding "No." The process of selecting long-lived assets, projects, and programs according to financial criteria is known as **capital budgeting**.

Capital budgeting is part of the budgeting process. It is based on the organization's overall operating plan. Capital budgeting is different from expense and revenue budgeting, however, in that it is based on operating plans for future periods. It is in future periods that the newly acquired assets and projects will be "on-line" and will generate revenues. Most capital projects will be financed with external funds. Therefore most organizations treat the capital budget separately from the operating components (expense and revenue) of the budget. The total amount to be allocated, the rules for allocation, and the information flows in the capital budgeting process are separate from those of operational budgeting.

Capital budgeting is also a part of the strategic management process. Whenever one selects a major item of equipment (a magnetic resonance imaging device, for example) or uses capital budgeting procedures to decide for or against a product line (will we have a cardiology program?), one is making strategic choices. It is through the capital budgeting process that the financial team participates in the determination of the organization's overall strategy.

Capital budgeting is (or should be) where the fun is for financial managers. It is always more fun to acquire new "stuff" than to pay for it or take care of it. It is no wonder that this area occupies so much of the professional and academic literature of finance. Capital budgeting practice draws on accounting, economics, mathematics, statistics, and strategic management. Good capital budgeting requires creativity, judgment, sound analysis, and careful information management.

After completing this chapter, the reader should be able to choose and apply an appropriate asset selection criterion, distinguish among the relevant types of cash flows, compute after-tax cash flows, and recognize the major limitations of the capital budgeting process. The reader should also be prepared to proceed to the more advanced capital budgeting topics presented in Chapter 11.

CRITERIA AND CONSTRAINTS

Capital budgeting is a multistep process for selecting long-lived assets, projects, and programs. Although one cannot ignore the many nonfinancial criteria that influence capital and product line acquisition decisions, this chapter and the one that follows are concerned with the application of financial criteria. Applying those criteria is not necessarily a mercenary process, and one cannot be so narrow-minded in their application as to ignore obvious nonfinancial costs and benefits.

If an organization is to survive, it must have cash inflows that at least equal its cash outflows. It is not necessary that inflows balance outflows in every period; some years' cash outflows (exaggerated by capital acquisition or extraordinary items) will be greater than cash inflows. Long-term survival, however, demands that the present value of all future cash inflows be at least as great as the present value of all future cash outflows.

The statement above makes three important points. First, survival depends on cash flows. Accumulated accounts receivable cannot pay bills. Cash is necessary, un-ambiguous, and available to meet obligations. It is on cash flow that survival de-pends. Second, although cash inflows need not meet outflows in each year, all future cash inflows must be adequate to meet all future outflows. To evaluate a future in-flow's sufficiency to meet some outflow (and the interest expenses that an accumu-lated outflow excess will generate), one must consider the time value of that inflow. To compare a stream of inflows to a stream of outflows, one must compare their time value at some common date (see Chapter 5). Third, it is all cash inflows and outflows that must be considered. Donations, government appropriations, and interest income are cash flows just as much as collections of revenue.

The basic question that any capital budgeting system must ask, then, is "Does this asset or project, in a time value sense, at least pay for itself? If not (if it requires a subsidy), is there a subsidy forthcoming?" If the answer is yes, then the project is worth doing. If the answer is no, from a financial perspective, it is not.

MULTIPLE STEPS

Pinches (1982) discussed the asset selection in terms of four stages. First, someone must recognize that an asset is worth evaluating for acquisition. That is the identi-fication stage. In that stage one isolates, from the many assets or projects that are available, those that have promise of meeting the financial tests described below. The tools used in this stage are creativity, imagination, and knowledge of the tech-nological environment.

The second stage is development. In this stage one develops (forecasts) the potential cash flows expected from the assets or projects under review. It is the accuracy of the cash flow projections made in this stage that determines how use-ful the capital budgeting process will ultimately be. Knowledge of conditions in the markets for services is the principal tool used in this stage.

The third stage is the application of a decision rule to the cash flows projected in the development stage. Most financial professionals consider this stage to be *the* capital budgeting process. Rather, the selection and application of a quantitative decision rule is only the third of four steps in the process. Time-value-of-money calculations are the principal tools brought to bear in this stage.

The fourth stage in the process is the audit. In the audit stage, one asks, "Did our projections prove accurate? Were our expectations about the project's outcome borne out? What can we learn from this experience that will help us to improve the capital budgeting process?" Unfortunately, the audit stage is often ignored.

CASH FLOWS RECONSIDERED

Net cash inflow is the difference between cash inflows and cash outflows in any given period. Cash flows are not usually constant over the life of a project but change over time. Further, it is *after-tax* cash flows that are of interest to the organization, and as will be discussed, the effects of income tax on cash flows is not constant over the life of any asset or project. Cash flows before taxes in period t ($CFBT_t$) need to be modified to arrive at cash flows after taxes for the period ($CFAT_t$). Also, as we plan and make decisions, we cannot know the future with certainty. We always perform capital budgeting with expected cash flows.

Initial Cash-Flows

It is useful to distinguish among three types of cash flows in evaluating any project. First, every asset acquired or project begun involves **initial cash outflows**. These cash flows occur at the beginning of the project or at acquisition of the asset (at time = 0) and are usually denoted as $CFAT_0$. $CFAT_0$ is always negative. That is, one cannot have something for nothing; nature does not give "freebies." One acquires assets or initiates projects by spending money (having negative cash outflows). Also a part of initial cash outflows is the project's requirement of net working capital.

Operating Cash Flows

The second type of cash flow involved in any project or in the life of any asset is **operating cash flows**. These are the net flows that result from putting the asset on line or from carrying out the project. One hopes that operating cash flows are positive.

For investor-owned organizations, operating cash flows are subject to tax. Thus, for every period, one must multiply $CFBT_t$ by one minus the applicable tax rate. That is not the end of the story on tax effects, however. Initial cash flows do not usually have direct tax consequences. Although they represent negative cash flows, they are not usually tax-deductible expenses. Rather, these flows set up fixed assets that can be depreciated (see Chapter 3) over their useful lives. Depreciation is a tax-deductible expense. Therefore, in organizations that are subject to income taxation, depreciation expense is deducted from net income in calculating taxable income. The amount of depreciation expense multiplied by the applicable income tax rate (federal plus state) is a **tax shield**, the amount of tax (that would apply in absence of deductibility of depreciation) that need not be paid.

CFAT_t, then, has two components: adjusted CFBT_t *plus* the relevant tax shield:

$$\text{CFAT}_t = [\text{CFBT}_t \times (1-T)] + [(\text{Dep}_t) \times T]$$

where CFAT_t and CFBT_t are cash flow after tax and cash flow before tax, respectively, in period t; Dep_t is depreciation expense in period t; and T is the tax rate, expressed as a decimal.

Terminating Cash Flow

The third type of cash flow is the **terminating cash flow**. These flows are primarily the capture of the salvage value of the equipment in place. For projects that are likely to be continued indefinitely, there is no expectation of salvage value. As discussed later, the tax status of terminating cash flows is complex.

A component of both initial cash flows and terminating cash flows is **net working capital commitment**. Working capital consists of cash, marketable securities, accounts receivable, inventory, and a few other items. Usually a new project will require the commitment of some resources for inventory and additional cash on hand. Those are resources that must be raised along with the other initial commitments to the project. They are very much a part of initial cash outflows. Similarly, upon termination the working capital commitment is released. Release of working capital should be treated as a cash inflow upon termination. Figure 10–1 shows the various types of project cash flows and the time periods in which they are incurred.

Financing Cash Flows

Conspicuous by their absence from the list of types of cash flow, above, is **financing cash flows**. These are not considered in developing cash flows for capital budgeting purposes. Financing cash flows are the payments that must be made to

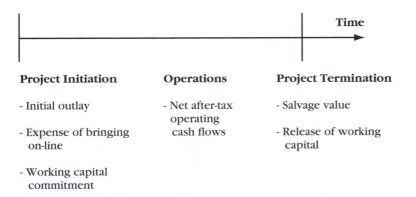

Figure 10-1 Timing and types of cash flow.

those who provide the funds to acquire the assets under consideration or to initiate the project being proposed. These interest payments are very real and, often, very large. Even when the necessary funds are generated internally rather than being acquired in financial markets, financing cash flows are important. By using funds on one project, the organization gives up the opportunity to invest them at some interest rate. Thus financing costs cannot be ignored, even when they are opportunity costs.

The reason that financing cash flows are not included in cash flow development lies in the time value of money. Remember from Chapter 5 that it is the accumulation of interest that gives rise to the time value of money. Therefore the selection of a discount rate for time-value-of-money calculations in capital budgeting takes account of the financing cash flows that the project requires. Because these financing flows are accounted for in time-value-of-money calculations, to include financing flows in operating cash flow calculations would be to double-count the effects of market interest rates.

Also note that depreciation is not a cash flow item. According to Generally Accepted Accounting Principles, the expense associated with any item of capital equipment is the annual depreciation expense assigned to it (see Chapter 3). That depreciation involves no cash outflow, however, and has no direct effect on the project's or asset's operating cash flows. The only effect depreciation expense has on project cash flows is indirect, through the tax shield discussed earlier (and therefore is only important to organizations subject to income taxation).

Taxes do not move the world. Managers and financial planners who allow the tax effects of their actions to dominate their decisions can do their organizations great harm. Taxes, however, do involve substantial cash outflows (or cash outflows saved) and ought not to be ignored. As shown earlier, it is the cash flow after taxes that is important in capital budgeting decisions. Terminating cash flows must be adjusted for tax effects, for organizations that have income tax exposure, just as operating cash flows must.

A terminating cash flow consists of two parts: salvage value and the release of working capital. The release of working capital normally generates neither a tax liability nor a tax shield. The recovery of salvage value can, for organizations subject to income tax, have complicated tax consequences. Every health care organization should have access to the services of an attorney or accountant who understands current income tax regulations (federal and state) so that they will not be caught unawares by changes in those laws. The sale of any asset generates revenue and that revenue is used in the computation of taxable income. If the sale price of an asset exceeds its depreciated book value, the difference is taxable. Every organization should be aware of possible changes in the treatment of salvage value for tax purposes.

Interest expense is a tax-deductible item under corporate tax law. That is, interest expense is subtracted from profit in computing taxable income. The deduction of interest expense, however, should not be considered in computing after-tax cash flows in capital budgeting analysis. The reason is related to the reason for not counting financing cash flows among operating cash flows. Just as the financing cash flows are "counted" in the discounting process, the organization should account for the tax-deductibility of interest expense by using its *after-tax cost of capital* as its discount rate.

When evaluating an asset or project, one should consider *only* incremental cash flows. That is, cash flows that would occur without the asset or project's being online should not count for (or against) the project under review. When considering mutually exclusive projects, only the cash flows that are different between the two need to be reviewed. For example, if two pickup trucks are being evaluated for the same purpose, the cash inflows can be expected to be the same for both. Therefore one need only consider the cash flows that are different, the cash outflows associated with operating each of the two alternatives. The choice with the lower present value of cash outflows is the better of the two.

A NOTE ON EXPECTED INFLATION

As the future unfolds, and as cash flows are received, prices will change. Most likely, a service whose price is $50 today will be much more expensive by the time the service is terminated. That raises a question for cash flow forecasters: should cash flows be projected using today's prices, or should expected inflation be factored into expected cash flows?

One should factor expected inflation into one's cash flow projections. The reason is that market interest rates, used to discount future cash flows, include market participants' best assessment of future inflation. As discussed in Chapter 9, a market interest rate will consist of a real rate of interest and an inflation premium. Lenders demand such inflation premiums in order to maintain the purchasing power of the returns they receive (Fisher, 1930). Therefore one ought to use inflation-adjusted cash flows when one's discount rate is a market rate of interest (Bierman & Smidt, 1993).

DECISION PROBLEMS AND DECISION RULES

There are three types of problems into which capital budgeting decision rules fall: accept/reject, mutually exclusive choice, and capital rationing. For each of these, there is a single decision rule that is "best" in that it will generate the optimal (most wealth-enhancing) decision consistently. These decision rules are shown in Table 10.1.

Accept/Reject

The simplest type of decision is the **accept/reject** decision. In accept/reject decisions, one is considering whether or not to acquire an asset or to initiate a project. No other alternatives are under review. One might ask, "Do we or don't we set up an outpatient clinic in the town's new shopping mall?" or "Do we or don't we purchase a pickup truck?"

If such a project or asset adds value to the organization, then it is worth initiating or acquiring. The best measure of whether or not a stream of future cash flows actually adds value to the organization is the **net present value** of the stream. Thus

Table 10-1 Decision problems and decision rules. Adapted from Long, H. W. (1982). Asset choice and program selection in a competitive environment (Part I). Health Care Financial Management 36(7), 40-55.

	Investor-Owned	Not-for-Profit	Government
Accept/reject	NPV greater than or equal to zero	NPV greater than or equal to zero	Expert decision, based on need
Mutually exclusive choice	Select alternative with the largest NPV of at least zero.	Select alternative with the greatest NPV of at least zero.	Select alternative with the lowest present value of cash outflows.
Capital rationing	Select highest profitability index, then next highest profitability index, and so on until budget is exhausted.	Select highest profitability index, then next highest profitability index, and so on until budget is exhausted.	Expert decision, based on need

Adapted from Long, H.W. (1982). Asset choice and program selection in a competitive environment (Part I). *Health Care Financial Management* 36(7), 40-55.

the best decision rule for accept/reject decision problems is "Is its net present value at least zero?" If the net present value is greater than zero, the project adds value to the organization. If the net present value is exactly zero, it neither adds nor subtracts value from the organization. In either case, the project is acceptable. If the net present value is less than zero, the project subtracts value from the organization and, according to purely financial criteria, should not be undertaken.

Long (1982a, 1982b) proposed modifying the net present value–based rules for accept/reject decision rules, depending on the ownership of the organization making the decisions. His results are still thought provoking and controversial. For investor-owned organizations, Long proposed that the decision rule be exactly as just described. Such organizations, after all, exist to maximize the wealth of their equity investors. Private not-for-profit organizations, which figure so heavily in the health care sector, however, are somewhat different. These organizations, although constrained in what they can do by their need to survive, exist to provide services. Thus Long proposed that private not-for-profit organizations accept or reject projects on the basis of nonnegative net present values. He also suggested, however, that those organizations, when they identify projects with nonnegative net present values, reduce the prices that they charge for their services so that, after the fact, their realized net present values would be exactly zero. Thus the gains from nonnegative net present values would accrue to consumers, not to the organizations themselves.

Long made an equally controversial argument with respect to government-owned organizations (VA medical centers, county-owned hospitals, local public health departments). These, he suggested, exist to turn tax dollars into services. They are meant to be consumers of capital. Therefore government organizations should make their accept/reject decisions on the basis of need, regardless of net present values.

Mutually Exclusive Choice

In **mutually exclusive choice** situations, more than one alternative is on the table, but only one can be selected. One might ask, "Do we put an outpatient emergency in the new shopping mall, in the old shopping mall, or nowhere?" or "Do we acquire the Chevrolet pickup truck or the Ford, or no truck at all?" The "none at all" alternative is almost always one of the alternatives in a mutually exclusive choice situation.

In choosing among mutually exclusive alternatives, one seeks the option that adds the most value to the organization. Therefore the best decision rule to employ in these situations is to select the alternative with the highest net present value, so long as that net present value is at least zero. Long modified that rule for private, not-for-profit, and government organizations. As for accept/reject decisions, Long would retain the basic decision rule for not-for-profit organizations' project selection. He would, however, have those organizations reduce their prices so that, after the fact, their realized net present values were zero. Government organizations, according to Long, exist to turn tax revenues into services. Therefore he would have them ignore net present values in selecting projects and assets but select the mutually exclusive alternatives that have the lowest present values of cash outflows. With the lowest present values of cash outflows, government organizations select the alternative that allows them to provide the most service with the least cash outlay. Both customers and taxpayers would benefit from adoption of such a decision rule.

Capital Rationing

Capital rationing is the decision problem in which a fixed dollar amount is to be invested in a given period. Among all of the projects available, the best subset must be selected. Financial theory says that there should never be capital rationing problems. Any project whose net present value is at least zero is worth doing. Therefore, theory argues, organizations ought never to limit their value by failing to invest in positive-NPV projects. In real life, however, capital rationing is quite common. Boards of trustees often set limits on annual capital spending. Governmental bodies always set annual capital appropriations limits that are binding on government-owned institutions. There are also limits on managers' abilities to manage new projects. Those limits set behavioral limitations on the number of initiatives begun in any one year and may necessitate capital rationing.

Profitability Index

Table 10–2 shows why the **profitability index** method is superior to the net present value method in making choices under capital rationing. The governing board has set a limit of $50 million in capital spending for the year. The staff has identified $100 million in worthwhile projects (projects with NPV at least zero). The appropriate discount rate is 8 percent. Which $50 million should the organization

Table 10–2 Capital rationing: Net present value versus profitability index

Total amount to be invested: $50 million
Discount rate: 8%

Year	Project A	Project B	Project C	Project D	Project E
0	($15,000,000.00)	($25,000,000.00)	($25,000,000.00)	($17,500,000.00)	($17,500,000.00)
1	2,251,000.00	3,745,000.00	3,750,000.00	2,625,500.00	2,626,500.00
2	2,251,000.00	3,745,000.00	3,750,000.00	2,625,500.00	2,626,500.00
3	2,251,000.00	3,745,000.00	3,750,000.00	2,625,500.00	2,626,500.00
4	2,251,000.00	3,745,000.00	3,750,000.00	2,625,500.00	2,626,500.00
5	2,251,000.00	3,745,000.00	3,750,000.00	2,625,500.00	2,626,500.00
6	2,251,000.00	3,745,000.00	3,750,000.00	2,625,500.00	2,626,500.00
7	2,251,000.00	3,745,000.00	3,750,000.00	2,625,500.00	2,626,500.00
8	2,251,000.00	3,745,000.00	3,750,000.00	2,625,500.00	2,626,500.00
9	2,251,000.00	3,745,000.00	3,750,000.00	2,625,500.00	2,626,500.00
10	2,251,000.00	3,745,000.00	3,750,000.00	2,625,500.00	2,626,500.00
NPV @ 8%	104,393.23	129,254.84	162,805.25	117,318.71	124,028.79
PI @ 8%	1.006959486	1.0051701936	1.00651220841	1.006703926453	1.00708735675

Choice by NPV	NPV
C	$162,805.25
B	129,254.84
Total	292,060.09

Choice by PI	NPV
E	$124,028.79
A	104,393.23
D	117,318.71
Total	345,740.74

select? One approach would be to take the projects with the highest net present values, moving from highest to lowest until the $50 million is spent. To do so in this case would be to select project C (NPV = $162,805.84) and project B (NPV = $129,254.84). Those two projects would exhaust the $50 million in allowable spending and provide a combined net present value (addition to the value of the organization) of $292,060.09.

A better way to select the subset of possible projects in a capital rationing problem is to use the profitability index method. The profitability index is defined as the present value of all future cash flows divided by the absolute value of the initial cash outlay. In equation form,

$$\text{Profitability index (PI)} = \left[\sum_{t=1}^{N} (\text{CFAT}_t / (1 + r)^t) \right] / |\text{CFAT}_0|$$

where r is the discount rate and N is the last year of the project's life. Note that if a project's net present value is at least zero, its profitability index will be at least one.

To use the profitability index method, one calculates the profitability indexes for the projects under review and arrays them in descending order by profitability index. One then selects projects until the budget is exhausted, or until the profitability indexes fall below 1.0. In the case shown in Table 10–2, one would select projects E, A, and D, completely exhausting the $50 million allowed. The total net present value of the three projects is $345,740.74, substantially greater than the combined NPV of the two projects with the largest individual NPVs.

Why the anomaly? In selecting among mutually exclusively choices, one wants big projects that add large amounts of value to the organization. That is what the net present value test identifies. In capital rationing, however, one wants to maximize the payoff per dollar invested. That is precisely what the profitability index measures.

The profitability index method has limitations, however. It will identify the best subset of projects if and only if three conditions are met: (1) projects are not divisible (one is considering only whole projects), (2) the optimal subset of projects identified exactly exhausts the budget allowed, and (3) only one period's capital budget is under review. If any of those conditions is violated, the optimal solution to capital rationing requires the use of linear programming. That method is discussed in Chapter 11.

Also note the circularity in reasoning involved in capital rationing: one must calculate the profitability index using a discount rate without knowing the riskiness of the projects to be selected (because one does not yet know which projects will be selected). Unless each project's profitability index is calculated using its own risk-adjusted discount rate (discussed in Chapter 11), however, the discount rate for the decision problem is not well defined.

Long's decision-making framework provides guidance on the solution of capital rationing problems in government-owned organizations. As for accept/reject decisions, Long would have capital rationing decisions made on the basis of expert judgement, based on the needs of the organization and the population it serves.

In determining which decision rules to include in Table 10–1, one class of rules can be eliminated immediately: those that ignore the time value of money. Such rules, including the calculation of the payback period and analysis of the accounting rate of return, will provide valid decisions only by accident. Because the after-tax cash flows from long-lived assets and projects are received over time, one cannot ignore their timing. Table 10–3 illustrates a case in which the use of payback period calculation will provide an inferior solution.

Payback Method

One of the most often-used methods of evaluating long-lived projects is the payback method (Kamath & Elmer, 1989). In the payback method, one calculates how long it takes for a project or asset to pay back, in after-tax cash flows, its initial cash outlay. Short payback periods are preferred to long payback periods. In Table 10–3 project A has a payback period of exactly 4 years. The $50,000 initial outlay is exactly paid back by the two $25,000 cash flows. Project B, however, has a payback period of 4.09 years. At the end of 4 years, it has paid back only $44,000 of its original $45,000 outlay. The payback method says that A is preferred to B. Any reasonable decision method says the opposite. Do not use the payback method to evaluate investment choices.

WHAT ABOUT INTERNAL RATE OF RETURN?

One set of decision rules that does incorporate the time value of money is that set based on the **internal rate of return (IRR)** to the investment. The internal rate of return to a project or asset is defined as the interest rate that makes the net present value of the project or asset equal to zero (makes the present value of future net cash inflows exactly equal to the initial cash outflow). Figure 10–2 illustrates the calculation of the internal rate of return for an initial investment of $100,000 that generates after-tax cash flows of $12,000 per year for 12 years. The figure shows the net present value of the project falling as the discount rate rises. At one value of the discount rate (6.11 percent in this case), the net present value is zero. That value of the discount rate is the internal rate of return to the project or asset. In equation form,

Table 10–3 Comparing payback periods for mutually exclusive choices.

Year	CFAT Project A	CFAT Project B
0	($50,000)	($45,000)
1	0	11,000
2	0	11,000
3	25,000	11,000
4	25,000	11,000
5	0	11,000
Payback period	4.00 years	4.09 years
NVP at 5%	– $7,836	$2,624

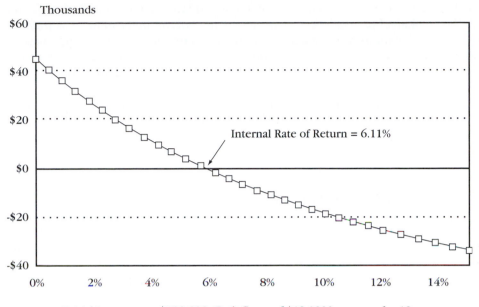

Thousands

Initial investment: $100,000; Cash flows of $12,0000 per year for 12 years

Figure 10-2 Net present value at various interest rates.

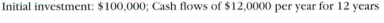

$$\sum_{t=0}^{N}[CFAT_t \, / \, (1 + IRR)^t] = 0$$

There are several advantages to using decision rules based on the internal rate of return. It is intuitively appealing. The internal rate of return is the rate of return that investment in the project or asset produces. It can therefore be compared to the cost of capital that one incurs in investing in the project. If, in an accept/reject situation, the IRR is greater than the cost of capital incurred (if the project generates a greater return than it costs), the project is worth undertaking. In mutually exclusive choice situations, the project with the greatest IRR (at least as great as the after-tax cost of capital) is the one to select.

There are, however, enough problems associated with decision rules based on the IRR that it is better to avoid its use than to risk its drawbacks and uncertainties (Feldstein & Fleming, 1964). First among the problems with the IRR is the implicit assumption it makes about reinvestment opportunities. Remember from Chapter 5 that the discounting process assumes that cash can be reinvested at the discount rate during the project's life. When one calculates the IRR and uses it to make investment decisions, one assumes that one can reinvest at the IRR. That may not be the case, especially for good projects.

The second problem with the IRR is the fact that a project can have more than one IRR. Notice, in the equation just given, that any project's IRR is the solution to an *n*th-degree polynomial expression; if the project is to last for 12 years, finding the internal rate of return requires solving an equation containing $(1 + r)^{12}$. From high school algebra, recall that a second-degree polynomial can have as many as two distinct, valid solutions; a third-degree polynomial can have as many as three distinct, valid solutions; and an nth-degree polynomial can have as many as n distinct, valid solutions. When multiple solutions exist for IRR, comparison with the cost of capital is particularly tricky.

The third complication with the use of IRR is related to the second. Sometimes one or more of the solutions to an nth-degree polynomial are not a real number but involve the imaginary unit, i, (defined as the square root of negative one). Imaginary internal rates of return cannot be compared to a cost of capital expressed in real numbers (real lenders require that returns be measured in real numbers).

Another problem with the internal rate of return arises in comparing mutually exclusive choices of substantially different scales. A small project may have a relatively high internal rate of return but contribute very little to the value of the organization (have a lower NPV), whereas the larger project, by its very size, may contribute much more to the value of the organization yet have the lower internal rate of return. Because enhancing the value of the organization is the objective, the higher-NPV project should be selected over the higher-IRR project.

A way to rescue the IRR as a decision model for mutually exclusive choices of unequal scales is to consider the IRR of the "incremental project" (Bierman & Smidt, 1993, pp. 89–90). Subtract the cash flows of the smaller project from those of the larger project and call the remainder the incremental project (an imaginary project that represents an add-on to the smaller alternative). If the smaller project has an IRR at least as great as the cost of capital, it is worth doing, when considered in isolation. If the incremental project has an IRR at least as great as the cost of capital, it is worth doing, too. One does the smaller project and the incremental project by doing the larger project. Thus, if the IRR of the incremental project is at least as great as the cost of capital, the larger project is the choice to make. That's a lot of work just to rescue the IRR model.

Finally, IRR may present problems in evaluating mutually exclusive projects that have different cash flow patterns. Figure 10–3 illustrates the changes that take place in the NPVs of two projects with different cash flow patterns. Projects A and B have the same initial cash outflow ($100,000) but have different patterns of expected cash inflows. Project A has higher cash flows early, followed by lower cash flows late in its project life. Project B has lower expected cash flows in its early years, followed by higher cash flows in later years. The mathematics of present value make project B's net present value more sensitive to changes in the discount rate than project A. Note that project A has the higher IRR. That is, the discount rate at which project A's NPV is zero is higher than is that for project B. At every interest rate below about 4.5 percent, however, project B has the higher NPV.

What is one to do if A and B are mutually exclusive alternatives and the relevant discount rate is 4 percent? IRR says to select A, but NPV says to select B. Because one is concerned with increasing the value of the organization, B is better than A *at the prevailing rate of discount*. When the timing of cash flows is substan-

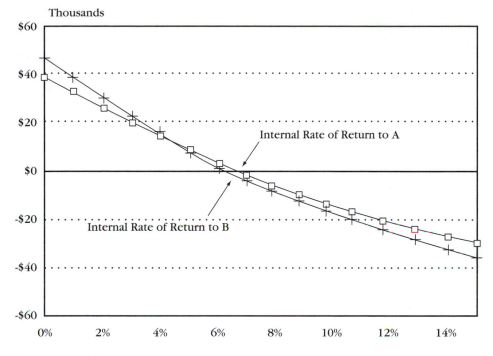

Thousands

Initial investment: $100,000

Figure 10-3 Net present values of two projects with different cash flows.

tially different for two mutually exclusive alternatives, using IRR can lead to the wrong answer.

Most of the time, using IRR-based rules (accept if IRR is at least as great as the cost of capital; select the alternative with the higher IRR at least as great as the cost of capital) will lead to value-maximizing decisions. In some cases, however, especially in mutually exclusive choice decisions, IRR can lead one astray. It should be used with caution.

SELECTING THE DISCOUNT RATE

The mathematics of the time value of money and the discussion about the effects of cash flow timing above illustrate that the selection of the discount rate is critical in making capital investment decisions (Wheeler & Smith, 1988). Selecting a discount rate that is too low will allow poor projects to pass muster. Selecting a discount rate that is too high will mean that worthwhile projects will not be adopted. As shown in Figure 10–2, selecting an inappropriate discount rate can also mean selecting the wrong choice from among mutually exclusive choices.

Consider a very simple world. There are no market "frictions"; that is, one can borrow and lend at the same interest rate without having to pay any intermediaries; and there are no taxes. In this simple world, there is also no risk; all out-comes can be predicted with certainty. Bonds can be issued without any flotation cost. Also, in this simplified world, there is only one source of funding for capital projects, the sale of bonds, which differ from one another only in their amount.

In a world like the one just described, the "correct" discount rate for every capital budgeting decision is the rate of interest on the bond that is used to finance the acquisition of the capital. Why? Remember why one discounts future cash flows. Discounting is important because funds have alternative uses. Excess cash can be used to acquire assets, or it can be lent at interest. If cash must be borrowed in order to make an acquisition, interest must be paid on the loan. That earning or paying of interest makes the timing of cash in and cash out important. It necessitates consideration of the time value of money and selection of a discount rate.

The simplifying assumptions, taken together, mean that there is only one interest rate prevailing at any one time. That interest rate is the appropriate discount rate. It is both the opportunity cost of internal funds and the market cost of external funds. It is a before-tax, after-tax, and tax-free discount rate. It applies to all projects regardless of risk. In the real world, where these simplifying restrictions do not apply, there is more than one interest rate; there are intermediaries who take a cut from financing activities; and, alas, there are taxes.

There is a substantial body of literature on the selection of the discount rate, given the complexity of the world (Mishan, 1976; Wheeler & Smith, 1988). For the decisions of private, not-for-profit, and investor-owned organizations, scholars agree that the appropriate discount rate should be the organization's after-tax, weighted average cost of capital (adjusted for flotation costs), where the weights used are the market-value percentages of each financing source in the target capital structure (Chapters 13–15 discuss the cost of capital and capital structure in greater detail).

What does all of that mean? First, just as it is after-tax cash flows that matter, so it is the after-tax cost of capital that is important. Because interest payments to bond holders (but not dividend payments to equity holders) are tax-deductible expenses, the after-tax rate of interest is given by

$$R_{d,a\text{-}t} = R \times (1 - T)$$

where $R_{d,a\text{-}t}$ is the after-tax interest rate on debt, R is the before-tax cost of debt, and T is the marginal income tax rate. Because payments to equity holders are not tax deductible, there is no comparable adjustment for the cost of equity. Also note that, for many health care organizations, the marginal income tax rate is zero (they are exempt from both federal and state income tax).

The discount rate should also be adjusted for the flotation cost of securities. These are the expenses associated with issuing new equity or debt, expressed as a percentage (F) of the amount issued. They include payments to attorneys, accountants, investment bankers, and bond trustees, and any regulatory fees. Brigham and Gapenski (1991) show that the appropriate way to adjust for flotation costs is to divide $R_{d,a\text{-}t}$ or R_e (the cost of equity) by $(1-F)$ in the discounting calculations.

Organizations can finance their capital acquisitions in any of several ways. Investor-owned organizations can use equity finance, by selling shares of common and/or preferred stock. Both not-for-profit and investor-owned organizations can use cash on hand as a form of equity financing. Virtually all health care organizations can use debt finance, either by selling bonds or by taking on bank debt. Each of those forms of financing is available at its own cost. An organization's capital structure is the mix of financing forms. The target capital structure is the mix toward which the organization is moving. Every target capital structure has a **weighted-average cost of capital (WACC)** given by

$$WACC = W_e R_e' + W_d R_{d,a-t}'$$

where W_e is the weight of equity financing in the capital structure (market value of equity divided by the total market value of claims, debt, and equity) and R_e' is the cost of equity, adjusted for flotation costs.

No matter how one expects to finance an asset or project, one should use the WACC as the discount rate. Otherwise one might use the cost of debt to evaluate weak projects and the higher cost of equity to evaluate strong projects. To do so is to compare financing sources rather than to compare projects. When new projects are more or less risky than the firm as a whole, new complications arise (see Chapter 11).

The discount rate, like most interest rates, is usually expressed as an annual rate. If one is given cash flows on a semiannual basis, convention dictates that one divide the annual rate in half to obtain a discount rate for 6-month periods.

Some have argued that the net present value of government projects ought not to be calculated using market discount rates (Mishan, 1976; Wheeler & Clement, 1990). Mishan advocates the use of the "social opportunity cost of public investment," the rate at which private investment is given up to allow government investment. Wheeler and Clement advocate dividing the benefits from government and not-for-profit investment into two parts: cash flow and social output. There may be social outputs (the value of inoculating child A that accrues to child B, who comes into contact with his, otherwise contagious, playmate). Cash flows, they argue, are captured by the organization and should be discounted at a market-based rate of interest. Social outputs should be discounted at a social discount rate. The measurement of the volume of social outputs and of the social discount rate create problems for the practical analyst.

A SIMPLE EXAMPLE

Consider a not-for-profit hospital faced with a familiar choice: to open or not to open a emergency center in a new suburban shopping mall. The mall's developers claim that referrals alone will make the center a financial winner for the hospital. Cautious analysts in the comptroller's office argue that the startup costs of the center, and its annual cash outflows (including insurance), will be a major drain on the hospital's overall cash flow.

Initial cash outflows for the center are projected as follows: $225,000 for equipment, furniture, and fixtures; and $75,000 for new working capital (inventory, accountants receivable, cash on hand). Analysts in the planning department estimate that the center will generate 10 visits per day, 7 days per week, 52 weeks per year, with average cash inflow per visit of $50. The planning analysts also estimate $150,000 per year in net cash flows from increased admissions to the hospital. Annual operating expenses of the center will be $250,000. The hospital's weighted average cost of capital is 6 percent. As a not-for-profit provider, the hospital has a zero income tax rate. The center has an expected life of 10 years and no expected salvage value. Table 10–4 shows the calculations necessary to answer the question, "Is the emergency center a wise use of the hospital's limited funds?"

The initial cash outflow is the outfitting requirement plus the net new working capital commitment, a total of $300,000. In each year following, anticipated net cash inflows are $82,000, the sum of the incremental cash inflows (direct and indirect) and incremental cash outflows. In the tenth year, there is an additional cash inflow of $75,000, the release of the required working capital.

The sixth column in Table 10–4 shows the present value factor, at 6 percent, for each of the years in the center's life. These are taken from Table 5–2. Multiplying the annual net cash flows by the associated present value factors yields the stream of discounted cash flows. The sum of all of the discounted cash flows, including the initial cash outflow, yields the net present value of the emergency center, $345,406.75.

With a net present value of $345,406.75, the emergency center is well worth undertaking. That amount represents the addition to the value of the overall organization that will come, if all of the assumptions used in the calculations are borne out, from equipping, opening, and operating the center. So long as the net present value is at least zero (so long as the proposed project does not detract from the organization's value), the project is worth doing.

CAPITAL BUDGETING AND ITS DISCONTENTS

The example just given illustrates several of the pitfalls of the capital budgeting process. First, the development stage is critical. Decisions based on net present

Table 10–4   Analysis of an emergency center

Year	Cash Outflow	Direct Cash Inflow	Indirect Cash Inflow	Net Cash Flow	PVF at 6%	Discounted Cash Flow
0	$300,000			($300,000)	1.0000	($300,000.00)
1	250,000	$182,000	$150,000	82,000	0.9434	77,358.49
2	250,000	182,000	150,000	82,000	0.8900	72,979.71
3	250,000	182,000	150,000	82,000	0.8396	68,848.78
4	250,000	182,000	150,000	82,000	0.7921	64,951.68
5	250,000	182,000	150,000	82,000	0.7473	61,275.17
6	250,000	182,000	150,000	82,000	0.7050	57,806.76
7	250,000	182,000	150,000	82,000	0.6651	54,534.68
8	250,000	182,000	150,000	82,000	0.6274	51,447.81
9	250,000	182,000	150,000	82,000	0.5919	48,535.67
10	250,000	257,000	150,000	157,000	0.5584	87,667.98
NPV						345,406.75

value (or internal rate of return or profitability index) can be no better than one's cash flow projections. "Garbage in, garbage out" is a useful rule to remember. Unfortunately, in only a few, rare situations can one predict future cash flows with any semblance of certainty. Also, the decision is very sensitive to one's choice of discount rate.

If time-value-of-money calculations are so sensitive to uncertain projections and to discount rate choices, can they be a reasonable basis for making important decisions? That concern has led some observers to suggest that capital budgeting, as taught to management students (including health care management students) and as practiced in many large organizations, leads to underinvestment and to declining competitiveness (Hays & Abernathy, 1980; Hayes & Garvin, 1982; Porter, 1992).

The arguments of these analysts and others come down to a few points. American firms use discount rates that are artificially high. These high discount rates ensure that none but the strongest projects will be approved, protecting the careers of the managers who propose projects. These artificially high "hurdle rates" also mean that American organizations don't adopt enough innovations, restrict their capital stocks, and become inefficient and uncompetitive. Our capital markets are also, they argue, loathe to finance any but the safest capital expansions, further restricting innovation, efficiency, and competitiveness.

Meyer (1985) observed that, in hospitals, the capital budgeting process was often used as a ceremonial step to justify decisions already made on political or clinical grounds. In fact, casual observation suggests that once service lines are selected, simple accept/reject decisions become foregone conclusions. For example, if one is in the obstetrics business, one is going to have an ultrasound lab. It is the mutually exclusive choice decision (ultrasound A or ultrasound B) that becomes important, and that is a decision over which obstetricians and ultrasound technicians like to have substantial influence. Cleverly and Felkner (1984) found that the use of sophisticated capital budgeting techniques was not associated with improved hospital financial performance.

Capital budgeting, done incorrectly, can lead to the suboptimal outcomes observed by Hayes, Abernathy, and others. The task of the innovative manager must be to lead the capital budgeting decision wisely, to organize data well, and to recognize and adjust to the organizational politics that are paramount in the acquisition of health care technology.

SUMMARY

This chapter has presented the basic model for the selection of long-lived assets and projects. That model involves four steps: identification, cash flow development, calculation and application of a decision rule, and an audit after the fact. The preferred decision rules, except for capital rationing situations, are those based on the project's net present value.

The capital budgeting process yields outcomes that are only as good as the assumptions used and the judgment of the analyst. Cash flows are notoriously difficult to predict. The decisions made in net present value models are particularly sensitive to the choice of the discount rate. Several knowledgeable observers believe that, in their choices of discount rates, American firms have sacrificed innovation and competitiveness for organizational safety.

Chapter 11 will extend the basic capital budgeting model to some more complex situations, including unequal project lives, the lease-or-buy decision, and the analysis of projects involving risk.

Discussion Questions

1. When the net present value and the internal rate of return decision rules provide conflicting answers to mutually exclusive choice problems, which should be followed? Why?

2. What makes the profitability index better than the net present value as a guide for capital rationing decisions? What does it take into account that net present value does not?

3. What investment criterion does Hugh Long recommend for accept/reject decisions in not-for-profit organizations? Do you agree or disagree? Explain.

4. Is there ever a valid reason for ignoring the results of financial capital budgeting analysis? Explain.

5. Capital budgeting using discounted cash flow methods looks like a scientific process, yielding exact solutions. Is it? Explain.

CONTINUING CASE

Billy Bob Ferguson was trying to explain his dilemma to the board of Lone Star Home Health Services. The organization needed to replace a station wagon, money was tight, and choices had to be made. Just to complicate matters, two local automobile dealers had offered to make "special deals" on wagons ("If they're so generous, why don't they just donate a station wagon?"). Each of the deals was to be tied to a special advertising campaign.

"So what's the problem?" John Tyler asked. Tyler was a steady supporter of LSHHS and owner of Jamestown's only chain of dry cleaning establishments. "Just select the one with the best offer."

"That's not so simple," Billy Bob explained. "Buck Jones has offered us one model for $22,500. For that price, he's thrown in the modifications we need for home infusion visits. Bill Johanson offered us a different model, but with modifications it will run $30,000."

"It *is* simple, Billy Bob, just go with Buck's offer," replied Tyler. Tyler often condescended to Ferguson.

"It's not so simple. I went through school with Bill, and he's a big giver at Jason's [the Reverend Jason Cooper, chair of LSHHS's board] church. His car has lower operating expenses, too. *Consumer's Journal* says it would run us $2,000 every 6 months (fees, insurance, operating expenses, repairs) for 6 years and $2,700 every 6 months for 4 years. After 10 years, we'd have to scrap either car." Billy Bob had been in banking for a long time and he trusted *Consumer's Journal* when it came to cars.

"Well, what's the deal on Buck's offer?" asked Irv Mason. Irv was an accountant at Central Agri-Products and always looked for numbers to compare.

"*Consumer's Journal* says that Buck's model would cost us $2,500 every 6 months for 5 years and $3,000 every 6 months for the next 5 years. Neither one of these clunkers would have any resale value after we finished with them." (In a stage whisper, John Tyler asked Nan Brust why Billy Bob always bought "clunkers" from his old pals.)

Irv was on a roll now. "Is anything the same about these two?"

"We'd put them to the same use. We already have a cash emergency fund set aside, so we don't have to worry about that. No matter which one we get, we can finance it for 6 percent at CCB Bank." Billy Bob still kept track of interest rates.

"How do you do depreciation?" was Irv's last question.

"Just like everybody else, we use the MACRS system." [See Chapter 3.]

"That's all I need to know. I'll have the correct answer for you in 5 minutes." Irv had his calculator out of his pocket already.

CASE QUESTIONS

1. What cash flows does the board need to consider? Lay out a worksheet of cash flow estimates.

2. What, if anything, does Irv need to do to take account of taxes?

3. How does Irv need to treat depreciation in his calculations? How does he need to treat interest expense?

4. Select a method for selecting between the two station wagons. Perform the necessary calculations and determine the "correct" answer.

5. Would your answer be different if the discount rate were 15 percent? If it were 2 percent?

REFERENCES

Bierman, H., Jr. & Smidt, S. (1993). *The capital budgeting decision* (8th ed.). New York: Macmillan.

Brigham, E.F. & Gapenski, L.C. (1991). Flotation cost adjustments. *Financial Practice and Education, 1*(2), 29–34.

Cleverly, W.O. & Felkner, J.G. (1984). "The association of capital budgeting techniques with hospital financial performance. *Health Care Financial Management, 9*(3), 45–55.

Feldstein, M.S. & Fleming, J.S. (1964). "The problem of time-stream evaluation: Present value versus internal rate of return rules. *Bulletin of the Oxford University Institute of Economics and Statistics, 26*, 79–85.

Fisher, I. (1930). *The theory of interest.* New York: Macmillan.

Gapenski, L.C. (1993). Capital investment analysis: Three methods. *Healthcare Financial Management, 47*(8), 60–66.

Hayes, R.H. & Abernathy, W.J. (1980). Managing our way to economic decline. *Harvard Business Review, 58*(4), 67–77.

Hayes, R.H. & Garvin, D.A. (1982). Managing as if tomorrow mattered. *Harvard Business Review, 60*(3), 70–79.

Kamath, S.R. & Elmer, J. (1989). Capital investment decisions in hospitals: Survey results. *Health Care Management Review, 14*(2), 45–56.

Long, H.W. (1982a). Asset choice and program selection in a competitive environment (Part I). *Healthcare Financial Management, 36*(7), 40–55.

Long, H.W. (1982b). Asset choice and program selection in a competitive environment (Part II). *Healthcare Financial Management, 36*(8), 34–50.

Meyer, A.D. (1985). Hospital capital budgeting: Fusion of rationality, politics and ceremony. *Health Care Management Review, 10*(2), 17–28.

Mishan, E.J. (1976). *Cost-benefit analysis.* New York: Praeger.

Pinches, G.E. (1982). Myopia, capital budgeting and decision making, *Financial Management, 11*(3), 6–19.

Porter, M.E. (1992). Capital disadvantage: America's failing capital investment system. *Harvard Business Review, 70*(5), 65–82.

Wheeler, J.R.C. & Clement, J.P. (1990). Capital expenditure decisions and the role of the not-for-profit hospital: An application of a social goods model. *Medical Care Review, 47*(4), 467–486.

Wheeler, J.R.C. & Smith, D.G. (1988). The discount rate for capital expenditure analysis in health care. *Health Care Management Review, 13*(2), 43–52.

SELECTED READINGS

Bierman, H., Jr. & Smidt, S. (1993). *The capital budgeting decision* (8th ed.). New York: Macmillan.

Mishan, E.J. (1976). *Cost-benefit analysis.* New York: Praeger.

CHAPTER

11

Special Topics in Capital Budgeting

Learning Objectives

After reading this chapter, the student should be able to:

1. Use linear programming to solve a complex capital rationing problem.
2. Define and measure total and systematic project risk.
3. Adjust the discount rate in a net present value calculation to account for differential project risk.
4. Make a "lease or buy" decision.

Key Terms

Equivalent annual amount

Equivalent annual cost

Certainty-equivalent

Decision tree

Least common
    multiple

Linear programming

Net advantage of leasing

Option

Pure play

Risk-adjusted discount rate
    (RADR)

Set of feasible
    solutions

Simplex theorem

State-preference
    theory

Chapter 10 developed the basic capital asset selection model: develop cash flows; calculate net present values and select assets based on present value rules or, in the capital rationing case, on profitability index rules. This chapter develops the basic model further. Real life is not always so neat as to allow the use of the simple models. In particular, the conditions for the use of the profitability index are usually violated in capital rationing, cash flow projections are risky, mutually exclusive choices may have unequal useful lives, and projects may embody options apart from their expected cash flows. Also, leasing has emerged as a useful alternative to purchasing assets. After reading this chapter, the reader should be able to adapt the basic capital budgeting model to a variety of complex circumstances.

CAPITAL RATIONING: THE GENERAL CASE

Chapter 10 introduced capital rationing as the decision problem in which a limited capital budget is to be divided among a large number of projects so as to maximize the value of the firm. Selection on the basis of profitability indexes will provide the best solution to the capital rationing problem if (1) only one period's budgeting is under review, (2) no partial projects are allowed, and (3) the set of projects selected exactly exhausts the budget. Unfortunately, in real life, all of those three conditions are unlikely to be met. Particularly when one allows for planning over several periods, partial projects are the norm, not the rare exception. One might, for example, spread the initial cash outflow for a new facility over 2 years (paying the general contractor on a percentage-of-project-completed basis). Thus two-thirds of the facility could be on year 1's capital budget and one-third on year 2's budget.

Linear Programming

What an organization wants, when forced to engage in capital rationing, is the subset of all available projects that maximizes the organization's value. One needs, then, to use a decision rule that identifies the best mix of projects, including partial projects, subject to the available resource constraints. One can think of projects as variables, with various amounts of each variable to be chosen for each year over a planning horizon. Selecting the combination of variables that maximizes a function is the problem for which **linear programming** was developed (Dorfman, Samuelson, & Solow, 1958). Using the linear programming model, one can solve for the optimal solution to capital rationing problems, even if the three conditions just cited are not met.

In linear programming, one seeks to maximize an objective function (in linear form), subject to a family of linear constraints. In capital rationing, the objective function is the net present value of all new projects chosen. The constraints are that every project under review receive no less than zero investment (the nonnegativity constraint) and that total spending in each period be no greater than that period's budget. If one were considering three projects and one had two periods' budgets to consider, one would look at a problem like the following:

$$\text{Maximize: NPV} = A_{1,1}\text{NPV}_1 + A_{2,1}\text{NPV}_2 + A_{3,1}\text{NPV}_3 + A_{1,2}\text{NPV}_1\text{PVF}_1 + A_{2,2}\text{NPV}_2\text{PVF}_1 + A_{3,2}\text{NPV}_3\text{PVF}_1$$

Subject to:
$$A_{1,1} \geq 0$$
$$A_{2,1} \geq 0$$
$$A_{3,1} \geq 0$$
$$A_{1,2} \geq 0$$
$$A_{2,2} \geq 0$$
$$A_{3,2} \geq 0$$

$$\text{Budget}_1 \geq A_{1,1}\,\text{CFAT}_{0,1} + A_{2,1}\,\text{CFAT}_{0,2} + A_{3,1}\,\text{CFAT}_{0,3}$$

and

$$\text{Budget}_2 \geq A_{1,2}\,\text{CFAT}_{0,1} + A_{2,2}\,\text{CFAT}_{0,2} + A_{3,2}\,\text{CFAT}_{0,3}$$

In that formulation, Budget$_1$ and Budget$_2$ are the expenditure limits for periods 1 and 2, respectively. These are set in advance and are known to the decision makers. They are the principal constraints in the problem. There are also constraints ensuring that the values of $A_{i,j}$ are positive (that nature is not providing something for nothing). NPV = ⋯ is the objective function to be maximized.

$A_{i,j}$ is the proportion of project i to be undertaken in period j. Thus, if $A_{1,2}$ takes a value of .75, then 75 percent of project 1 is to be undertaken in period 2. These values of $A_{i,j}$ are the solutions to the decision problems; they are the unknowns for which one is solving. The net present values of all period 2 investments must be discounted one period (multiplied by the present value factor for one period at the relevant discount rate), as those investments will be made, and their NPVs enjoyed, one period later.

The linear programming formulation can appear daunting to those unfamiliar with it, and it has some limitations. For example, it assumes that all projects are divisible. Plane & Trifts (1993), focusing on the limitations of the method advocate an alternative method based on spreadsheet calculations.

Figure 11–1 shows, for a very simple case, how linear programming problems are solved. For the case shown, there are two inputs that determine the value of a single objective function. As inputs increase, the objective function also increases. The lines running diagonally across the figure show levels (fixed values) of the objective function. Along any one of those "contour" lines, one can substitute input 1 for input 2 without changing the value of the objective function. As one moves up and to the right (northeast on the map), contour lines represent progressively higher values of the objective function. The problem to be solved is to determine the highest level of the objective function possible given the constraints on the two inputs.

The constraints on the two inputs are shown by the dotted lines. These are simple constraints, merely that the level of each input not exceed some predetermined limit. The area bounded by the input constraints (the area within the "fence" formed by the axes and the two constraints) is the **set of feasible solutions**.

In this case, the solution, the highest level of the objective function possible, is determined by using all of the available amounts of input 1 and input 2. In linear programming terminology, the two constraints are both *binding*. In more complicated cases, in which there are multiple constraints, one or more constraints may not be binding in the optimal solution. Such a situation is shown in Figure 11–2.

In the case shown in Figure 11–2, there are constraints on the levels of inputs 1 and 2 used (just as in Figure 11–1), and there is a constraint on the total input (1 plus 2) used (the diagonal dotted line). As a result, the set of feasible solutions is the area bounded by points A, B, C, and D. The highest feasible value of the objective function is reached by using the inputs in the amounts implied for point B.

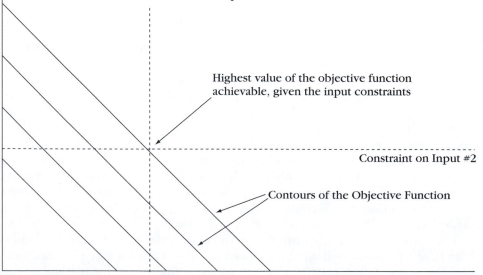

Figure 11-1 Solution to a linear programming problem.

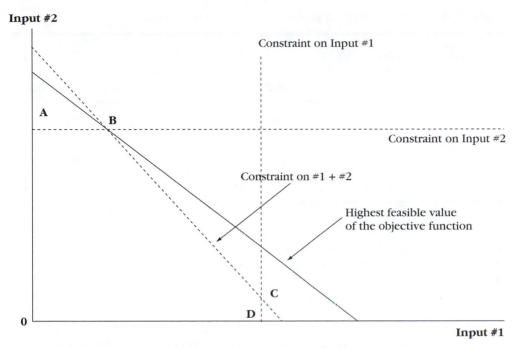

Input #2

A

B

Constraint on Input #1

Constraint on Input #2

Constraint on #1 + #2

Highest feasible value
of the objective function

C

D

0

Input #1

Figure 11-2 A linear programming problem with a nonbinding constraint.

The Simplex Theorem

At B, the constraint on input 2 is binding, as is that on total input use. At B, however, one is well within the constraint specified for input 1. The **Simplex theorem** for the solution of linear programming problems states that the optimal solution will always occur at critical points, points at which two or more constraints are binding (Dorfman, Samuelson, & Solow, 1958, pp. 74–78). The simplex method searches for critical points and identifies the one critical point at which the objective function takes its highest value.

Fortunately, software is now available that allow one to perform Simplex calculations easily with a modest microcomputer. Some of these programs are available commercially or as part of classroom packages, and some are in the public domain. One need no longer be an expert in matrix algebra to do linear programming.

Consider an example. The trustees of Neighborhood Clinic have adopted a capital budget for $1,000,000 for the coming year and a capital budget of $1,500,000 for the following year. Neighborhood Clinic's weighted average cost of capital is 6 percent. Five possible projects are under consideration; their initial cash outlays and (projected) net present values are shown in Table 11–1.

The manager's task, in Table 11–1, is to select the set of projects, including partial projects, that maximize the organization's total incremental net present value. The objective function (the function to be maximized), then, is

Table 11–1   A capital rationing problem: Neighborhood Clinic

Year 1 Budget = $1,000,000
Year 2 Budget = $1,500,000

Project	Initial Cash Outlay	Net Present Value
A	$750,000	$155,000
B	150,000	75,000
C	400,000	75,000
D	400,000	100,000
E	125,000	35,000

No project may be replicated more than once in each period.

$$\text{Maximize NPV} = A_{A,1}155{,}000 + A_{B,1}75{,}000 + A_{C,1}75{,}000 + A_{D,1}100{,}000 +$$
$$A_{E,1}35{,}000 + (A_{A,2}155{,}000 \times \text{PVF}_{.06,1}) +$$
$$(A_{B,2}75{,}000 \times \text{PVF}_{.06,1}) + (A_{C,2}75{,}000 \times \text{PVF}_{.06,1}) +$$
$$(A_{D,2}100{,}000 \times \text{PVF}_{.06,1}) + (A_{E,2}35{,}000 \times \text{PVF}_{.06,1})$$

The uppercase $A_{i,j}$'s in the objective function represent the "amount" of each project (A through E) to be acquired in year 1 and year 2. That is, $A_{C,2}$ is the amount (the percentage) of project C to be acquired in year 2. These $A_{i,j}$'s are the unknowns for whose solution the analyst is searching. Again, note that the linear programming approach assumes that all five of the projects are divisible in each of the 2 years. If any one of the projects is not divisible ($A_{i,j}$ must be either 0 or 1), then the analyst must use integer programming, an alternative technique.

The amount of each project multiplied by the net present value of that project represents the amount that the investment would contribute to the organization's net present value. For example, if the optimal value of $A_{D,1}$ is .75, then the organization should acquire 75 percent of project D in year 1, contributing $75,000 to the value of the organization.

For year 2 investment, the projects' contributions must be discounted. Because the investment is delayed 1 year, so is the realization of their net present values. Delayed net present values must be discounted (in this case, for 1 year at 6 percent) to bring them back to the present. Just as in the profitability index method presented in Chapter 10, the linear programming approach requires that each project be evaluated using its own discount rate.

The constraints faced by Neighborhood Clinic in its decision are

Subject to:
$$A_{A,1},\ A_{B,1},\ A_{C,1},\ A_{D,1},\ A_{E,1} \geq 0$$

$$A_{A,2},\ A_{B,2},\ A_{C,2},\ A_{D,2},\ A_{E,2} \geq 0$$

$$1{,}000{,}000 \geq A_{A,1}750{,}000 + A_{B,1}\,150{,}000 + A_{C,1}\,500{,}000 +$$
$$A_{D,1}450{,}000 + A_{E,1}\,200{,}000$$

$$1{,}500{,}000 \geq A_{A,2}\,750{,}000 + A_{B,2}\,150{,}000 + A_{C,2}\,500{,}000 +$$

$$A_{D,2}450,000 + A_{E,2}200,000$$

$$2 \geq (A_{A,1} + A_{A,2}), (A_{B,1} + A_{B,2}), \cdots, (A_{E,1} + A_{E,2})$$

The first two of those constraints state that Neighborhood Clinic cannot have negative investment. It can invest nothing in project A in year 1, or it can invest some positive amount in it; but it cannot get any of project A back from nature. The second two constraints state that the total amount invested in each period cannot exceed that period's budget. The formulation of this problem has one additional constraint: no project can be "done" more than twice in a single year (it cannot be replicated more than once in a given budget period). That constraint is added to avoid the trivial solution of identifying the "best" project and investing in it over and over again until the budget is exhausted. (In real life, however, that may be the best solution for many organizations: stick to the one type of investment, outpatient diagnostic centers or skilled nursing facilities, that works best, especially if one defines the geographic market widely enough). In the case of Neighborhood Clinic, however, where acquiring one CAT scanner might have substantial payoff, acquiring a second may add no incremental cash flows at all. Within a single facility, constraints on how many times a project or asset can be replicated make good economic (and managerial) sense.

Table 11–2 shows the solution to the problem, calculated via the Simplex method. Neighborhood Clinic should divide its investment in year 1 between investments B (2 of them), D (1.125 of them), and E (2 of them). The table also shows that investment will exhaust the first year's budget. For year 2, Neighborhood should share its capital budget among investments A (0.2 of it), B (2 of them), D (2 of them), and E (2 of them). Again, the full capital budget is expended.

In a sense, linear programming (or related, situationally appropriate methods) is a viable approach to solving all capital budgeting decisions. Whether one is dealing with accept/reject, mutually exclusive choice, or capital rationing decisions, one is seeking the best use of the organization's resources. Those resource allocation decisions are just what linear programming (and other optimizing) methods are designed to do.

Table 11–2   Solution to a capital rationing problem: Neighborhood Clinic

Project	Year 1 Investments	Year 2 Investments	Year 1 Cash Outflows	Year 2 Cash Outflows
A	0.000	0.200	$0.00	$150,000.00
B	2.000	2.000	300,000.00	300,000.00
C	0.000	0.000	0.00	0.00
D	1.125	2.000	450,000.00	800,000.00
E	2.000	2.000	250,000.00	250,000.00
Total cash flows			1,000,000.00	1,500,000.00

ADJUSTING FOR PROJECT RISK

A basic fact of life in strategic management, financial planning, and marketing analysis is that the future is not certain. No matter how carefully and realistically one project's cash flows, those projections are only expectations. There is a range of possible outcomes (perhaps a wide range), and the projected cash flow is but one point in that range. Some projects and assets involve greater risk than others (the range of possible outcomes is wider or the probability of extreme deviations from the expectation is greater). How to take account of differences in the riskiness of projects in capital budgeting has been a subject of great debate for many years (Aggarwal, 1993; Bierman & Smidt, 1993). As in Chapter 9, *risk* and *uncertainty* are used interchangeably here.

Figure 11–3 shows the distributions of possible outcomes for first-year cash flows for four projects. The first project has no risk at all. Its expected outcome is the only possible outcome. The second has a very low level of risk, because most of its possible outcomes are clustered tightly about the expected cash flow, and the outcome with the greatest probability is the expected outcome. The third shows more risk than the second, because the dispersion of possible outcomes is greater. The fourth shows the greatest degree of risk. Not only is

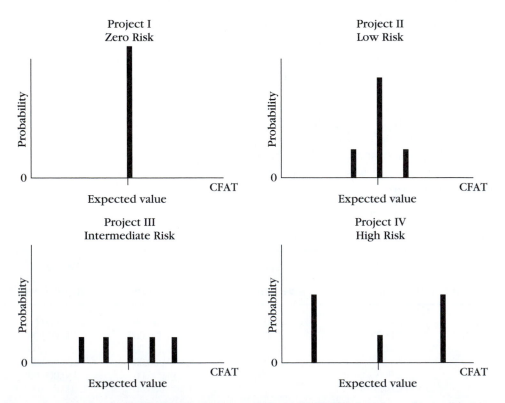

Figure 11-3 Four degrees of project risk: possible first-year cash flows.

its dispersion of possible outcomes great, but the probabilities of the outlying possibilities are greater than those for project III.

The measure that best captures the riskiness of a project is the standard deviation of possible outcomes about their expected value. This is not the standard deviation over time, but the standard deviation of possibilities, within each project year, about that year's expected cash flow. Unfortunately, before the fact (when one makes capital budgeting decisions), one can't observe those standard deviations. After the fact, when one audits capital budgeting decisions, all risk has been resolved; one only observes realized cash flows, not the dispersion of possible outcomes.

State-Preference Theory

Three methods have been advanced for dealing with risk in capital budgeting. The most theoretically appealing is based on **state-preference theory** (Bierman & Smidt, 1993). In state-preference theory, possible outcomes in each time period are associated with various "states of the world," each of which has a probability of occurring. Individuals and organizations have preferences for one state of the world over another and attach a different utility to each state's outcome. The outcomes (for each period) that matter are the expected utility, given the possible states, and the probability and utility of each. The state-preference approach is theoretically sound, but very difficult to implement. To describe all the possible states of the world for each period, for even a simple, short-lived project, is virtually beyond human capacity.

Certainty-Equivalent Method

A second method for dealing with risk, also theoretically appealing, is the **certainty-equivalent** method. Any expected cash flow (subject to risk) can be associated with a certainty equivalent. The certainty equivalent is the smallest amount that the decision maker would accept, with certainty, in place of the expected outcome, which is subject to risk. In effect, the certainty equivalent of any amount of any expected outcome is the expected outcome minus a penalty associated with the riskiness of the outcome (Friedman & Savage, 1948).

Under the certainty-equivalent method of adjusting for risk, one uses not the expected cash flows for each period in a project's life but the certainty equivalents of those cash flows. The appropriate discount rate to apply to the certainty equivalent cash flows, then, is the risk-free rate. The problem with applying this method is there is no objective way to determine what the certainty equivalent of any expected cash flow is.

Risk-Adjusted Discount Rate

The problems involved in putting the state-preference and certainty-equivalent approaches to work have led almost all who adjust for risk in capital budgeting to employ the **risk-adjusted discount rate** (RADR, pronounced "radar") method. As discussed in Chapter 9, riskier organizations have higher costs of capital than do safer organizations. Therefore many believe that riskier projects should be assessed at higher discount rates (costs of capital) than safer projects.

In a sense, the RADR method is simple to apply; one need only increase the discount rate to adjust for the riskiness of the project under review. In practice, however, the RADR method exposes one to the same problem as the other methods of risk adjustment: how to determine the appropriate degree of risk adjustment objectively.

Decision Trees

The total risk associated with a project can be defined as the standard deviation of possible outcomes, or the standard deviation of possible net present values associated with the project. Figure 11–4 and Table 11–3 show how a **decision tree** can be used to measure that standard deviation (Magee, 1964).

The project depicted in Figure 11–4 requires an initial cash outlay of $100,000 and has an expected life of 2 years. For the first year, there are three possible values for cash flow after taxes: $75,000 (with probability of 0.5), $50,000 (with a probability of 0.3), and $25,000 (with a probability of 0.2). In the figure, the probability of any outcome is shown next to the arrow pointing to that outcome. Given any realized cash flow after taxes at the end of year 1, there are two possible values for cash flow after taxes at the end of year 2. Moving from $CFAT_0$ to a particular value of $CFAT_1$ and then to a particular value of $CFAT_2$ defines a path within the decision tree. Each path (each set of cash flows) has a net present value. The probabil-

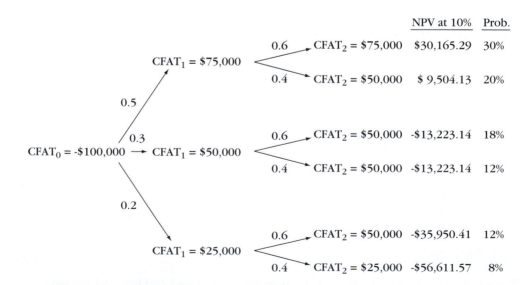

Figure 11-4 Measuring project risk with a decision tree.

Table 11–3 Calculating expected NPV and its standard deviation

Year	Path 1 CFAT	Path 2 CFAT	Path 3 CFAT	Path 4 CFAT	Path 5 CFAT	Path 6 CFAT
0	($100,000)	($100,000)	($100,000)	($100,000)	($100,000)	($100,000)
1	75,000	75,000	50,000	50,000	25,000	25,000
2	75,000	50,000	50,000	50,000	50,000	25,000
NPV at 10%	30,165.29	9,504.13	(13,223.14)	(13,223.14)	(35,950.41)	(56,611.57)
Probability	30.00%	20.00%	18.00%	12.00%	12.00%	8.00%
Weighted NPV	$9,049.59	$1,900.83	($2,380.17)	($1,586.78)	($4,314.05)	($4,528.93)

Expected NPV =   ($1,859.50)

Std. dev. = $4,694.63

ity of achieving that particular net present value is the product of the probabilities of moving along that path in year 1 and in year 2. Thus, at a 10 percent discount rate, the net present value of the first path (identified as path 1 in Table 11–3) is $30,165.29. The probability of realizing that net present value is 0.30 (0.50 × 0.06).

The expected net present value of the project shown in Figure 11–4 is calculated in Table 11–3. That expected value is the sum of the weighted net present values of each possible outcome. That is, one multiplies each of the possible net present values by its probability (to calculate the probability-weighted net present value) and finds the sum of those weighted net present values. For the project shown in Figure 11–4, that expected net present value is negative, −$1,859.50. Note that −$1,859.50 is the expected net present value in the statistical sense only. It is not the most likely value; in fact, there is no possible outcome whose net present value equals −$1,859.50.

The total risk of the project shown in Figure 11–4 is the standard deviation of the possible weighted net present values about the expected net present value (the weighted standard deviation). In this case, that standard deviation is $4,694.63. This is a very risky project. One can use the standard deviation of weighted outcomes as a criterion for adjusting the discount rate for risk. The higher the standard deviation (or, to adjust for project size, the standard deviation divided by $CFAT_0$), the greater is the risk-adjusted discount rate to use. This method has the advantage of being based on an objective criterion: the total risk of the project.

Using decision trees as a basis for risk-adjusting the discount rate has several drawbacks. First, the standard deviation of weighted possible net present values depends on the discount rate chosen. Thus one's selection of an initial discount rate will, in part, determine by how much to adjust the discount rate for risk. Ideally, one should avoid that sort of circular analysis. Second, although the method is less subjective than its alternatives, the probabilities used to weight the possible cash flows can only be guesses. Third, as the number of periods and the number of possible outcomes in each period grows, the number of possible realized net present values becomes very large. For a 5-year project, with only two outcomes per year, there are 32 (2^5) paths. If there are three outcomes in each of 5 years, there are 243 (3^5) paths.

If one's goal in using the RADR approach is to simulate the risk-adjusted yield that investors would demand to fund the project in question, using decision trees poses another problem. With a decision tree, one can measure the total risk of the project (subject to the limitations just discussed), but one has little guidance as to how much to adjust the discount rate for any given level of project risk.

Capital Asset Pricing Model

An alternative to the decision tree method is the use of the capital asset pricing model (CAPM) discussed in Chapter 9. CAPM has the advantage of considering only a project's systematic risk, which is the only risk about which the suppliers of capital are concerned. When using the CAPM, one's estimated RADR is determined by

$$RADR_i = R_f + \beta_i [E(R_M) - R_f]$$

where $RADR_i$ is the risk-adjusted discount rate for the ith project, R_f is the risk-free rate of interest, $E(R_M)$ is the expected return to the market, and β_i is the ith project's beta.

The trick to using the CAPM model in estimating the RADR is the selection of the project's beta. Individual projects do not have betas. One must, then, select a firm whose shares are publicly traded (and that does, therefore, have an observable beta) and that only (or almost only) engages in the activity being analyzed. Such a firm is called a **pure play**. If, for example, one were deciding whether or not to set up a free-standing imaging center, one would look at the market beta of a firm that operates free-standing imaging centers.

Wheeler and Smith (1988) show that the pure play beta must be modified only for differences in the degrees of leverage between the pure play firm and the firm doing the analysis. That is, one first removes the effect of the degree of financial leverage of the pure play firm. One then relevers the unlevered beta, using the degree of financial leverage of the firm in question.

If, as is usually the case, the beta of the pure play firm's debt is zero, then its unlevered beta is given by

$$\beta_U = \beta_L / [1 + (1-T)(1-C)(D/E)]$$

where β_L is the pure play's levered (actual) beta, T is the pure play's marginal tax rate, C is the percentage of the pure play's interest expense reimbursed on a cost basis (see the discussion of reimbursement issues, below), D is the market value of the pure play's debt financing outstanding, and E is the market value of its equity financing outstanding.

To relever β_U to reflect the financial leverage of the firm doing the analysis, again assuming the beta of debt securities to be zero, use the following formula:

$$\beta_L = \beta_U [1 + (1-T)(1-C)(D/E)]$$

where T, C, D, and E reflect the situation not of the pure play firm but of the firm doing the analysis. Using the CAPM has advantages of theoretical consistency and objectivity, but it can be very cumbersome to apply.

ADJUSTING FOR UNEQUAL LIVES

Often, mutually exclusive alternatives have different expected useful lives. In fact, it may be that the difference in their expected lives is what makes them interesting choices. Volvos are more expensive than Chevrolets, but they are widely believed to last longer. A desktop computer based on the most recently developed microprocessor is more costly than one based on last year's chip, but will serve for a longer time before being pronounced obsolete.

When comparing two alternatives with unequal lives, one must adjust for their difference in expected replacement frequency. When comparing a delivery vehicle that will last for 3 years to one that will last for 6 years, the 6-year vehicle will appear, at first blush, to be more costly, everything else equal. The reason is that its operating cash outflows continue for 6 years. Table 11–4 illustrates the problem of unequal project lives for two such vehicles for a not-for-profit health care provider.

The two vehicles will be used in the same activity, so that only cash outflows are different between them. Neither of the two has any expected salvage value. Because the decision maker is not subject to income tax, there is no depreciation tax shield. The information in Table 11–4, naively applied, suggests that vehicle A (present value of cash outflows = $25,154.19) is superior to vehicle B (present value of cash outflows = $39,708.05) at an 8 percent discount rate. In fact, one can easily verify that, using only the information in Table 11–4, vehicle A would appear to be the better choice *at any discount rate*. Vehicle B has the greater present value of cash outflows for three reasons: it is more expensive at the outset, its annual operating cash outflows are greater, and it will remain in service longer. Remaining in service longer, however, is a positive attribute for vehicle B and ought not to count against it. There are two methods that will adjust this problem for the unequal lives of the alternatives.

Least Common Multiple Method

Table 11–5 shows the adjustment using the **least common multiple** method. Given the expected useful lives of vehicle A (3 years) and vehicle B (6 years), one finds the least common multiple of those lives. The least common multiple is the smallest whole number that is evenly divisible by both expected useful lives. The least common multiple of 3 and 6 is 6; of 3 and 4, 12; of 3 and 5, 15; of 6 and 9, 18; and so on. One then finds the present value of cash outflows for each of the two alternatives for the least common multiple of years and compares those two.

Table 11–4 Choosing between two vehicles with unequal lives

Year	Vehicle A Cash Outflow	Vehicle B Cash Outflow	Discount Factor @ 8%	Discounted Vehicle A Cash Outflow	Discounted Vehicle B Cash Outflow
0	$20,000	$30,000	1.000	$20,000.00	$30,000.00
1	2,000	2,100	0.926	1,851.85	1,944.44
2	2,000	2,100	0.857	1,714.68	1,800.41
3	2,000	2,100	0.794	1,587.66	1,667.05
4		2,100	0.735	0.00	1,543.56
5		2,100	0.681	0.00	1,429.22
6		2,100	0.630	0.00	1,323.36
Present value of cash outflows				25,154.19	39,708.05

Table 11–5 Choosing between two vehicles with unequal lives: least common multiple adjustment

Year	Vehicle A Cash Outflow	Vehicle B Cash Outflow	Discount Factor @ 8%	Discounted Vehicle A Cash Outflow	Discounted Vehicle B Cash Outflow
0	$20,000	$30,000	1.000	$20,000.00	$30,000.00
1	2,000	2,100	0.926	1,851.85	1,944.44
2	2,000	2,100	0.857	1,714.68	1,800.41
3	22,000	2,100	0.794	17,468.00	1,667.05
4	2,000	2,100	0.735	1,470.00	1,543.56
5	2,000	2,100	0.681	1,361.17	1,429.22
6	2,000	2,100	0.630	1,260.34	1,323.36
Present value of cash outflows				45,126.04	39,708.05

Using the least common multiple adjustment, one finds vehicle B to be the superior choice at a discount rate of 8 percent. As in almost all capital budgeting problems, the decision is now sensitive to the choice of discount rate.

When using the least common multiple method, be careful of the treatment of "rollover" outflows and inflows that will occur as projects are replicated. Using the least common multiple adjustment also involves the use of a hidden assumption: that one would replace vehicle A with an exact duplicate at the end of year 3. Any expected differences in working capital commitment or in replacement cost should be built into these calculations.

Equivalent Annual Cost Method

Table 11–6 shows the other commonly accepted adjustment method, the calculation of **equivalent annual cost** (Ross, Westerfield, and Jordan, 2003, pp. 338–339). When cash inflows are different between the two alternatives (so that net present values must be considered), the adjusted figures are known as **equivalent annual amounts**.

To find the equivalent annual cost, one seeks the annual annuity of cash outflows that has the same present value as the actual stream of cash outflows. By so doing, one converts the outflow stream to an annual equivalent. Outflow streams of unequal length can then be compared on an annual equivalent basis.

To find the equivalent annual cost, remember that the present value of a stream of cash outflows is

$$\text{PV of cash outflows} = \sum_{t=1}^{N} (\text{Cash outflow}_t)(\text{PVF}_{t,r\%})$$

Table 11–6 Choosing between two vehicles with unequal lives: equivalent annual cost adjustment

Year	Vehicle A Cash Outflow	Vehicle B Cash Outflow	Discount Factor @ 8%	Discounted Vehicle A Cash Outflow	Discounted Vehicle B Cash Outflow
0	$20,000	$30,000	1.000	$20,000.00	$30,000.00
1	2,000	2,100	0.926	1,851.85	1,944.44
2	2,000	2,100	0.857	1,714.68	1,800.41
3	2,000	2,100	0.794	1,587.66	1,667.05
4		2,100	0.735	0.00	1,543.56
5		2,100	0.681	0.00	1,429.22
6		2,100	0.630	0.00	1,323.36

Present value of cash outflows	25,154.19	39,708.05

Present value factor for an annuity, 3 years at 8% = 2.577
Present value factor for an annuity, 6 years at 8% = 4.623

Equivalent annual cost, vehicle A = $9,760.67
Equivalent annual cost, vehicle B = $8,589.46

Given the present value of outflows, one is seeking the constant annual cash outflow that has the same present value. With a little rearranging, one derives

$$\text{Equivalent annual cost} = \text{PV of cash outflows}/ \sum_{t=1}^{N} (\text{PVF}_{t,r\%})$$

Remember that $\sum_{t=1}^{N} (\text{PVF}_{t,r\%})$ is the present value factor for an annuity.

Thus the equivalent annual cost is the present value of cash outflows divided by the present value factor for an annuity for the life of the project. One compares equivalent annual costs and selects the alternative with the lower value. (If one is considering projects with differing cash inflows, one looks at equivalent annual amounts and selects the alternative with the greater equivalent annual amount.)

LEASE OR BUY?

The lease-or-buy decision is one of the most frequently encountered in the health care sector, and one of the least well understood. Strictly speaking, the lease-or-buy decision is not a capital budgeting decision at all. It is a decision made after one has decided to acquire a piece of capital. It is, really, a financing decision: which of the alternatives, lease or buy, is the least costly?

Gapenski and Langland-Orban (1991) explain the motivation for leasing. The advantages of leasing may arise from several sources. A leasing company (a lessor) may have access to capital at lower rates of interest than does a potential lessee. Similarly, a leasing company may have better access to channels for selling previously leased equipment than a lessee. The lessor, then, is better able to deal with the obsolescence of the equipment (often by selling it abroad) than a potential lessee, who would be stuck with an obsolete but unsalable piece of equipment.

The simplest, and most widely used, means of evaluating a potential lease is the calculation of the **net advantage of leasing (NAL)** (Mukherjee, 1991). The NAL is the present value of the annual cash savings due to leasing, calculated using the cost of borrowed funds as the discount rate. If the NAL is positive, then leasing is the desired alternative. If the NAL is negative, then purchasing the asset is superior to leasing. The cost of borrowed funds is the appropriate rate of discount because the lease is itself a form of debt.

The formula for NAL is

$$\text{NAL} = I_0 - \sum_{t=0}^{N} [L_t(1-T) + \text{Dep}_t(T)]/(1 + r'_d)^t$$

The formula requires some explanation. I_0 is the initial cash outlay necessary to make the purchase. I_0 represents what the lessee saves, at time $= 0$, by not having to purchase the asset. From that initial cash outlay, one subtracts the present value of the cost of leasing. The result is the net advantage of leasing rather than purchasing the asset. There are two components of the cost of leasing. L_t is the lease payment due at time t. The summation runs from 0 to N to allow the possibility of a lease payment at time 0. Lease payments are tax deductible, so one takes only the after-tax lease payment, $L_t(1-T)$, where T is the potential lessee tax rate.

The second component of the cost of leasing is the opportunity cost of forgone depreciation expense. A lessee does not take depreciation as a tax deduction. Thus the annual depreciation shield forgone is also a cost of leasing.

The two components of the cost of leasing (lease payment and forgone depreciation shield) are added together for each year of the lease and are discounted by the after-tax cost of debt, r'_d. The after-tax cost of debt is the interest rate on borrowed funds, multiplied by $(1-T)$.

STRATEGIC OPTIONS

Projects and assets bring with them cash flows, direct and indirect. If a medical group is considering establishing a walk-in clinic in a shopping mall, the direct cash inflows are the revenues that might be collected in the clinic for services rendered in that location. The indirect cash flows are the additional revenues generated by referrals of walk-in patients back to the main practice site ("Your blood glucose seems high. Why not come to our main clinic on Monday for a full workup?") and by the advertising value of having a visible facility. One should subtract any cash flows drawn away from pre-exiting facilities.

Many projects and assets also bring with them **options**, the right to take advantage of favorable circumstances at a later time (Magiera & McLean, 1996). Thus an option is valuable in strategic positioning. An asset or project's embedded options indicate how the asset can contribute to a change in overall strategy rather to current cash flows alone.

An option is the right to purchase or sell some asset at a specified price within some specified time period. The most familiar example is the stock option, the right to purchase or sell 100 shares of common stock at a set "strike price" any time prior to the option's expiration date.

Assets used in health care organizations bring options as well. A mobile x-ray unit allows the option to take the unit on the road and the option to bid to provide imaging services in distant sites. Those options are valuable, even if they are not exercised.

There are three types of options that one must consider in capital budgeting. First, there is the time-to-wait option. That is the option to delay entering a market until some opportune moment. Suppose, for example, one elects not to build an outpatient facility on a parcel of land across town. Ownership of the parcel, however, provides a time-to-wait option, the right to construct and open the clinic if and when market conditions are favorable.

Similar is the add-on option. When putting up a three-story clinic, one may wish to lay in a foundation adequate for five stories. The additional stability provides the option of putting up more square footage should the situation require. The additional strength of the foundation requires additional cash outlay in the present. If, however, the value of the add-on option is at least as great as the additional cash outlay, the added expense was worthwhile.

The third type of option to be considered is the abandonment option. In any net present value analysis, one assumes a useful life for the asset. Owning the asset allows one to end the asset's life at the optimal time. In fact, at every moment in time, one should ask, "Is the salvage value I could realize today at least as great as the net present value of continuing to use the asset?" If the answer is yes, it is time to abandon. The option to abandon is valuable, from the first day of ownership to the last.

Option valuation is a complex topic beyond the scope of this text. Generally, options increase in value as the value of the underlying asset rises, as the time remaining until option expiration rises, and as the variance of the value of the underlying asset increases. Sophisticated users of capital budgeting need to consider the values of the options embedded in their assets and projects.

SUMMARY

The process of allocating scarce resources among competing capital investments is more complicated than it may appear at first. As one removes the simplifying assumptions, the capital budgeting process is both more powerful and more difficult to employ. Each of the methods presented in this chapter extends capital budgeting one more step. It is important that the process can be adapted to cover a wide variety of circumstances and to yield subtle distinctions between potential endeavors.

The simple models of capital budgeting can, as their critics point out, seldom be applied directly. There is always risk associated with projected cash flows. One must adjust accordingly. Capital rationing, even if disfavored by financial theory, is common. Leasing is an increasingly common alternative. Options of all types are ever more important in capital acquisition.

Discussion Questions

1. If linear programming is such a great method for capital budgeting, why does it sometimes yield such silly allocations?

2. What is a pure play? How would you identify one?

3. Surveys indicate that few health care organizations actually adjust their net present value estimates for project risk. Why do you think they do not? Why should they?

4. What are the advantages of leasing?

CONTINUING CASE

Roger Jackson was in a foul mood that August morning. It had been unusually hot for several weeks, and the compressor on the central air conditioning system at home would have to be replaced. He and Mrs. Jackson had planned a week at their favorite Rocky Mountain getaway, and this was another source of pressure on his time. He had agreed to chair the local Boy Scout council's effort to raise money to refurbish the camp prior to next summer ("They expect me to get the pledges in before Labor Day!"). Too much to do, and now this car thing again.

PCI, Inc. leased a Ford Expedition for Dr. Jackson (much like the one Henry Kirk wished the corporation leased for him; see the Continuing Case for Chapter 2). He needed a vehicle for his business-related travels, and the SUV gave him extra room to carry corporate belongings (files, equipment). Once he had even had to pick up an order of supplies in Ft. Worth and haul them into the clinic. "Good car, that Expedition." The only trouble was that every 3 years, Bill Johanson over at the dealership presented him with a complicated new decision problem. "Get me that Fowler woman!"

The task Dr. Jackson assigned Janet Fowler was not particularly complicated: decide if it's better for PCI, Inc., to lease the SUV or to buy it for Dr. Jackson's use. Bill Johanson came up with the following alternatives. PCI could buy the Expedition (Dr. Jackson had already picked one out; it was on the floor, and ready for the planned trip to Colorado) for

$52,000. At the end of a 3-year useful life, Johanson predicted ("but no guarantees, mind you") that the trade-in on the SUV would be $20,000.

PCI could lease the Roadmaster for $3,500 down and $10,000 due on the first, second, and third anniversaries of the lease contract. Whether purchased or leased, PCI would be responsible for registration, tax, license, and (in order to keep the warranty in force) scheduled maintenance.

Janet Fowler looked at the figures. She was having a quiet snit of her own. Her automobile air conditioner had just gone out ("hottest time of the year") and she resented having to spend extra time in the office so that Dr. Jackson could have a new car "for corporate purposes exclusively." Nonetheless, she began to put the pieces together. She estimated PCI's tax rate for the coming year to be 20 percent. She knew that PCI would use the MACRS depreciation tables (see Chapter 3) to depreciate any items it purchased. Any depreciation expense not taken prior to sale would simply be lost.

CASE QUESTION

Should PCI lease or buy, assuming a cost of capital of 4 percent? 6 percent? 8 percent?

REFERENCES

Aggarwal, R. (1993). *Capital budgeting under uncertainty*. Englewood Cliffs, NJ: Prentice Hall.

Bierman, H., Jr. & Smidt, S. (1993). *The capital budgeting decision* (8th ed.). New York: Macmillan.

Dorfman, R., Samuelson, P.A., & Solow, R.M. (1958). *Linear programming and economic analysis*. New York: McGraw-Hill.

Friedman, M. & Savage, L.J. (1948). The utility analysis of choices involving risk. *Journal of Political Economy, 66*(1), 279–304.

Gapenski, L.C. & Langland-Orban, B. (1991). Leasing capital assets and durable goods: Opinions and practices in Florida hospitals. *Health Care Management Review, 16*(3), 73–81.

Magee, J.F. (1964). How to use decision trees in capital budgeting. (1964). *Harvard Business Review, 42*(5), 79–96.

Magiera, F.T. & McLean, R.A. (1996). Strategic options in capital budgeting and program selection under fee-for-service and managed care. *Health Care Management Review 21*(4).

Mukherjee, T.K. (1991). A survey of corporate leasing analysis. *Financial Management, 20*(3), 96–107.

Plane, D.R. & Trifts, J.W. (1993). Capital budgeting under resource rationing: Explicit enumeration using Lotus 1-2-3 as an alternative to linear programming. *Financial Practice and Education, 3*(2), 47–55.

Ross, S.A., Westerfeld, R.W., and Jordan, B.D. (2003). *Fundamentals of corporate finance* (6th ed.). New York: McGraw-Hill/Irwin.

Wheeler, J.R.C. & Smith, D.G. (1988). The discount rate for capital expenditure analysis in health care. *Health Care Management Review, 13*(2), 43–52.

SELECTED READINGS

Aggarwal, R. (Ed.). (1993). *Capital budgeting under uncertainty*. Englewood Cliffs, NJ: Prentice Hall.

Bierman, H., Jr. & Smidt, S. (1993). *The capital budgeting decision* (8th ed.). New York: Macmillan.

Managing Long-Term Financial Assets: The Endowment

CHAPTER

12

Managing the Endowment

Learning Objectives

After reading this chapter, the student should be able to:

1. Explain the nature of an endowment and its role in subsidizing the organization.
2. Identify an endowment's assets and claims on the balance sheet.
3. Articulate an endowment's investment goals and constraints.
4. Prepare a written investment policy for an endowment.

Key Term

Endowment

Popular mythology holds that the majority of the financial needs of not-for-profit hospitals are met by donations and the incomes from their endowments. In fact, that is not the case, with only a tiny part of most providers' needs being met from those sources (there are well-known exceptions, such as the Shriners' Crippled Children's Hospitals and Burn Centers, St. Jude Hospital, and a few others). It remains true, however, that a well-managed endowment can provide income to supplement operating revenues and, for an organization with a small operating margin, provide the cushion that means survival. It is also true, in an era of third-party payor parsimony, that shifting the cost of uncompensated care to paying patients is not a viable strategy. A healthy endowment can provide the resources necessary to care for those who cannot pay.

An **endowment** is, at its heart, just a portfolio of assets. Although the manager of a charitable endowment must be aware of the special constraints and goals of the endowment, he or she is managing according to the same principles as a pension fund manager or a mutual fund manager. This chapter outlines those principles.

THE ENDOWMENT CONCEPT

Any health care organization that has assets held (more or less) permanently for the purpose of producing income to supplement operating revenues has an endowment. The "investments" entry on the asset side of the Mayo Foundation's Year-2000 balance sheet was over $1.6 billion, one of the largest health care endowments in the United States. Although not so large as Mayo's holdings, many organizations have such assets (on the balance sheet they are usually listed under "marketable securities"), even though they may not consciously manage them as an endowment portfolio.

The balance sheet treatment of endowment portfolios varies enormously. On the asset (left-hand or debit) side of the balance sheet, such assets may be listed only as a general category (marketable securities), or they may be listed separately under "restricted assets" or "board-designated assets."

On the liabilities-owners' equity (right-hand or credit) side of the balance sheet, there may be no separate accounting of the portfolio at all, its being subsumed under "net assets" (assuming one is looking at a not-for-profit organization). Alternatively, the fund balance may be subdivided into "net assets, unrestricted" and "net assets, restricted," the latter being the endowment. Remember from Chapter 3 that "net assets" are actually claims against the organization, not assets at all.

At the extreme, the endowment may be reported on a separate balance sheet, with its assets matching its own liabilities and fund balance. Although that strict treatment of the endowment portfolio may be most revealing from an accounting perspective, it is the decisions governing investment of the endowment and the disposition of the income generated therefrom (investment income, nonoperating income, interest income) that are most important from the financial management perspective.

SOME PRINCIPLES REMEMBERED

Chapter 9 developed some of the guidelines of which a rational portfolio manager must be aware in a world of competitive, relatively efficient, capital markets. These include holding a diversified portfolio; not trying to "beat the market" by trading on "hot tips" (everybody has the same hot tips); and recognizing that the risk that financial markets reward is the systematic risk of the portfolio, measured by the portfolio's beta. Endowment managers, no less than any other portfolio managers, need to be aware of those rules. Space does not allow a full treatment of investment finance in this chapter. Those wishing to explore the topic further should consult a standard textbook on the subject (Bodie, Kane, & Marcus, 2002).

The Capital Asset Pricing Model (CAPM) works well for equity investments (ownership claims: common stock, preferred stock, limited partnership and master limited partnership shares) but is less often used for debt investments (bonds, bills, notes). For such securities, one looks to the bond rating agencies' assessments of the creditworthiness of the issuing organization. One sets a minimum acceptable rating level and invests accordingly.

Relatively little has been written about the special investment needs of health care endowments (Kittell, 1987; Ambachtsheer, Maginn, & Vawter, 1990). Traditionally, endowment assets have been invested conservatively, advancing little beyond the investment rules laid down by Graham and Dodd in their classic treatise on investing to capture fundamental value (Graham, Dodd, & Cottle, 1962). At least one observer has said, "Rule number 1: never lose the corpus (the principal of the endowment); rule number 2: never forget rule number one." Recent developments in portfolio management allow endowment managers to contribute more actively to the health of their organizations (McLean, 1990).

Ambachtsheer et al. (1990, pp. 4-26–4-36), building on a framework originally laid down by Vawter, approach the management of any institution's portfolio by describing expectations for market returns, portfolio objectives, and portfolio constraints. They identify the major portfolio constraints as (1) the investor's degree of risk aversion, (2) the investor's need for liquidity (being able to turn the portfolio into cash quickly), (3) the investor's cash flow needs, (4) tax considerations, (5) legal and regulatory restrictions, and (6) the investor's unique needs and circumstances. They provide a brief description of the investment situation of a typical endowment (health care or other) within their framework.

A general framework is an important point of departure, but no two endowments are alike, and the endowment manager must assess the organization's unique situation in order to be of value.

THE RETURN OBJECTIVE

The return objective of any endowment portfolio is simple to state: earn the greatest total return consistent with the portfolio's constraints. The last part of that objective, "consistent with the portfolio's constraints," is especially important, as the risk aversion, cash flow, regulatory, and unique constraints of most endowments are significant. The total return to a portfolio, like the return measure introduced in Chapter 9, is current income (dividends, interest, and other distributions) plus capital gains (whether realized as cash or not). Unrealized capital gains are as important a component of total return as current cash flow. Those gains represent the value of the endowment that could be realized (by selling assets) in times of financial distress.

CONSTRAINTS

Risk Aversion

The investment portfolios of most health care organizations have usually been managed very conservatively. One need only speak with a sample of chief financial officers to get a sense of their reluctance to take on market risk. However, a high degree of risk aversion is not necessary for good endowment management in every case.

Any endowment's willingness to take on market risk should depend on the specific circumstances of the organization the endowment is to serve. If the organization needs the annual proceeds of the endowment to meet a substantial part of its fixed cost, then the appropriate degree of risk for the portfolio is low. If, however, the endowment serves an organization that has steady cash flows from operations, serving an economically healthy market area with a well-insured population, earning a reasonable rate of return from operations, then it can take on more market risk and remain prudent.

Why would an endowment want to take on more risk, especially if the parent organization does not need the funds for current operations? Remember from Chapter 9 that investors (suppliers of funds) are, almost universally, risk averse. They have to be induced to accept market risk by the promise of higher expected returns. Therefore investing in a relatively risky diversified portfolio (a portfolio with a beta of 1.3, for example) will, in the long run, produce higher returns (and greater portfolio value) than investing in a relatively safe diversified portfolio (a portfolio with a beta of 0.8, for example). Having followed the riskier course over time, the sponsoring organization will have greater resources with which to build and maintain facilities or to provide care for the uninsured (although the portfolio will have to "take a few hits" from time to time).

Time Horizon

Endowments held for general support have a perpetual time horizon. Because the organization is perpetual (it has no anticipated date of liquidation), so does its endowment. The absence of a finite time horizon allows the investment manager greater flexibility than he would otherwise have. There is no terminal date on which the value of the endowment must equal some prespecified amount.

Special-purpose endowments, however, often have defined time horizons. A building fund, for example, has a time horizon determined by building plans. The presence of a definite time horizon makes investment in equity securities, whose market values vary widely over time, unwise. Rather, those assets should be invested in fixed income securities, whose maturity (and therefore return of par value) can be timed to coincide with the horizon. Another, somewhat more complicated, strategy is to invest the special-purpose endowment in fixed income securities and to set the duration (a measure of the sensitivity of a fixed income portfolio's value to changing interest rates) of the portfolio equal to the time horizon (McLean, 1990). That process is called *immunizing* the portfolio and, barring the borrowers' defaulting on their obligations, guarantees a fixed terminal value.

Cash Flow Needs

The cash flows that health care organizations need from their endowments vary widely. Some organizations require investment income to meet their operating expenses. Others have positive operating margins and look to their endowments only for extraordinary needs or for long-term capital formation.

Needs for current cash flow dictate the types of securities that belong in the endowment portfolio. Bonds that pay interest annually or semiannually (as distinguished from zero-coupon bonds that pay no current interest) and the stock of public utility companies are more suited for endowments that must produce cash flows than are other types of securities. Endowments that need not produce substantial cash flows can invest in securities that produce little current income. Among those are real estate, venture capital funds, and the common stock of firms that pay little or no dividends.

Tax Status, Law, and Regulation

The tax status of the endowments of health care organizations is more complicated than it first appears. It is tempting to say that, because it is not-for-profit organizations that are most likely to have endowments, and because they are exempt from federal (and, by extension, state) income tax under Section 501(c)(3) of the Internal Revenue Code, their endowments are also exempt from all tax requirements. It is tempting, but it may be wrong.

There are several ways, legally, to structure an endowment, and each of those structures has its own tax implications. If structured as a separate foundation, the endowment will be subject to a new realm of regulations under the Internal Revenue Code. In particular, nonoperating foundations are subject to minimum spending requirements and taxes on their investment gains.

A foundation structure may, however, be useful for investor-owned health care organizations who find themselves holding endowments. Suppose that, in Central City (a fictitious town), the only hospital is owned by a national investor-owned corporation. Mrs. Smith bequeaths $1 million to the hospital to be used for the care of the indigent in the community. How does the parent corporation handle the funds? To avoid commingling the bequest with the parent corporation's assets, and commingling the investment income with its taxable income, Mrs. Smith's attorney, and those of the corporation, might establish a foundation to hold and manage the gift. The purpose of the gift could be preserved and the income, subject to federal and state requirements and taxes, reserved for its intended use.

The not-for-profit status of most endowments makes certain types of securities inappropriate for their portfolios. Municipal bonds, for example, pay interest that is exempt from federal (and often state) income tax. For $1 of interest on a corporate bond, a tax-paying investor is able to keep only $1(1−T), where T is the tax rate the investor faces. For $1 of interest on a municipal bond, however, the tax-paying investor keeps the entire $1. In equilibrium, then, the municipal bond will pay less interest than an otherwise equivalent corporate bond. Specifically,

$$r_{\text{municipal}} = r_{\text{corporate}} (1-T)$$

where $r_{\text{municipal}}$ is the municipal bond's equilibrium interest rate, $r_{\text{corporate}}$ is the interest rate applying to an otherwise equivalent corporate bond, and T is the tax rate of the marginal investor.

Because health care endowments do not pay income tax on current cash income (if minimum spending requirements are met), they should not accept the lower interest rates paid by municipal bonds. They can invest in corporate bonds, receive the higher interest rates, and keep all of the proceeds (their tax rates being zero).

Similarly, the market for preferred stock is largely manufactured by the peculiarities of the tax code. To avoid triple taxation of corporate dividends (tax laws already provide for the double taxation of corporate dividends, once as corporate profits and a second time as personal income) corporations can exclude a large percentage of any dividends they receive from other corporations. That exclusion applies to dividends only, not to interest received. Preferred stock pays a regular, fixed cash flow, like a bond, but pays it as a dividend, making it largely tax excluded. Tax-paying corporations are willing to give up some yield to receive the tax exclusion benefits of holding preferred stock. Because not-for-profit endowments cannot use the tax exclusion benefits of preferred stock, they ought not to invest in it.

Unique Needs

Endowments often have special needs that most other investment portfolios do not face. Many endowments, because they represent the material wealth of charitable organizations, feel the need to hold only the securities of corporations whose products and conduct are consistent with the precepts of the endowments' parents. Thus securities issued by makers of alcohol and tobacco producers, retailers who deal in pornography, and, in an earlier time, corporations that did business in South Africa may be excluded from the portfolios of many health care endowments (Domini, 1987).

The effect on returns of limiting the portfolio's investment universe in this way is a matter of some controversy. Grossman and Sharpe (1986) found that eliminating South Africa–related stocks from a portfolio had not hurt returns, because it limited the portfolio to the stocks of smaller firms at a time when such firms did well relative to the market as a whole. Ennis and Parkhill (1986), on the other hand, challenged social investing for reducing the opportunities for diversification. Reid (1987), again looking at South Africa-free portfolios, found that they had severely limited ranges of stocks from which to choose and were exposed to much greater price volatility than portfolios that were not South Africa–free.

The requirements of social investing are, however, very real for portfolios sponsored by philanthropic, particularly religious, organizations. They usually have mission-driven, not return-driven, motivations. Portfolio managers constrained by social investment criteria need explicit guidance on those criteria and need to make the sponsoring organizations aware of the possible effects of the constraints on investment performance.

INSIDE OR OUTSIDE MANAGEMENT

Portfolio managers command high salaries and require substantial support services. Portfolio management services, on the other hand, are available in the external market, with fees, usually based on the volume of assets under management (Seidner & Cleverly, 1990). Which is the better approach to management?

There are several nonmonetary advantages to having an in-house manager. One is the greater accountability that an employee has to the organization, to his or her supervisor (the treasurer), and to the trustees. Another is that the outside managers, even if they are both honest and conscientious about reporting portfolio performance, are difficult to supervise. An employment relationship is a good substitute for time-consuming and imperfect monitoring (again, agency problems are important; see Chapter 2).

On the other hand, skillful money managers often seek the greater independence and rewards of working in their own firms. It may be possible to hire better management outside than can be hired internally. Also, the fixed costs of managing even a modest portfolio are substantial, and a specialist firm can spread those costs over many clients.

On the purely monetary side, one should compare the present value of the costs of internal management of the portfolio to the present value of the costs of external management. An outside manager might charge 1 percent of the value of assets under management per year. An internal manager, clerical staff, support, and fixed cost might have an equivalent annual cost of $200,000. It would follow, then, that an endowment facing those numbers should hire an external manager unless its asset value is at least $20,000,000.

Portfolios also need custodians, banks that hold the securities for the endowment. The role of the custodian is both as a check and balance on the portfolio manager and as a matter of convenience. One should ask whether or not an outside manager (with many client portfolios) can obtain custodial services less expensively than a single portfolio could. One should also ask whether an external manager can negotiate lower transactions fees (brokers' commissions) than could a single portfolio. If so, those cost differences should be incorporated into the decision as to whether or not to hire an external manager.

SAMPLE INVESTMENT POLICY

Imagine a small (120-bed) community hospital, Regional Medical Center (RMC), with $1,500,000 in "board-designated assets" (its endowment). The $1,500,000 is held as cash and marketable securities (the right-side entry, "net assets, board-designated" is matched by the left-hand entry "cash and securities, board-designated"). Increases in the value of common stock since the early 1980s have made the current market value of the endowment almost $3,000,000.

The trustees of RMC believe that they should develop a written investment policy to guide their outside money manager. They have adopted the framework suggested by Ambachtsheer et al. (1990). Seidner and Cleverly (1990, pp. 178–181) provide a sample investment policy based on a different framework. RMC's investment policy is shown in Table 12–1.

SUMMARY

The investment policy statement in Table 12–1 is only illustrative and is necessarily brief. One may question the wisdom of some of the provisions, such as the low level of risk allowed or the exclusion of any derivative securities. What is important for the endowment, however, is that there be such a statement of policies that it give useful guidance to whoever will manage the portfolio.

Endowments can provide the margin for survival in a competitive environment. They can also provide seed money for new ventures and building projects. An endowment that generates annual cash flow can subsidize those activities (care of the indigent, burn centers, neonatal intensive care, health education) that do not produce adequate revenue to cover their costs, but that are important to the public's health. Good portfolio management, then, is a part of good health care financial management.

Discussion Questions

1. What elements should be covered in an endowment's written investment policy?

2. The line between holding marketable securities as working capital and holding them as an endowment is quite fuzzy. What elements determine when assets constitute an endowment?

3. What qualities and qualifications should one look for in an outside investment manager?

4. Is "social investing" good investing? Explain.

5. Some health care organizations, seeking to preserve principal, invest only in government bonds. Is this a wise investment strategy? Explain.

Table 12–1   Regional Medical Center investment policy for board-designated funds

Mission

The mission of Regional Medical Center is to provide the finest quality of health care services to the citizens of our city and county. RMC will maintain a setting that is conducive to the highest-quality practice of medicine and that elicits the best efforts of its administrators, trustees, employees, and volunteers.

The mission of Regional Medical Center's board-designated assets is to support the mission of RMC by providing cash, beyond that available from continuing operations, for capital improvement, community outreach, new program initiation, the care of indigent patients, and such other uses as the Board of Trustees may determine.

Objective

The objective that will govern the management of the assets associated with board-designated funds is to earn the highest possible total return consistent with the constrains enumerated below.

Constraints

Risk Exposure

The corpus of the board-designated funds is to be maintained. To that end, only U.S. Treasury securities, mortgage-backed securities issued by the Government National Mortgage Association, investment-grade corporate bonds (those rated BBB or higher), and the common stock of corporations with consistent records of profitability will be included in the portfolio. At no time will the common stocks comprise more than 45 percent of the total portfolio and at no time will the beta of the common stock component (as measured against the Standard and Poor's 500 Index) be greater than 0.80.

Time Horizon

Board-designated assets are to be maintained in perpetuity.

Cash Flow Needs

The annual income from board-designated assets will be used to support the operations of RMC to the extent that RMC provides uncompensated care and to the extent that new initiatives require support before they begin to produce cash flows. Therefore the portfolio should produce no less than 5 percent of its total value in annual cash flows without the requirement of sale of any assets.

Tax Status

Regional Medical Center is a private not-for-profit entity, exempt from federal income taxation under Section 501(c)(3) of the Internal Revenue Code. Tax-favored investment vehicles are therefore inappropriate for inclusion in the board-designated funds' portfolio.

Legal and Regulatory Constraints

The endowment will be managed in accordance with all applicable federal, state, and local laws.

(continues)

Table 12–1 (continued)   Regional Medical Center investment policy for board-designated funds

The trustees will ensure that the designated fund manager will adhere to all applicable fiduciary requirements, managing the assets solely in the interest of RMC.

Unique Constraints

The trustees, administration, medical staff, and employees of Regional Medical Center are keenly aware of their role in promoting the health and well-being of the citizens of our city and county and beyond. To that end, no assets associated with board-designated funds will be invested in the securities of corporations that engage in processing, manufacturing, or fabrication of tobacco products, alcoholic beverages, firearms, ammunition, or pornographic films or literature. The funds manager will report all holdings to the trustees on a quarterly basis, and both the manager and the trustees will ensure that this constraint is met at all times.

The securities associated with the board-designated funds will not be lent to investors for short sales. The portfolio will not engage in trading options contracts, futures contracts, or other "derivative" securities.

CONTINUING CASE

"A surprise, but a happy surprise." That was how Billy Bob Ferguson described Lone Star Home Health Services' recent windfall to Jason Cooper, chair of LSHHS's board. "Mrs. Guenther's will gives us $400,000 (give or take) in stock and jumbo CDs (certificates of deposit)." Mrs. Guenther had been a paying client of LSHHS for the last 5 years of her life and she wanted services extended to "Clearwater County's less fortunate senior citizens."

The Reverend Cooper saw this as an opportunity to extend the mission of LSHHS, to really live up to the promise that the founders of the organization had in mind. It was a promise that lack of funds had always prevented being fulfilled. "Billy, of course you will see to the investment details." Ferguson had been a lending officer at Clearwater County State Bank (now CCB Bank) from his return from Korea in 1960 until his retirement in 1992. Everyone on the board assumed that he was an expert in all things financial.

"Oh, Lord," he complained to Alice later that evening, "this will be just like that cost accounting thing Joleen Garza made me do (see the Continuing Case for Chapter 7). I don't know anything about investments. The bank never even had a trust department. I'm sure not going to turn that kind of money over to Jack. He doesn't even know the word *fiduciary*." Jack Elliott was a broker for a national firm's Jamestown office and had handled William and Mary Ferguson's college funds for years. "Jack will get us into some harebrained thing like oil well drilling or shopping malls in Waco (two of Jack's favorite investments)."

"All right, Billy," Alice, once again, calmed her husband, "what do you need to get started?"

A week later, Ferguson was ready for a meeting. He and Jason Cooper had made an appointment with John Stevens, a money manager (*not* a broker) in Fort Worth who came highly recommended. They were impressed by Stevens's oak-paneled offices, the subdued lighting, the books and reports on the shelves, and the Bloomberg news service terminal humming in the background. Stevens's Chartered Financial Analyst® certificate was displayed prominently in the outer office.

The board had agreed that the Guenther Endowment (as they were now calling it) would be treated as "net assets, restricted" on the right-hand side of the balance sheet and matched by "assets, restricted" on the left-hand side. That much agreement had required two hours at a special meeting of the board. They also believed that the $400,000 (give or take) should produce at least $30,000 per year in cash in order to have an effect on LSHHS's ability to provide services to those who cannot pay. The Reverend Cooper had spent about half an hour convincing the board of the need to get rid of some tobacco stocks that were among the assets bequeathed.

Mr. Stevens said some pleasant things about the bird hunting in Clearwater County and then got down to business. His fee would be 1 percent of assets under management per year. LSHHS needed to take possession of the stock as soon as possible (Jack Elliott had been Mrs. Guenther's broker, too) and pass it on to the custodian Stevens recommended. The custodian would charge 0.25 percent of assets held per year. "Of course, the portfolio will have to bear all of its own transactions costs. Now, may I see your investment policy statement?" Stevens asked.

"Our what?" Billy Bob inquired. "We don't have a policy statement, whatever that is."

Stevens explained the need for a written investment policy statement and loaned the pair a thick book on portfolio management. "Let's meet again a week from today."

"More work, more work." Once again Ferguson was plunging into unknown waters.

CASE QUESTIONS

1. Prepare an investment policy statement for the Guenther Endowment.

2. Given the level of expenses involved in its administration, is it reasonable to expect the endowment to generate $30,000 per year in cash

flow? How might a reasonable cash flow requirement statement be written?

About the same time that Mrs. Guenther's stock portfolio was providing a special opportunity for LSHHS, the Clearwater County Health Department was facing an opportunity of its own. John (Big John) Garza's recent death had been a great personal shock to Joleen Garza and her family, but one provision of her father's will provided a professional shock as well. The elder Mr. Garza had left shares in Garza Oil Company to a trust fund whose only beneficiary was the County Health Department. The voting rights of those shares were to be exercised by the Health Director (currently Joleen), who would act as co-trustee (along with a designated officer at CCB Bank).

All of the above sounded fine to Joleen. The income from her father's shares would allow her to undertake some initiatives, such as a mobile vaccination clinic, that had been on hold for a long time. She felt secure in knowing that she would have additional votes in corporate matters. All seemed right until her first meeting with Tom Land at CCB (her co-trustee).

After expressing his condolences on her father's death (Tom had once worked the all-night shift at the original Garza Texaco station), and assuring her of his interest in working together productively, Tom dropped a bombshell. CCB's attorneys insisted that the Garza Trust (as it was to be known) diversify its holdings. As Garza Oil was not registered as a publicly traded corporation, a value would have to be assigned and a buyer found who was willing to pay at least the "fair market value" for the shares. Garza Oil was to be no more than 25 percent of the total value of the Garza Trust.

Joleen, other members of her family, and the current minority shareholders (a few long-time employees and the First Presbyterian Church) could bid for the shares, but the Trust could give no one preferential status. Proceeds from the sale of the Trust's shares would be reinvested in the shares of publicly traded corporations.

Joleen found the CCB Bank's proposals to be personally insulting and damaging to the Trust. "Garza Oil is the best company in Clearwater County, and one of your best customers!"

"Yes, Joleen, but the law is the law. If the Bank is to act as a fiduciary, we have to follow the rules."

CASE QUESTIONS

1. Explain the logic of diversifying the Trust's assets.

2. Outline a process for establishing the "fair market value" of the shares in Garza Oil (refer to Chapter 6).

3. What potential agency costs does the Trust avoid by not having Dr. Garza voting both her own shares and those of the Trust?

4. Prepare an investment policy statement for the Garza Trust. Make sure that your statement covers, inter alia, the maximum portion of the Trust that may be held in any one asset (e.g., Garza Oil Company).

REFERENCES

Ambachtsheer, K.P., Maginn, J.L., & Vawter, J. (1990). Determination of portfolio policies: Institutional investors. In J.L. Maginn & D.L. Tuttle (Eds.), *Managing investment portfolios* (2nd ed., pp. 4-1–4-77). Boston, MA: Warren, Gorham & Lamont for the Institute of Chartered Financial Analysts.

Bodie, Z., Kane, A. & Marcus, A.J. (2002). *Investments* (5th ed.). New York: McGraw-Hill/Irwin.

Domini, A.L. (1987). The significance of social investing. In C.E. Kittell (Ed.), *The challenge of investing for endowment funds* (pp. 71–73). Homewood, IL: Dow Jones-Irwin for the Institute of Chartered Financial Analysts.

Ennis, R.M. & Parkhill, R.L. (1986). South African divestment: Social responsibility or fiduciary folly? *Financial Analysts Journal, 42*(4), 30–38.

Graham, B., Dodd, D.L, & Cottle, S. (1962). *Security analysis* (4th ed.). New York: McGraw-Hill.

Grossman, B.R. & Sharpe, W.F. (1986). Financial implications of South African divestment. *Financial Analysts Journal, 42*(4), 15–29.

Kittell, C.E. (Ed.). (1987). *The challenges of investing for endowment funds.* Homewood, IL: Dow Jones-Irwin for the Institute of Chartered Financial Analysts.

McLean, R.A. (1990). A strategic planning framework for endowment management. *Health Care Management Review, 15*(2), 53–60.

Reid, J.E., III. (1987). The impact of social issues on the investment process. In C.E. Kittell (Ed.), *The challenges of investing for endowment funds.* (pp. 74–83). Homewood, IL: Dow Jones-Irwin for the Institute of Chartered Financial Analysts.

Seidner, A.G. & Cleverly, W.O. (1990). *Cash and investment management for the health care industry.* Rockville, MD: Aspen.

SELECTED READINGS

Kittell, C.E. (Ed.). (1987). *The challenges of investing for endowment funds.* Homewood, IL: Dow Jones-Irwin for the Institute of Chartered Financial Analysts.

Maginn, J.L. & Tuttle D.L. (Eds.). (1990). *Managing investment portfolios* (2nd ed.), Boston, MA: Warren, Gorham & Lamont for the Institute of Chartered Financial Analysts.

Seidner, A.G. & Cleverly, W.O. (1990). *Cash and investment management for the health care industry*. Rockville, MD: Aspen.

Sherrerd, K.F. (Ed.) (1996). *Managing endowment and foundation funds*. Charlottesville, VA: Association for Investment Management and Research.

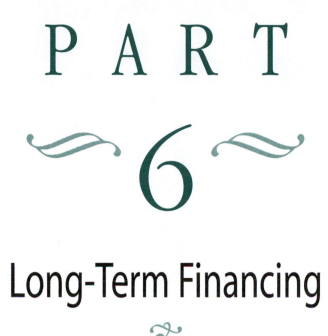

PART

6

Long-Term Financing

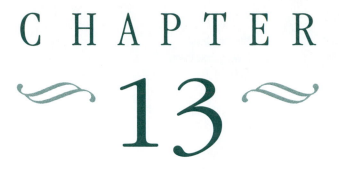

CHAPTER
13

External Financing: Sources

Learning Objectives

After reading this chapter, the student should be able to:

1. List the choices for external financing faced by health care organizations.
2. Explain the requirements placed on the organization by each external financing option.
3. Discuss the issues involved in optimal capital structure decisions.

Key Terms

Bankruptcy costs	Mortgage bond
Capital structure	Pecking order theory
Common stock	Preferred stock
Debenture	Senior
Free cash flow	Tax-exempt revenue bonds
General obligation bond	
Hospital revenue bond	

Those who have read the previous chapters understand much about how financial markets work and about how the external financial environment, by determining the cost of capital, influences the decisions of health care organizations. The costs of debt and equity (and the returns that are possible from investing the organization's own assets in debt and equity) influence what projects can be undertaken (by affecting the discount rate in capital budgeting) and, therefore, influence the very nature of the services that can be provided. The Capital Asset Pricing Model, discussed in Chapter 9, forms the basis for understanding the financial market's assessment of risk and its expectation of return.

Many issues remain unexplored, however. Among them are (1) how an organization can go about tapping the financial market, (2) with whom it must deal in that market, (3) what financing alternatives are available, (4) how to decide among those financing alternatives, and (5) what the experiences of other health care organizations have been in obtaining external funds. This chapter and the two that follow deal with these interrelated questions. After completing Chapter 13, the reader should be able to discuss the natures of equity and debt financing, to describe their advantages and disadvantages, and to design an optimal capital structure.

EXTERNAL FINANCING: KEY TO SUCCESS

In the 1980s large health care organizations experienced the need for external capital as never before. Funding for hospital construction under the Hill-Burton Act had lapsed. The need for capital financing had increased with the developments of new, effective, but very expensive, technologies (such as CAT scanning, MRI, organ transplantation, and lithotripsy). Cohodes & Kinkead (1984, p. 48) wrote that access to external financing was a key element in organizational success, and, in fact, in organizational survival. To respond to their needs for external financing, many organizations sold securities.

EXTERNAL FINANCING: THE CHOICES

The organization that decides to seek funds by selling securities has a multitude of alternatives from which to choose. Although all of those alternatives will provide cash for the organization, each brings with it a unique right-hand-side entry on the balance sheet and a unique obligation to the provider of funds. Figure 13–1 shows the major types of securities that one might consider selling to raise external funds. Note that not every alternative is available to every organization.

Investor-owned organizations can issue equity securities, raising external financing and imposing a particular type of obligation on the organization. The holders of **common stock** securities have no legal claim to an annual dividend, making common stock financing the least obligating form of external financing in terms of required cash flow. Equity holders, however, are the owners of the organization. They have a residual claim, the ownership of all that is left over after other suppliers of funds are paid off. Common stock holders almost always have a voice in the governance of the organization as well, although holders of small percentages of equity may be unable to exercise their voices effectively. Issuing common stock, then, is quite safe in terms of required cash payments, but quite risky in terms of possible dilution of ownership, claim on future profits, and loss of control. Common stock finance also requires a higher cost of capital than does any other type of financing. That cost of capital is masked by the fact that corporations need pay no annual dividend to common stock holders. Those stock holders, however, stand behind all debt holders and preferred stock holders in their claims against

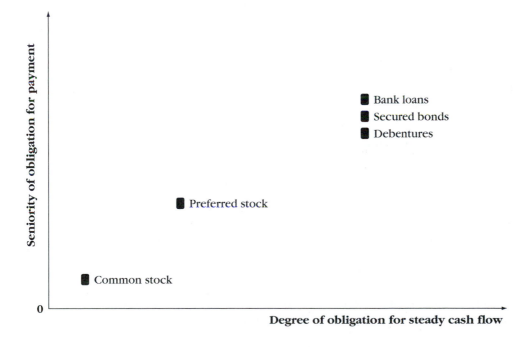

Note: Not every alternative is available to every organization.

Figure 13-1 External financing alternatives.

the firm (they own what is left over). In financial distress, debt holders are entitled to their claim in full (they seldom receive payment in full) before common stock holders receive anything. Because investors view it as risky, due to its low seniority of payment, stock holders demand higher *total* returns than do debt holders, and, failing to receive it, sell their shares.

Preferred stock is **senior** to common stock in that its holders must receive their dividends prior to any dividends' being paid to the holders of common stock. The purchasers of preferred stock are entitled to a fixed annual dividend in perpetuity. Usually, preferred stock holders either have no voting rights or have voting rights only when their dividends are not paid. Preferred stock is like a debt security in the fixity of its required payment. It is not, however, debt in the legal sense, and the payments made to its holders are, legally, dividends, not interest. Thus preferred stock is a desirable asset for taxable corporations, which can exclude a large percentage (varying with the degree of ownership held in the issuing corporation) of their dividend income from corporate income tax liability. Investors view preferred stock as less risky than the same firm's common stock but riskier than that firm's debt. Because of the tax exclusion of preferred stock dividends, however, the cost of capital for preferred stock financing is usually lower than the cost of capital for most debt financing.

Both not-for-profit and investor-owned organizations can obtain external financing by issuing debt. Not-for-profit organizations are limited in their external financing activities in that they can acquire external financing only by taking on debt. Investor owned organizations often prefer debt financing to equity financing. The claims of debt holders are always senior to those of equity holders. Taking on debt does not dilute the ownership of the organization. It does, however, obligate the organization to disburse cash to the lenders on the schedule specified in the loan contract (or the bond's trust agreement).

In the health care sector, government/nonfederal and not-for-profit organizations have the advantage of being able to obtain funding through the issuance of **tax-exempt revenue bonds** (Feldstein & Fabozzi, 1991). In every state, properly constituted units of government (in some states, a state financing authority; in others, cities and counties; and in others, special hospital districts) can issue bonds promising the holder interest backed by the revenues of specific not-for-profit and public providers. That interest, subject to a variety of restrictions and regulations, is not subject to federal income taxation for the recipient. In most states, the interest is not subject to state income taxation, if the bond is issued in the state in which the bond holder resides.

Because these bonds pay interest that is not subject to federal (and usually state) income tax, tax-paying investors are willing to accept lower rates of interest on them than they would on otherwise equivalent taxable bonds. Specifically, the equilibrium interest rate on a municipal bond (r_m) will be

$$r_m = r_c (1 - T_p)$$

where r_c is the rate of interest on an otherwise equivalent (same term to maturity, liquidity, and risk) corporate bond, and T_p is the tax rate of the investor at the margin. Government/nonfederal and not-for-profit health care providers should exploit every opportunity to gain tax-exempt financing before they attempt to obtain financing at taxable interest rates (either through issuing bonds paying taxable interest or through taking on bank debt).

There is debt and there is debt. Not all debt holders stand in equal seniority in terms of receipt of payments. **Debentures** are unsecured bonds, bonds not backed by any specific asset. **Mortgage bonds** are backed by claims on specific assets. Mortgage bonds are senior to debentures.

In the government and not-for-profit arena, bonds backed by the full faith and credit of a unit of government (**general obligations bonds**) are backed by the taxing power of the issuer. **Hospital revenue bonds**, on the other hand, are backed only by the revenues of the organization for which the bonds were issued. General obligation bonds, then, carry less risk for their holders but more risk for their issuers than hospital revenue bonds.

THE WEIGHTED AVERAGE COST OF CAPITAL ONCE AGAIN

Chapter 10 briefly discussed the weighted average cost of capital (WACC) in the context of selecting the appropriate discount rate in capital budgeting. The WACC is simply the average cost (in percentage terms) of a dollar of new financing for the organization, given some target mix of debt and equity financing. If an investor-owned firm were completely financed with equity (if it had no debt whatsoever), its WACC would be its cost of equity. As the share of debt financing in the organization's capital structure rises, the cost of debt becomes more important in its overall WACC.

The formula for WACC is

$$\text{WACC} = W_e r_e + W_{d,l-t} r_{d,l-t}{}' + W_{d,s-t} r_{d,s-t}{}'$$

where W_e, $W_{d,l-t}$, and $W_{d,s-t}$ are the weights (percentages of financing) of equity, long-term debt, and short-term debt, respectively. Those weights should be based on the market values of securities outstanding, not on the values recorded in the firm's books.

r_e, $r_{d,l-t}{}'$, and $r_{d,s-t}{}'$ are the relevant costs, expressed as percentages, of equity, long-term debt, and short-term debt, respectively. The costs of long-term and short-term debt are adjusted for the tax-deductibility of interest payments. If $r_{d,l-t}$ is the before-tax (nominal) cost of long-term debt, then the after-tax cost of long-term debt is

$$r_{d,l-t}{}' = r_{d,l-t} \times (1 - T_c)$$

where T_c is the firm's marginal tax rate.

When the weights used to compute WACC reflect the values of the securities currently outstanding, WACC reflects the current cost of capital. When the weights reflect a target capital structure that is different from the current capital structure, WACC reflects the cost of new financing.

DEBT AND EQUITY CHOICES: THE CAPITAL STRUCTURE DECISION IN THEORY

Students of finance have puzzled over capital structure for a long time (Myers, 1984). **Capital structure** is the mix of debt and equity that finances the organization. Every organization, except those financed purely by annual government appropriations, must make choices about capital structure. Given a certain level of net assets (equity), the managers of government-owned organizations must decide whether increasing their level of debt (taking out a bank loan, for example) would increase their debt/equity ratio too much. This section will show that "too much" debt is a very murky concept indeed.

Recall, from Chapter 4, that capital structure can be measured by any of several ratios, including the debt/equity ratio, the asset/equity ratio, and the equity financing ratio. Those financial statement measures take accounting values into account. In the analysis in this chapter, the mix of debt and equity should be understood to refer to market values (the current value of equity and debt securities in financial markets) rather than to accounting values.

Prior to about 1960, textbooks in financial management agreed that there was an optimal capital structure and that every corporation could identify it and adjust its financing percentages accordingly. That capital structure was the one that minimized the weighted average cost of capital and that therefore maximized the value of the organization (the value of the organization being the sum of all future cash flows discounted at the weighted average cost of capital). Figure 13–2 is a picture of that view of the world.

The logic behind the pre-1960 view of optimal capital structure is appealing. When the debt/equity ratio is zero (there is no outstanding debt), the weighted average cost of capital is simply the cost of equity. That is, when the weight of debt in total financing is zero and the weight of equity is 1.00,

$$\text{WACC} = W_d r_d + W_e r_e = r_e$$

Because the cost of debt (r_d) is less than the cost of equity (r_e), as the weight of debt increases, WACC declines. After some point, the rising weight of debt causes bond rating agencies to doubt the organization's ability to meet its debt obligations, ratings decline, and the cost of debt rises. As the cost of debt rises, with the weight of debt in the capital structure rising, the WACC must rise as well. The result is a single debt/equity ratio that minimizes the WACC and maximizes the discounted value of the organization. Even today, some textbooks in health care financial management adhere to this view, often identifying the optimal debt/equity ratio as 1.00.

The Modigliani-Miller Result

In 1958 Franco Modigliani and Merton Miller published mathematical results showing that the old view of optimal capital structure was wrong (Modigliani & Miller, 1958). The basic Modigliani-Miller (MM) result is shown in Figure 13–3.

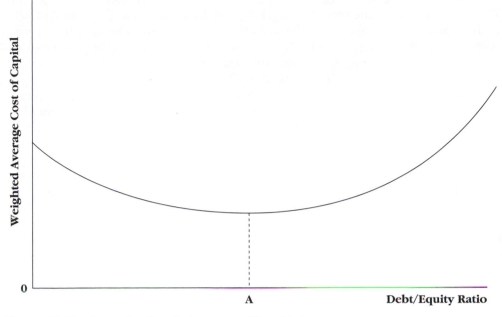

Figure 13–2   An optimal capital structure: The old view.

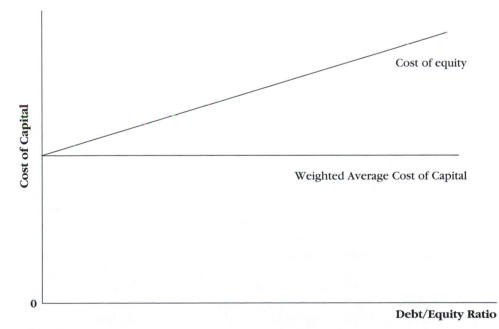

Figure 13–3   Capital structure and cost of capital: The Modigliani-Miller view.

As in Figure 13–2, when the debt/equity ratio is zero (when there is no debt), the WACC is the same as the cost of equity. MM also deduced that as the weight of debt in the capital structure increases, the cost of equity (r_e) increases linearly (consistent with the later-developed CAPM, which states that systematic risk rises with the degree of financial leverage). At the same time that the cost of equity is rising, the weight of equity in the WACC (W_e) is falling and the weight of debt (W_d) is rising. Because the cost of debt is well below the cost of equity, the effect of increasing the debt share of total financing while the cost of equity is rising causes the weighted average cost of capital to stay constant. MM's result, then, was that the weighted average cost of capital (and therefore the value of the firm) was constant at all capital structures. Thus, WACC, and the value of the firm, was based on the riskiness of the organization's expected future operating cash flows and was independent of the capital structure. Stated another way, the MM result is that the value of the organization depends on the cash flows that it expects to produce, *not* on how it is financed.

MM made yet another supporting argument. Suppose everyone had equal ability to borrow and lend in the capital market. Suppose further that there were an optimal capital structure. One could easily identify firms that did not have the optimal structure and purchase all of their debt and equity. That debt and equity would have less than its optimal value (at a nonoptimal capital structure, the value of the firm's securities would be less than their potential). One could then issue equity and debt in the optimal ratio and receive, from the market, the maximum value of the firm. The difference between the purchase price of the nonoptimal firm and the sale price of the securities of the now-optimal firm would be a pure profit (an arbitrage profit). Such an arbitrage opportunity cannot exist for long. Traders seeking arbitrage profits must be bidding up the prices of nonoptimally structured firms right now. The bidding for such firms will stop only at the firms' optimal values. Thus, in a world in which "homemade leverage" is possible, every observed capital structure must be an optimal capital structure.

The MM propositions were shocks to academic and practicing finance specialists. Debate on their analysis began soon after the publication of their initial article and has continued into the present (Miller, 1988; Weston, 1989). Modigliani and Miller weren't finished with their analysis, however. Following initial criticism, they revised their analysis to account for the fact that interest payments to debt holders are tax deductible for investor-owned enterprises (Modigliani & Miller, 1963). That tax deductibility further increases the difference between the cost of equity and the cost of debt. Under that tax deductibility, the WACC is a constantly declining function of the debt/equity ratio and the optimal capital structure is 100 percent debt. Miller (1977) later produced a subtle argument whose conclusion was that there was no optimal amount of debt for any one firm, but that there is an optimal amount of debt for the economy as a whole.

The idea that one can issue as much debt as one wishes without any effect on one's WACC flies in the face of what bond raters say they take into account (bond rating is covered in detail in Chapter 14). The links between debt levels and the cost of capital may lie in two effects not considered in MM's original work: bankruptcy costs and agency costs. Those links are shown in Figure 13–4.

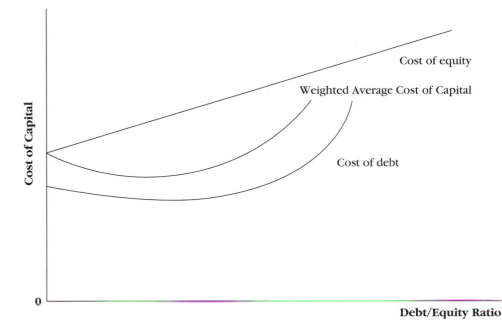

Figure 13–4   Capital structure and cost of capital: Including agency costs and bankruptcy costs.

Bankruptcy Costs

Bankruptcy costs are losses in the value of the organization that occur during the process of declaring bankruptcy and liquidating. They include payments to attorneys and accountants and failure to obtain full value for assets sold. If there were no bankruptcy costs, lenders would have no fear of bankruptcy, as they would receive the full par value of their loans plus accrued interest after liquidation was complete.

Agency costs are reductions in the value of the organization that occur as suppliers of capital recognize the ability of agents to gain at the expense of the organization (see Chapter 2). One type of agency problem (leading to agency costs) is that the greater the amount of debt in the capital structure, the greater is the incentive for the owners of equity (and their agents, management) to undertake risks.

As the percentage of debt in the capital structure grows, management *may* expose the organization to unwarranted risks. These risks expose the organization to an increased probability of bankruptcy, making potential bankruptcy costs more and more important. These expected bankruptcy costs eventually increase the cost of debt, causing the WACC to rise. As Figure 13–4 shows, the WACC *may*, then, have a unique minimum value, or a range of asset/equity ratios over which WACC takes on its minimum value. The value of the organization will be maximized when the WACC takes on the value(s) of asset/equity.

Such an optimal capital structure, if it exists, is very difficult to identify and will not be the same for every firm. McCue (1992) studied the capital structures of

California hospitals and found that smaller hospitals tend to have higher total debt/equity ratios than larger hospitals, but that larger hospitals have greater long-term debt than smaller hospitals.

THE CAPITAL STRUCTURE DECISION IN PRACTICE

It seems that there is no optimal capital structure that applies to all organizations everywhere at all times. The question of whether or not there is an optimal capital structure for any given firm is unresolved. In practice, health care organizations have a wide variety of capital structures, ranging from very little debt to virtually all debt financing. Table 13–1 illustrates, for a small sample of health care organizations, the range of debt/equity choices.

The first three organizations listed in Table 13-1 are investor-owned organizations. The last provider on the list, Rush-Presbyterian-St. Luke's Medical Center, is a large, not-for-profit academic medical center. All financial statement data are from their fiscal year 2000 annual reports. Stock prices for the investor-owned organizations are for the last trading days of their fiscal years (December 29, 2000 for HCA and HealthSouth, and May 31, 2000 for Tenet).

Not-for-profit organizations do not have market values for their equity, so one cannot calculate market asset/equity for them. Using the market value of equity (and assuming that the book value and the market value of debt are the same) significantly changes the investor-owned firms' asset/equity ratios. Because the market values of the firms' equity is higher than their book values, the market asset/equity ratios are lower than the book-value ratios. Note, however, that, even on a market value basis, the ratios vary substantially from firm to firm. Clearly, in practice, there is no unique "gold standard" for capital structures.

Gapenski (1993) and McCue (1992) studied capital structure decisions of hospitals. Gapenski found that a majority of both the not-for-profit and the in-

Table 13-1 Debt/equity ratios of selected health care organizations

Provider	Book Equity	Market Equity	Book Debt	Book Asset/Equity	Market Asset/Equity
HCA	$4,405,000	$24,229,887	$13,163,000	3.9882	1.5384
HealthSouth	$3,526,454	$ 6,291,176	$ 3,853,986	2.0929	1.6126
Tenet Healthcare	$4,066,000	$ 8,128,627	$ 9,095,000	3.2368	2.1189
Rush-Presbyterian-St. Luke's Medical Center	$ 736,000	N/A	$ 1,256,200	2.7068	N/A

All dollar figures are in thousands

All figures are for the 2000 fiscal years; market prices are for the last trading day of the providers' fiscal years.

Sources: HCA Corporation, 2000 Annual Report; HealthSouth Corporation, *2000 Annual Report*; Tenet Healthcare Corporation, *2000 Annual Report*; Rush-Presbyterian-St. Luke's Medical Center, *2000 Annual Report*; http://www.bigcharts.com; http://www.sec.gov/edgar.shtml

vestor-owned hospitals studied had target capital structures toward which they were moving. McCue found that several variables that represent financial strength (belonging to a system, for example) were positive predictors of the debt/equity ratio. That is, financial strength is related to the use of debt. Very small hospitals in McCue's study tended to use short-term borrowing a great deal, perhaps to cover cash shortfalls.

Myers (1993) described several possible explanations for organizations' strong support of one capital structure over another and for the distribution of capital structures among firms. One explanation is the **pecking order theory**. According to the pecking order theory, organizations prefer to finance their capital purchases with cash provided by operations. Their second choice is to incur debt, and their last choice is to dilute their ownership by issuing equity securities. The pecking order theory predicts that weak organizations will have more debt than strong organizations (as McCue found) because they generate less cash internally. The pecking order theory also predicts that growing organizations will have high debt/equity ratios, because they will outrun their internal cash capacity and will be reluctant to issue stock.

Consider again the possibility of bankruptcy costs that may drive up the cost of debt as the debt/equity ratio rises. Why do bond buyers, facing such possibilities, accept the risk inherent in very high levels of financial leverage? One explanation for investor-owned organizations is that debt requires organizations to pay out their **free cash flow** and, thus, is a way of reducing agency costs (Jensen, 1986). Jensen defined free cash flow as cash flow from operations above that needed to meet debt service requirements *and* to engage in all projects with positive net present values. Thus defined, free cash flow is cash whose best use is distribution to shareholders.

When management exercises substantial discretion as agents, they can retain free cash flow and use it to provide perquisites for themselves. In so doing, they impose agency costs on shareholders, because potential shareholders observe free cash flow's being hoarded. Investors as a group, then, would prefer that firms with substantial free cash flow substitute debt for equity. Taking on greater debt puts more debt service obligation on management. Cash that was free before increasing the debt/equity ratio is now owed to bond holders. Investors as a whole are better off with the higher debt/equity ratios.

Jensen further argued that one can easily identify the firms that are candidates for the debt-for-equity exchanges. These are firms that produce lots of cash but are in industries in which growth opportunities (and thus positive NPV projects) are limited. One can argue that the hospital industry fits that description nicely. Investors' desire to obligate free cash flow, according to Jensen, is one of the motivations for the leveraged buyout wave of the 1980s.

SUMMARY

Health care organizations have a wide variety of external financing options. These include common stock (investor owned only), taxable debt, and tax-exempt debt (government and not-for-profit only). The choice of mix of those financing alternatives is the capital structure decision. In practice, organizations adopt an enormous range of capital structures.

The choice of capital structure is complicated in several ways. First, the choice is important because it influences the organization's cost of capital and, therefore, overall market value. Second, there may be no clearly defined cost-minimizing capital structure. Modigliani and Miller's work, and the research that followed, showed that there may be only a vaguely defined range of optimal capital structures.

Third, the relationship between the cost of capital and the debt/equity ratio depends on the nature of the agency relationships within the organization and is not well understood. A wide range of capital structures can be consistent with organizational survival and success.

Discussion Questions

1. What external financing options are open to investor-owned health care organizations? To private, not-for-profit health care organizations?

2. What are the advantages of debt financing over equity financing? Of equity financing over debt financing?

3. What would determine the optimality of a capital structure (debt/equity mix)?

4. Explain Modigliani and Miller's justification of their basic proposition.

5. What factors might give rise to an optimal capital structure that is not 100 percent debt?

CONTINUING CASE

Henry Kirk and Janet Fowler were in a quandary. Dr. Jackson was interested, once again, in raising cash, both for PCI, Inc., and for himself. He thought that selling new shares of PCI would raise cash, incur no new fixed obligations of cash flow, and provide an opportunity for him to sell some of his own PCI shares. Dr. Jackson held 40 percent of the existing shares in the corporation. No other shareholder held more than 12 percent.

Kirk's instincts told him the move was not in PCI's best interest. "Dr. Jackson (no one in the firm called Dr. Jackson "Roger"), we're very near our ideal capital structure now, $16,370,000 in total liabilities and $18,968,000 in owners' equity, book value. If we sell new shares, or if you sell your own shares, you'll lose some of your control." Kirk, who made no secret of his desire to own equity in PCI, thought to himself that he would not mind either opening up ownership of the closely-held corporation or Dr. Jackson's losing some of his control over the firm.

Dr. Jackson was adamant. "PCI needs the money, and I need the cash. I'll always be in charge here; it will always be my company. Besides, equity is cheaper than debt. Didn't they teach you anything in hospital management school?"

CASE QUESTIONS

1. In what sense is (or is not) PCI, Inc.'s current capital structure optional?

2. Is Dr. Jackson correct about the relative costs of equity and debt?

3. Is Dr. Jackson correct about the permanency of his corporate control?

REFERENCES

Cohodes, D.R. & Kinkead, B.M. (1984). *Hospital capital formation in the 1980s.* Baltimore, MD: Johns Hopkins University Press.

Feldstein, S.G. & Fabozzi, F.J. (1991). Municipal bonds. In F.J. Fabozzi (Ed.), *Handbook of fixed income securities* (3rd ed., pp. 413–441). Homewood, IL: Business One Irwin.

Gapenski, L.C. (1993). Hospital capital structure decisions: Theory and practice. *Health Services Management Research, 6*(4), 237–247.

Jensen, M.C. (1986). Agency costs of free cash flow, corporate finance, and takeovers. *American Economic Review, 76*(2), 323–329.

McCue, M.J. (1992). Determinants of capital structure. *Hospital and Health Services Administration, 37*(3), 333–346.

Miller, M.H. (1977). Debt and taxes. *Journal of Finance, 32*(2), 261–275.

Miller, M.H. (1988). The Modigliani-Miller proposition after thirty years. *Journal of Economic Perspectives, 2*(4), 99–120.

Modigliani, F. & Miller, M.H. (1958). The cost of capital, corporation finance, and the theory of investment. *American Economic Review, 48*(3), 261–297.

Modigliani, F. & Miller, M.H. (1963). Corporate income taxes and the cost of capital: A correction. *American Economic Review, 53*(3), 433–443.

Myers, S.C. (1984). The capital structure puzzle. *Journal of Finance, 39*(3), 575–592.

Myers, S.C. (1993). Still searching for the optimal capital structure. *Journal of Applied Corporate Finance, 6*(1), 4–14.

Weston, J.F. (1989). What MM have wrought. *Financial Management, 18*(2), 29-38.

SELECTED READINGS

Brealey, R.A. & Myers, S.C. (1991). *Principles of corporate finance* (4th ed.). New York: McGraw-Hill.

Gapenski, L.C. (1993). Hospital capital structure decisions: Theory and practice. *Health Services Management Research, 6*(4), 237–247.

McCue, M.J. (1992). Determinants of capital structure. *Hospital and Health Services Administration, 37*(3), 333–346

Miller, M.H. (1988). The Modigliani-Miller proposition after thirty years. *Journal of Economic Perspectives, 2*(4), 99–120.

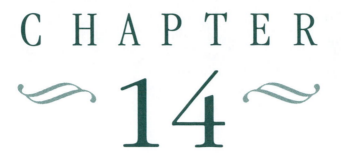

CHAPTER
14

Procedures for
Long-Term Financing

Learning Objectives

After reading this chapter, the student should be able to:

1. Interact effectively with investment bankers and other financing professionals.
2. Explain basic procedures and regulations involved in long-term financing.
3. List and explain the roles of the professionals involved in arranging long-term financing.
4. Explain the contents of a financing prospectus to a skeptical board of directors.

Key Terms

Best efforts basis	Mandatory
Bond counsel	registration
Bond insurance	Mezzanine financing
Due diligence	Specialist
Feasibility study	Trustee
Full disclosure	Underwrite
Insider trading	Underwriter's spread

External financing (funds obtained from outside the organization) has to come from someone and has to come through some channel. Those someones, individuals and institutions, are called *investors*, the suppliers of funds pictured in Figure 9–1. The channels through which funds flow from investors to users, the institutions who manage those channels, and the procedures that the users of funds must employ to tap external funds are the subjects of this chapter.

One chapter in a comprehensive textbook cannot make its reader an expert in external financing procedures. After reading this chapter, however, the reader will have a basic understanding of financing procedures and will be prepared to deal with experts in this area.

ACTORS AND FRICTIONS

The image of a market operating without interference, to serve the interests of buyers and sellers, lies at the heart of economic analysis. Economists are not so naive as to believe that market processes are really so ideal, in financial, or any other, markets. Rather, individuals and institutions (accountants, attorneys, auditors, brokers, custodians, dealers, investment bankers, printers, and trustees) stand between buyers and sellers. Not worthless drones or leeches, these actors facilitate exchange.

The payments made to these facilitators ("a cut off the top") are frictions in the market. In physics, theoretical motion is impeded by the presence of friction. Physical friction robs the motion of an object of energy, produces heat (sometimes a lot of heat), and causes the observed speed, acceleration, and distance traveled of the object to be less than it would be in a frictionless world. In financial markets, the frictions caused by the presence of facilitators deprives the parties to any transaction of some of the returns they would otherwise have received. These institutional frictions can produce a form of heat: legal and regulatory proceedings.

Why then, are all of these "unnecessary" actors involved in the process? In the exchange of securities, users of funds receive money now, in return for which they promise to pay cash flows in the future. The suppliers of funds will not enter into such contracts unless they believe that the user will be able to pay the contractual cash flows and that the contract is enforceable (that is, that in addition to being *able* to make the contractual payments, the user of funds *will*, in fact, make the payments). That is why accountants and auditors enter into the process and why legally binding documentation is necessary. Trustees and attorneys are introduced into the process to ensure that contracts are to be enforced.

If the contract implicit in a security's sale is enforceable, the security can be taken to market. Few issuers of securities have the network of contacts to be able to sell stocks or bonds to suppliers of funds (in fact, doing so is called "self-dealing," and is tightly regulated). Rather, specialists in bringing securities to market (brokers, dealers, and investment bankers) offer their services, taking a fee for their trouble. Someone must guarantee the possession of the securities, either in paper form or, more common today, in electronic form. That custodianship is the role of yet other specialists, individual custodians and depository institutions.

Chapter 2 dealt with a recurring theme in health care financial management, agency problems and agency costs. Financial market facilitators are agents of the users of funds who hire them, and agency problems abound when one obtains external financing. One should understand the roles of those facilitators, so that one can manage the agency problems they bring with them and mitigate the agency costs that can decrease the value of the organization.

Anyone who has ever taken out a mortgage, borrowed to finance an automobile or a college education, or leased a computer or television knows that there are strict procedures one must follow to obtain financing. In general, the greater the amount to be borrowed, the more complex are the procedures involved. In general, any issuance of securities, debt, or equity must include **full disclosure** of all relevant information. The requirement of full disclosure in securities offerings long predates the passage of the federal Truth in Lending Act, which extended such requirements to consumer and mortgage loans.

The process for determining that one has followed the appropriate procedures, obeyed all applicable laws, and made all necessary disclosures is called **due diligence**. Performing due diligence can protect one from certain types of liability; failure to perform due diligence can expose one to substantial legal liability.

REGULATORS AND REGULATION

Regulators are critical players in securities markets and therefore in external financing. American securities law, as it affects the issuers of securities, is based on the Securities Act of 1933, the Securities Exchange Act of 1934, the common law that has evolved in the courts, and applicable state laws. Securities sold in interstate commerce are subject to regulation under federal law and to registration in each state in which they are offered.

Securities law is a complex, technical field, well beyond the scope of this text. There are a few themes that underlie securities regulation in the United States. Under the separation-of-powers clause of the U.S. Constitution, the federal government has only limited power to oversee the issuance of bonds by state and local governments. Many of the provisions of the 1933 and 1934 acts do not apply at all to the municipal sector, and most provisions do not apply to very small issues of securities.

Mandatory registration is one of those basic principles of federal securities law (federal registration is not required of municipal securities, including hospital revenue bonds). Non-municipal securities that are to be offered for sale to the public must be registered with the U.S. Securities and Exchange Commission (SEC) and with state securities commissioners (Pointer & Schroeder, 1986). Registration does not imply that the SEC endorses or recommends the securities as investments but does guarantee that certain information is on file and that certain procedures have been followed.

Full disclosure is a duty of every securities issuer and of the agents of those issuers. Under the "general anti-fraud provisions" of the 1933 act, the duty of full disclosure *does* apply to municipal, as well as to corporate, securities. The duty of full disclosure requires that the issuers of publicly offered securities disclose, in their prospectuses, all materially relevant information about themselves to all who would consider purchasing their securities. Such warts-and-all disclosure can be embarrassing. Some hypothetical examples of facts that *must* be disclosed (if they be true) include the following: (1) Mr. Smith, the Chief Executive Officer of the Hospital, served a 6-month probated sentence for misappropriating funds from a previous employer; (2) the local health care market is becoming increasingly competitive, threatening the cash flows of the health system; and (3) local public officials have suggested that the hospital should provide more free care to the public, a requirement that could jeopardize the organization's ability to meet its debt obligations.

Once an organization has issued securities to the public, it must continue to disclose all materially relevant information about itself so long as those securities are in the public's hands. In the investor-owned sector, that disclosure takes the form of filing quarterly (form 10-Q) and annual (form 10-K) forms with the SEC. These are now available for all but the very smallest publicly traded firms in electronic form. The SEC's "Electronic Data Gathering and Retrieval" (EDGAR) system is available at no charge at http://www.sec.gov/edgar.shtml.

A related, and controversial, principle of securities regulation that affects every issuing organization is that of no **insider trading** (trading by insiders on the basis of material information gained through a position of fiduciary responsibility). Insiders have access to information prior to its disclosure to the public. Were they to sell (buy) securities the day before an announcement of bad (good) news, they could earn substantial profits at the expense of an uninformed public. To prevent this from happening, insiders (broadly defined to include managers, trustees, attorneys, accountants, investment bankers, and financial printers) may not trade for their own accounts, or for the accounts of others, on the basis of such information. They must hold securities of their organization for at least 6 months after purchase, and they may not breach their fiduciary duties by disclosing inside information to others who can use the information to make gainful trades.

An old adage, well worth remembering, says, "If you don't know the law, know a lawyer." When contemplating issuing securities, confer early and often with legal counsel, your own and that of your investment baker.

MIDDLEMEN

Health care organizations (and other types of nonfinancial organizations) are not equipped to sell their own securities. In fact, even if a health care organization could sell its own securities, it would risk running afoul of the "no self-dealing" restrictions embedded in securities regulation. Several types of specialized organizations have developed to bring new securities to market, and it is to one or more of them that a health care provider should turn to access the capital market. Among these middlemen are investment bankers, brokers, dealers, advisers, and exchanges. Those categories represent separate functions, but several of those functions may be performed by the same organization.

Investment bakers are specialists in bringing securities to market (Bloch, 1986). Investment banking firms (such as Merrill Lynch and Goldman Sachs) are distinct from commercial banking organizations (such as Citibank), separated by the Banking Act of 1937 (also known as the Glass-Steigel Act). Under Glass-Steigel, commercial banks may not underwrite securities except in the municipal sector. This prohibition is breaking down, as some commercial banks have set up independent subsidiaries to engage in securities underwriting.

Typically, an investment banking firm will act as the lead in the financing team (Shields, 1983). In that capacity, the investment banker will act as adviser to the issuer. The advisory service is usually performed for an hourly fee (although some investment banking firms will waive the advisory fee if they also serve as underwriter). Some small investment banking firms, including some specializing in serving the health care sector, limit their services to captaining the team and acting as an adviser.

Often the investment banker will, prior to the sale of the securities, agree to **underwrite** them. That means that the investment banker will guarantee a net proceed per share (or per bond) to the issuer. The difference between the gross price paid by the investor and the price guaranteed to the issuer is the **underwriter's spread**. The underwriter's spread, usually 1 or 2 percent of the gross price, is the source of profit for the underwriter. Some issues of securities are not underwritten but are sold on a **best efforts basis**. Under such an arrangement, the investment banker agrees to make his or her best effort to sell the securities for a fee. Often, especially for large issues of securities, one investment banker is unwilling to underwrite an entire issue alone. In such a case, the lead underwriter establishes a syndicate, with each of several underwriting firms taking a share of the total issue.

When marketing securities to the public, the investment banker is acting as a dealer. Securities dealers purchase securities for and sell securities from their own accounts. One of the most important functions of the investment banker is his or her willingness to "make a market" in the issue after it is sold to the public. That is, to bolster the confidence of investors, and to avoid having to pay a premium based on investors' fear that the issue will be illiquid (fear that they will be unable to resell their holdings), investment bankers announce their intentions to maintain an inventory of securities and to post *bid* (what they will pay) and *ask* (what they demand to be paid) prices for the securities for the foreseeable future. That willingness to make a market is unimportant for issues of stocks listed on the organized exchanges, but is very important for bonds and for stocks traded over the counter.

Dealers are distinguished from brokers in that brokers take orders from the public and fill them by acting as agents, making contact with dealers or other, on the floor of an organized exchange, finding another broker representing another member of the public. Virtually all dealers also act as brokers.

After securities are offered to the public, they can be traded (if they continue to meet the registration and reporting requirements) in secondary markets. There are two types of secondary markets in the United States, negotiated markets (over-the-counter transactions) and auction markets (organized exchanges). Most bond trading and much stock trading is done in the over-the-counter market. In that sector of the capital market, dealers post bid and ask prices. Brokers, representing individual investors, are required to seek the "best execution" of an order, usually meaning obtaining the lowest ask price or the highest bid price posted. Many stocks are traded in this way through the National Association of Securities Dealers Automated Quotation (NASDAQ) system.

Stocks of most of the largest American corporations, and a relatively small number of bonds, are listed on one or more organized stock exchanges. The best known of these are the New York Stock Exchange and the American Stock Exchange. A small number of regional exchanges (for example, the Chicago Stock Exchange, the Philadelphia Stock Exchange, and the Pacific Stock Exchange) offer trading in the shares of regionally important but smaller corporations.

To be listed on an organized exchange, a corporation must meet the exchange's listing requirements (number and geographic distribution of shareholders, corporate governance regulations) and must pay a listing fee. The exchange then assigns a member firm, a **specialist**, to make an orderly market in that corporation's stock. Trades are made when floor brokers, placing bids through the specialist, find willing sellers or buyers. The system is an auction market because prices are set by floor brokers' making their trading desires known through open outcry.

HANGERS-ON

In addition to the middlemen who bring securities to market, a great many other professionals and organizers participate in the financing process. For municipal bond financing (including hospital revenue bond financing), someone must verify that the bond does, in fact, qualify as tax-exempt (that the interest on the bond is not subject to federal and, in many cases, state income tax). That verification is the role of the **bond counsel**, an attorney hired for that purpose by the bond issuer.

Every security that is offered for sale to the public must, under the Securities Act of 1933, be described in a prospectus, providing full disclosure to potential buyers. Part of that full disclosure is provision of financial statements. Those statements must be audited by a certified public accountant.

Another role often, but not always, played by certified public accountants is that of conducting the **feasibility study**. Hospital revenue bonds must be issued for specific purposes. The feasibility study discloses what the expected financial position of the issuer will be after the specific purpose is complete. For example, if the purpose of a hospital revenue bond financing is to construct an outpatient diagnostic center, the feasibility study will describe the project; project the utilization of the center; and present a pro forma financial statement, forecasting the position of the organization after the center is functioning.

Someone, usually the investment banker acting as adviser, must check that all statements in the prospectus are true, that all numbers add up, and that all representations are accurate. That process is known as a due diligence review. Its performance is a mandatory part of securities issuance.

The prospectus must be printed. Although that sounds trite and obvious, financial printing is a major industry, highly concentrated, geographically, in lower Manhattan. The first printing of the prospectus, the preliminary statement or "red herring," is printed and placed in limited circulation without any yields or securities prices being included. The final prospectus includes the interest rate the securities will offer (for a bond) and the price at which the securities are offered (for stocks and for bonds). Those yields and prices are set at the close of the market on the day prior to the security's final SEC registration and offering to the public. The financing team must be able to enter those crucial numbers into their calculations and the printer must be able to deliver the final prospectus overnight.

Many financings involve several stages, and are not completed until several procedures are complete. In such cases, the sale of securities to the public is possible only after some intermediate transactions take place. Thus several business days transpire between the offering of securities and the collection of cash by the issuer. Commercial banks, or other intermediaries, often provide **mezzanine financing**, short-term financing to be repaid from the proceeds of the securities offering. One commercial bank trust department serves as the **trustee** of each bond offering, acting as the bond holders' representative, ensuring that all bond covenants (agreements between the bond issuer and the bond holders specified in the bond's terms of offering or trust indenture) are kept and suing the bond issuer if they are not.

One of the most important parties to the funding process is the bond rating agency. Bond rating agencies are private corporations that evaluate debt issues for their credit-worthiness. Among the best known of these firms are Standard and Poor's, Moody's Investors Services, and Duff and Phelps. The bond issuer pays a fee to have its new issue rated. The initial rating appears on the cover of the bond prospectus. Bonds not rated at the time of issue (and those rated below investment grade) bear an alluring nickname: *junk*. During the life of the bond, the rater follows the creditworthiness of the bond, upgrading or downgrading the issue as determined by the rater's staff of analysts. Investors are very sensitive to ratings, and the risk premium in required yield associated with a one-category change in rating is substantial.

Ratings categories differ from agency to agency, but generally run from AAA+ (the very best; no possibility of default) to D (already in default). Although the rating agencies insist that the rating process is not mechanistic, there are a few factors that are known to weigh heavily in rating decisions. These include bed size (larger hospitals tend to have better ratings), share of total bed days paid for by government payors (a higher Medicare and Medicaid share leads to a higher rating), financial liquidity (the more liquid, the higher the rating), and profitability (the more profitable, the higher the rating) (McCue, Renn, & Pillari, 1990).

A FINANCING TALE

To illustrate the roles of the players, including the regulators, in the external financing process, consider a hypothetical not-for-profit organization, Regional Health System (RHS), about to construct an off-site diagnostic center (Thomas Arthur discusses the financing process in detail in Shields, 1983, Chapter 10). After consideration by management, preliminary approval by the trustees, and discussion with a planning consultant, RHS is prepared to proceed with its financing and construction. As a not-for-profit organization, RHS will not issue common stock but will finance the facility with some type of debt security.

RHS would contact an investment banker to serve, first, in the financial adviser capacity. The financial adviser would meet with RHS's senior management, discuss the current and (expected) future state of financial markets, and gain approval for the composition of the financing team. In most states, the financial adviser would also help RHS to obtain approval from the state's Certificate of Need (CON) authority. The application for the CON would contain much of the same information as the prospectus for the bonds to be issued later, so the financial adviser is a key player in its preparation. The financial adviser is compensated for each hour of service.

Because RHS is a not-for-profit health care provider, it can use the municipal bond market to obtain financing. That is, an issue of tax-exempt hospital revenue bonds is probably the best way to finance the new facility. RHS, however, cannot merely decide that its bonds will be municipal bonds; only units of state or local government can issue municipal bonds. RHS's financial adviser must contact the appropriate bond-issuing authority (the identity of that authority varies from state to state) and obtain its cooperation (usually for a fee) in the issuing process. The financial adviser or the issuing unit of government must also bring onto the financing team a bond counsel, a specialist in determining whether or not the issue will, in fact, be tax-exempt. The bond counsel's statement in the bond prospectus has important implications for every tax-paying investor and is a crucial element in the marketing of the bonds.

The financial adviser will engage a consultant to prepare a feasibility study for the bond prospectus. That study, a part of full disclosure, informs potential investors of the type of facility to be built, its probable utilization, and of the projected financial position of RHS after completion of the project and assumption of the associated debt. Other members of the financing team are also brought into the process at this time. These include an auditor to audit the financial statements of RHS, a facilities consultant, and the financial adviser's attorney to ensure that all applicable regulations are followed.

The financial adviser will also take the RHS through the rating process. This will include preparing materials to submit to the agency or agencies chosen to rate the bond and making the presentation to the rater's analysts at their offices in New York or Chicago. This activity can be worth millions of dollars, as poor ratings mean high required yields, and knowledge of what the rater is looking for can mean the difference between a good rating and a bad one.

At this point, the term structure of the bond offering is determined; not all of bonds in a single issue must mature on the same date (and, when maturities vary, required yields will vary as well). The investment banker now steps out of the adviser role and into the underwriter's role. Some health care organizations prefer to pay a financial adviser who is not to be the underwriter. Increasingly, however, the same firm is both adviser and underwriter.

The financial adviser or the underwriter supervises the preparation of an initial prospectus, providing all of the information a potential investor needs, except the yield and price of the proposed bonds. This is the first step in which the parties must meet the requirement of due diligence, ensuring that all material statements are accurate. The preliminary prospectus (or preliminary statement) is known as a "red herring," because of the red ink that marks it as preliminary. Acting as a dealer, the underwriter circulates the red herring to potential investors during the offering period.

As a municipal issuer, RHS is not subject to federal registration. It is, however, subject to state securities laws, known as "blue sky laws" (because they prevent securities issuers from promising investors "the blue sky"). The underwriter's attorney has the responsibility of seeing that all applicable blue sky requirements are met.

As the offering date draws near, the underwriter, meeting with RHS (and keeping the municipal bond issuing authority informed), sets an interest rate (or rates, if maturities vary) for the bonds. This rate depends on market conditions, the riskiness of the bonds implied by the rating assigned to them, and their maturities. Ideally, the bonds' yield will be set so that the bonds sell at their par (face) value. The underwriter has agreed to turn over a set proportion of the par value to the issuer. The difference between the price of the bonds and the negotiated net proceeds to the issuer is the underwriter's spread and is the financial reward for underwriting.

If the underwriter places a yield higher than investors require on the bonds, the risk that bonds will go unsold, generating an unwanted inventory of bonds and a loss for the underwriter, declines. Underwriters, then, have an incentive to place higher-than-market yields on bonds, forcing unnecessarily high interest payments on the issuer (because yields and prices vary inversely with one another, this tendency of underwriters is also called *underpricing*; see Bloch, 1986, pp. 127–130). If the underwriter is successful in pursuing that interest, the present value of the additional interest expense borne by the issuer is an agency cost, reducing the value of the issuing organization (see Chapter 2).

With the interest rate set, and investors (who have examined the red herring) at the ready, the financing team is ready for the final session. Closing papers, obligating the issuer to the terms of the trust indenture, must be signed, just as they would in a private mortgage financing. In a final working session, often an "all-nighter," the yield(s) are entered into the prospectus and all pro forma (projected) financial statements are recalculated to reflect the effect of that specific interest rate. The data and projections are checked (due diligence again) for accuracy and given to the printer, who will produce the final prospectus (see Figure 14–1).

Were RHS required to do so, its would send its prospectus to the Washington offices of the U.S. Securities and Exchange Commission via courier on the morning after its printing. With a quick stamp-in registration, the bonds would be registered and ready, after a required delay, for sale. As RHS is making a municipal offering, federal registration is not required. State registration, however, may be necessary prior to formal offering.

With the prospectus printed and properly registered, closing documents signed, and trustee engaged, the underwriter, acting as dealer, can now call investors and offer the securities. If the underwriter has done its job, the bonds will be sold before the close of business on the first offering day. RHS will receive its funds a few days later, after transfers are completed.

TO INSURE OR NOT TO INSURE: AN NPV PROBLEM

A useful innovation in municipal bond financing has been the emergence of **bond insurance**. When an issue is insured, the insurer, usually a consortium of insurance companies, such as the Municipal Bond Insurance Association (MBIA), guarantees that the bond holders will receive all of their promised payments. It is the enormous potential liability of the insurer that has caused the formation of consortiums to issue bond insurance.

The issuer of the bond pays the insurer a premium for its services. In return, the issuer's creditworthiness is enhanced. Now, not only is the issuer standing behind the bond issue, but so is the insurer. Clearly, only highly stable and creditworthy insurers carry any weight in the market. Therefore a small number of well-capitalized consortiums dominate this market. Bonds insured by the major players in this market are almost always rated AAA by the major rating firms. The benefit to the issuer is the lower yield associated with the AAA rating. Carpenter (1991) found a substantial reduction in interest payments associated with taking out bond insurance. Note that the bonds whose prospectus is shown in Figure 14–1 were insured by the Municipal Bond Investors Assurance Corporation (see the upper right corner of the cover sheet).

When should one insure one's bonds? The solution is a simple application of net present value analysis. The premium payment to the insurer is an initial cash outflow ($CFAT_0 < 0$). Over the life of the bond, usually every 6 months, the issuer enjoys a cash savings ($CFAT_t > 0$). That savings represents the difference between the interest that the issuer would have to pay, given its credit rating, were the bonds not insured and the interest that the bond issuer has to pay, given that the bonds are insured. The net present value of the insurance purchase is the present value of the interest savings minus the initial insurance premium. If the net present value of the insurance is at least zero, then one enhances the value of the organization by insuring the bonds.

SUMMARY

External financing is a complex process, requiring the services of a large number of experts. One approaches the process only after a lot of preparation. The process of selling securities to the public requires months of effort and tens of thousands of dollars in expense. External financing, however, as discussed in Chapter 15, is often the key to organizational survival and growth.

OFFICIAL STATEMENT

Ratings: **Moody's: Aaa**
Standard & Poor's: AAA
Insured by Municipal
Bond Investors
Assurance Corporation
(See "Ratings" herein)

$32,308,281.35
County of Pitt, North Carolina
Pitt County Memorial Hospital Revenue Bonds,
Series 1989

Dated December 1, 1989   Due December 1, as shown below
(except Capital Appreciation Bonds, which are dated the date of delivery)

THE BONDS ARE LIMITED OBLIGATIONS OF THE COUNTY OF PITT, NORTH CAROLINA (THE "COUNTY"), PAYABLE SOLELY FROM AND SECURED BY A PLEDGE OF NET REVENUES (AS DEFINED HEREIN) FROM THE OPERATION UNDER LEASE FROM THE COUNTY BY PITT COUNTY MEMORIAL HOSPITAL, INCORPORATED, A NORTH CAROLINA NON-PROFIT CORPORATION (THE "CORPORATION"), OF PITT COUNTY MEMORIAL HOSPITAL LOCATED IN GREENVILLE, NORTH CAROLINA, AND CERTAIN FUNDS AND ACCOUNTS ESTABLISHED UNDER THE BOND ORDER AND THE SERIES RESOLUTION (BOTH AS DEFINED HEREIN) AND HELD BY FIRST-CITIZENS BANK & TRUST COMPANY, RALEIGH, NORTH CAROLINA, AS TRUSTEE. NEITHER THE FAITH AND CREDIT NOR THE TAXING POWER OF THE COUNTY OR THE STATE OF NORTH CAROLINA OR ANY POLITICAL SUBDIVISION THEREOF IS PLEDGED FOR THE PAYMENT OF THE BONDS, NOR WILL THE BONDS BE OR BE DEEMED TO BE AN OBLIGATION OF THE COUNTY OR THE STATE OF NORTH CAROLINA OR ANY POLITICAL SUBDIVISION THEREOF, OTHER THAN OF THE COUNTY TO THE EXTENT OF THE AFOREMENTIONED SOURCES.

The Bonds are issuable as fully registered bonds. When issued, the Bonds will be registered in the name of Cede & Co., as nominee of The Depository Trust Company ("DTC"), New York, New York. So long as Cede & Co. is the registered owner of the Bonds, principal and interest payments on the Bonds will be made to Cede & Co., which will in turn remit such payments to the DTC Participants (as defined herein) and DTC Indirect Participants (as defined herein) for subsequent disbursement to the beneficial owners of the Bonds. Interest on the Current Interest Bonds (as set forth below) is payable on June 1, 1990 and semiannually thereafter on each December 1 and June 1. Purchases of Bonds will be made in book-entry form only, and individual purchasers will not receive physical delivery of bond certificates. Interest on the Capital Appreciation Bonds is not payable semiannually but is payable at maturity or upon prior redemption. Individual purchases of Current Interest Bonds will be made in the principal amount of $5,000 or any integral multiple thereof. Individual purchases of Capital Appreciation Bonds will be made in the maturity amount of $5,000 or any integral multiple thereof. So long as Cede & Co. is the registered owner of the Bonds, references herein to the holders or registered holders of the Bonds shall mean Cede & Co. and shall not mean the beneficial owners of the Bonds. See "The Bonds — Book-Entry-Only System."

The Bonds are subject to optional and mandatory redemption prior to maturity as more fully described herein.

Payment of the principal of and interest on the Bonds when due will be guaranteed by a municipal bond insurance policy issued simultaneously with the delivery of the Bonds by

Municipal Bond Investors Assurance Corporation.

$2,000,000 Current Interest Serial Bonds
(plus accrued interest from December 1, 1989)

Year	Amount	Interest Rate	Price	Year	Amount	Interest Rate	Price
1990	$200,000	5.70%	100%	1995	$200,000	6.15%	100%
1991	200,000	5.80	100	1996	200,000	6.20	100
1992	200,000	5.90	100	1997	200,000	6¼	100
1993	200,000	6	100	1998	200,000	6.30	100
1994	200,000	6.10	100	1999	200,000	6.40	100

$1,458,281.35 Capital Appreciation Serial Bonds

Year	Amount	Approximate Yield to Maturity	Price Per $1,000 Maturity Amount	Year	Amount	Approximate Yield to Maturity	Price Per $1,000 Maturity Amount
2000	$112,079.25	6½ %	$498.13	2003	$433,160.50	6.65%	$402.94
2001	97,561.80	6.55	464.58	2004	445,367,40	6.65	377.43
2002	370,112.40	6.60	432.88				

$6,740,000 6⅝% Current Interest Term Bonds Due December 1, 2009 — Price 98%

$22,110,000 6⅝% Current Interest Term Bonds Due December 1, 2019 — Price 97%

(plus accrued interest from December 1, 1989)

In the opinion of Bond Counsel, assuming compliance with the provisions of the Internal Revenue Code of 1986, as amended (the "Code"), as described herein, interest on the Bonds is not includable in the gross income of the recipients thereof for federal income tax purposes. Interest on the Bonds may be included in the calculation of certain taxes, including the alternative minimum tax on corporations as described under "Tax Exemption" herein. See "Tax Exemption" herein for a description of certain provisions of the Code that may affect the tax treatment of interest on the Bonds for certain registered owners of Bonds and for exemptions from taxation under the laws of the State of North Carolina.

The Bonds are offered subject to prior sale, when, as and if issued by the County and accepted by the Underwriters, subject to the approval of Brown & Wood, New York, New York, Bond Counsel. Certain legal matters will be passed upon for the County by Speight, Watson & Brewer, Greenville, North Carolina, for the Corporation by Poyner & Spruill, Raleigh, North Carolina, and for the Underwriters by Robinson, Bradshaw & Hinson, P.A., Charlotte, North Carolina. It is expected that the Bonds will be available for delivery to DTC in New York, New York on or about January 9, 1990.

The First Boston Corporation

First Union Securities, Inc.	The Robinson-Humphrey Company, Inc.
Interstate/Johnson Lane Corporation	Wachovia Bank and Trust
J. C. Bradford & Co.	Company, N.A.
NCNB National Bank	Wheat, First Securities, Inc.

The date of this Official Statement is December 20, 1989.

Figure 14-1 The cover of the proposal for an issue of hoispital revenue bonds.

Attorneys, accountants, financial specialists, brokers, bond insurers, regulators, and state bond authorities all have roles to play in the financing process. Health care organizations should rely on advisers whom they trust to help them in financing. Health care organizations should also understand what they are getting into, so that their advisers don't burden them with many years of agency costs.

Discussion Questions

1. Given the procedural and regulatory nightmares involved in selling securities to the public, why would any organization want to do so?

2. Give (and explain) a rule for deciding when selling bonds to the public is preferable to obtaining a bank loan.

3. Give (and explain) a rule for deciding when to purchase bond insurance.

4. What are the three major roles of an investment banker? Can they be performed by separate firms for a single issue of securities?

5. What are some implications of the prohibition of trading on the basis of inside information? Is that prohibition, on balance, worth retaining?

CONTINUING CASE

Roger Jackson was as nervous as he had ever been. Discussions of PCI, Inc.'s potential issue of additional common stock (see the Continuing Case for Chapter 13) had progressed. Now he, Henry Kirk, Janet Fowler, and Jack Hernandez were having lunch at a small restaurant in Dallas. At 1:30, they would meet with a representative of NT Securities, an investment bank specializing in small firms.

Jack Hernandez is a dentist, a long-time tenant of Physicians Clinic, and the second-largest shareholder of PCI, Inc. Jackson and Hernandez, together, control exactly 51 percent of PCI's shares.

"Jack, old buddy, have another glass of wine?" Jackson patronized. Hernandez was calm and thoughtful, deeply distrustful of the deal they might make.

At 1:30, the group from Jamestown met with John Powers of NT Securities in a 30th-floor conference room. Powers outlined some issues to consider. The anticipated expenses of preparing a small issue would be $100,000. NT Securities would expect a 2 percent underwriters' spread. NT was prepared to make a market in the stock once it was sold to the public.

"You might even be better off going to a bank. A big bank," Powers offered. "And have you ever thought about the effects of making a public offering, and being listed on NASDAQ, on your status with regulators? The two of you stand to lose your control of the corporation."

"Regulators? What regulators?" Powers's last question took Dr. Jackson by surprise.

CASE QUESTIONS

1. What issues (cost, regulatory) should PCI, Inc., consider in its choice of a public offering versus bank financing?

2. If PCI, Inc.'s choice is between a bank loan (8 percent per year for 30 years, with zero origination fees) and the small issue Powers described, what cost-of-capital differential makes the equity issue the better choice? (Don't forget all of the costs of flotation and the tax deductibility of interest payments.)

REFERENCES

Bloch, E. (1986). *Inside investment banking*. Homewood, IL: Dow Jones-Irwin.

Carpenter, C.E. (1991). The marginal effect of bond insurance on hospital, tax-exempt bond yields. *Inquiry, 28*(1), 67–73.

McCue, M.J., Renn, S.C., & Pillari, G.D. (1990). Factors affecting credit rating downgrades of hospital revenue bonds. *Inquiry, 27*(3), 242–254.

Pointer, L.G. & Schroeder, R.G. (1986). *An introduction to the securities and exchange commission*. Plano, TX: Business Publications.

Shields, G.R. (Ed.). (1983). *Debt financing and capital formation in health care institutions*. Rockville, MD: Aspen Systems Corporation.

SELECTED READINGS

Brealey, R.A. & Myers, S.C. (2000). *Principles of corporate finance* (6th ed.). New York: McGraw-Hill.

Shields, G.R. (Ed.). (1983). *Debt financing and capital formation in health care institutions*. Rockville, MD: Aspen Systems Corporation.

CHAPTER

15

Access to Capital and Organizational Viability

Learning Objectives

After reading this chapter, the student should be able to:

1. Explain the role of external financing in organizational growth and survival.
2. Explain the role of reimbursement policies in health care organizations' access to capital.
3. Explain the factors that influence not-for-profit providers' costs of capital.
4. Explain the relationship between the cost of capital for a not-for-profit health care provider and that of an otherwise equivalent taxable corporation.

Early in the film version of Tom Wolfe's *The Right Stuff*, the press liaison at Edwards Air Force Base explains to a group of test pilots why they need media coverage. The attention of reporters, he explains, means public support, and public support means funding. "Funding, that's what makes your rockets go up. . . . No bucks, no Buck Rogers."

Modern health care delivery shares with space exploration and every other technologically based endeavor the need for external funding. Without access to external funding, organizations are starved for capital, denied emerging technologies, and doomed to obsolescence and failure. Without access to external capital, the miracles of modern medical intervention are impossible. It is not that concern for capital markets is the province of mercenary providers and the financial specialists who serve them; access to capital has serious consequences for the public's health. Cleverly (1990) found access to external financing to be one of the principal determinants of hospital survival. Those organizations that did not survive, that closed their doors, were those least able to obtain funds from the capital market.

Although the "no bucks, no Buck Rogers" dictum certainly holds in institutional health care settings, both federal and state governments have retreated from direct provision of external financing for health care organizations, both hospitals and others. In the post–World War II era, much of the nation's hospital construction and capital needs were met via federal grants under the Hill-Burton Act (the Hospital Survey and Construction Act of 1946). In that same era, many hospitals that were owned by local governments were heavily subsidized by them. In the 1960s many urban neighborhoods were the beneficiaries of grants for the construction and operation of Neighborhood Health Centers and of Community Mental Health Centers.

Today, average taxpayer support of city and county hospitals has declined; and federal funding of the Hill-Burton and Neighborhood programs has evaporated. As a result, health care organizations have had to go to the capital market for external funding. Although that is not all bad, it does impose special constraints on those organizations. In particular, when organizations seek funds in the capital market, they must accept the discipline of that market. One test of project feasibility, not present when funds were provided from the public treasury or from private charity, is that of the market's willingness to provide funds. Funds may be available, at attractive interest rates, to construct outpatient surgery centers but may not be available to establish neonatal intensive care units. Now financial considerations take an important place among the reasons to initiate or not to initiate a health care program.

After reading this chapter, the reader will have a better understanding of how the external financing process influences the ability of health care organizations to fulfill their missions. This chapter also discusses some public policy issues that bear on the abilities of health care organizations to finance their assets.

THE PROBLEMS

One of the most frequently cited changes in the health care arena is the rapid development of technology and the rapid spread of technological innovation.

Practicing physicians (and not very old ones at that) often comment that the three most widely used imaging technologies (ultrasound, CAT, and MRI) did not exist when they were graduated from medical school. The monitoring technology of intensive care is less than 40 years old. The tests used today to diagnose and monitor such common conditions as diabetes mellitus are both different from and more accurate than those available 20 years ago.

New technologies, by their very natures, require external financing. To acquire, install, and put to use costly, newly developed equipment often requires injections of funds. Existing product lines are, often, unable to generate sufficient cash flows to finance new product lines. That financing of new ventures and new technologies is the traditional role of the capital market.

Thus, with health care organizations impelled to seek funds in the capital market to acquire the physical capital they need to render services, they gain a new set of stakeholders, the providers of capital. As suggested in Chapter 9, every user of funds competes with every other user in the capital market. There is no such thing as "health care capital." Every organization seeking funds must pay the yield that the market requires, given the riskiness, tax status, term to maturity, and liquidity of the securities it offers. Being a health care provider or being a not-for-profit entity does not entitle one to pay a lower yield than one's capital market competitors. One's capital market competitors form a much larger and much more diverse group than one's service market competitors.

Investors, acting in their roles as investors, are not grantors of charity. They do not accept smaller yields from worthy organizations than they would from any other. That fact is, the reader may remember, one of the pillars of finance (maximizing behavior) discussed in the introduction of this book. In fact, investors who have fiduciary responsibility for the funds they oversee (pension advisers, trust officers) would violate that responsibility were they to accept lower yields from health care providers, everything else equal, than from other users of funds.

The users of funds and the discipline of the financial marketplace, then, influence and limit what services can be offered and what technology acquired by health care organizations (Wilson, Sheps, & Oliver, 1982).

THE SOLUTIONS

There was a time, so goes the conventional wisdom, when hospitals' capital needs were relatively small and they were met largely by internally generated cash, private philanthropy, and government grants (Cohodes & Kinkaid, 1984; Gray, 1986). By the beginning of the 1970s, however, debt had become a major source of funds for both not-for-profit and government-owned hospitals. By the end of that decade, the importance of investor-owned providers had begun to grow rapidly, introducing large volumes of equity capital to the hospital care sector. Investor ownership continued to be the norm in some health care settings, especially long-term care, medical equipment, medical and dental supplies, pharmaceuticals, medical and dental practice, and personal care products.

National policy recognized and facilitated both the increase in debt financing and the allocation of equity capital to health care. States (and their units of local government) were allowed to issue bonds whose interest is tax exempt on behalf of private health care organizations. For not-for-profit organizations, those became known as *hospital revenue bonds* (backed by the revenues of the organization on whose behalf they are issued). For investor-owned organizations, industrial development bonds were the tax-exempt vehicle. Although the use of industrial development bonds for investor-owned facilities was essentially eliminated by federal tax reform legislation in 1986, hospital revenue bonds are still issued every business day.

Access to borrowing using tax-free long-term bonds encouraged capital formation in health care organizations in several ways. Assume that a AA-rated corporate bond requires a yield to maturity of r_C (the subscript C is for *corporate*). If issued at par, r_C is also the bond's annual coupon rate (see Chapter 9). Because those coupon payments are taxable income for the investor, she keeps only $r_C \times (1-T_P)$, of annual return, where T_P is the personal tax rate.

The holder of a hospital revenue bond, however, keeps all of the interest she receives because that interest is not taxable (see Chapter 13). $r_C \times (1- T_P)$, then, is the lowest rate the investor would accept for purchasing a AA-rated hospital revenue bond. So long as the personal tax rate is greater than zero, tax-exempt financing is an encouragement for capital formation in health care.

Thus the true cost of debt capital for not-for-profit providers is

$$r_{D,N\text{-}F\text{-}P} = r_C\,(1-T_P)$$

Whether not-for-profit providers have an advantage over investor-owned providers in the capital market depends on the relation between the personal tax rate and the corporate tax rate. What is important here, however, is that public policy initiatives have substantially lowered the cost of debt for health care providers and thus encouraged both their assumption of long-term debt and their acquisition of physical capital and technological toys.

Bonds are notoriously expensive to issue (see Chapter 14). Various professional fees (which change little with the size of the issue) can be a prohibitively large share of a small issue of bonds. For that reason, most small organizations are unable to issue tax-exempt revenue bonds and must rely on bank debt, which is more costly because its interest is not tax-exempt. The effect is to grant a capital market advantage to large organizations. National tax policy and practice within states have varied, but one means of providing capital market access to small organizations has been to establish funding pools (usually called equipment pools) from which small organizations could borrow. At this writing, such pools are not common.

Brown (1988) advocated the establishment of such pools, but with a twist. He would have providers taking grants from the pools rather than taking out loans. Were such grant pools available, funds could flow to small providers at zero cost, avoiding the discipline and constraint decried by Wilson, Sheps, & Oliver (1982).

REIMBURSEMENT MODES AND ACCESS TO CAPITAL

The delivery of health care requires physical capital, which in turn requires access to external financing. Diagnostic imaging requires massive investment in facilities and equipment, not the installation of a simple x-ray room. How organizations are paid has (and will continue to have) serious implications for their access to capital. Some aspects of the payment schemes are matters of public policy, and others are determined by market forces (the degree of capitation in the market).

A serious constraint on access to capital is the health care sector's growing reliance on capitated payments. Under capitation, a provider agrees to offer some set of services to a defined population for a fixed monthly "per member per month" fee. As capitated contracts become larger shares of hospitals' (and clinics' and specialists' offices') revenues, the connection between volume of service and revenue will break down. Those who provide external capital will assume, along with the providers of capitated care, the risk of *excess utilization* (where excess utilization is defined as utilization above that expected by the actuaries who advise the providers in their contract negotiations).

Under capitation, then, one can expect bond buyers to scrutinize the abilities of health care providers to anticipate utilization and to price their services in the same way they now scrutinize providers' financial statements. Actuarial accuracy and utilization control will be as important as adequate cash flow (see Chapter 20).

SUMMARY

Access to external capital is a major factor in the survival of any organization, especially of organizations as heavily dependent on emerging technologies as health care providers. Health care providers must compete in capital markets with all of the other users of funds. In the absence of external funding, in the presence of funding only at exorbitant costs of capital, new technology is beyond the grasp of most providers. Any initiative that will generate cash flows or save cash outflows in the future (equipment, facilities, vehicles, office innovations) becomes unobtainable.

In the past, public policy has made external financing of hospital capital inexpensive. New policy initiatives (such as the elimination of the capital cost pass-through) and new competitive structures (such as capitation) may remove that advantage in the future.

Discussion Questions

1. "This mania for organizational survival will kill health care." Do you agree? Explain.

2. What advantages in the capital market accrue to those who can issue hospital revenue bonds?

3. Do charitable organizations enjoy greater or lesser access to capital, all else equal, than more mercenary organizations?

4. Imagine a world in which no outside financing is available (no capital market, no bank loans, no new equity investors). How would health care organizations be different in such a world when compared with those in the United States?

CONTINUING CASE

This would be Billy Bob Ferguson's greatest achievement, if only everything fell into place. He was in the executive conference room at Memorial Hospital, seated across the table from Mat Burford, Memorial's President and Chief Executive Officer. The board of Lone Star Home Health Service had sent Billy Bob on a sensitive mission: to negotiate a joint venture with Clearwater County's largest hospital (see the Continuing Case in the introduction to this book).

The details had emerged slowly over several meetings. Memorial and LSHHS would each own 50 percent of a new entity, Central Texas Durable Medical Equipment and Services (nicknamed "Durable"). Durable would be a not-for-profit organization and would own durable medical equipment (hospital beds, home infusion equipment, oxygen tanks) for lease to LSHHS's clients. The funds needed to acquire the initial stock of equipment would come from an issue of revenue bonds, issued by the Clearwater County Hospital Authority on behalf of Memorial. Memorial would provide access to tax-exempt financing, and LSHHS would provide a captive consumer base. Debt service money (flotation expenses, interest, and repayment of principal) would flow to the lenders and intermediaries through Memorial.

Burford was holding forth on the importance of his organization's access to capital in the grand scheme of things, as a negotiating point in claiming a 55 percent share of the joint venture. ("Self-important windbag," Billy Bob thought. He had little use for Burford. Their daughters had taken dance lessons together 10 years before, and Burford had mellowed little since then.)

"Our loyal supporters throughout the county will certainly want to subscribe to our issue of bonds, and the major banks in Dallas and Houston know our credit standing and will want to acquire sizeable positions for their trust accounts."

"We're only talking about a $3 million issue of bonds, Mat. How sizeable can these positions be? Besides, won't your loyal investors demand the same returns from this venture as from other risky deals?" Billy Bob countered. He was thinking about the consultants' report that durable medical equipment rentals had become a "commodity" business, with lots of participants, each with little name-brand recognition, and each earning just enough margin to stay in business.

"Nonsense," was the reply, "we have always had special access to capital."

CASE QUESTIONS

1. Assess Mr. Burford's claims of investor loyalty and of special access to capital. How will the end of Medicare's capital cost pass-through affect the joint venture's ability to raise funds?

2. What is the likely effect of the size of the total issue of bonds on its feasibility?

3. How might the joint venture, and its financing, be restructured to take account of emerging competitive and financial realities in the durable medical equipment market?

REFERENCES

Brown, J.B. (1988). *Health capital financing*. Ann Arbor, MI: Health Administration Press.

Cleverly, W.O. (1990). After the fall: Reasons behind 1989 hospital closings. *Healthcare Financial Management, 44*(7), 22–24.

Cohodes, D.R. & Kinkead, B.M. (1984). *Hospital capital formation in the 1980s*. Baltimore, MD: Johns Hopkins University Press.

Gray, B.H., (Ed.). (1986). *For-profit enterprise in health care*. Washington, DC: National Academy Press for the Institute of Medicine.

Wilson, G., Sheps, C.G., & Oliver, T.R. (1982). Effects of hospital revenue bonds on hospital planning and operations. *New England Journal of Medicine, 307*(23), 1426–1430.

SELECTED READINGS

Brealey, R.A. & Myers, S.C. (2000). *Principles of corporate finance* (6th ed.). New York: McGraw-Hill.

Cohodes, D.R. & Kinkead, B.M. (1984). *Hospital capital formation in the 1980s*. Baltimore, MD: Johns Hopkins University Press.

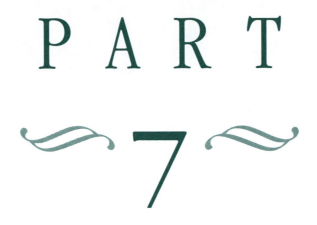

PART

7

Managing Short-Term Assets and Liabilities

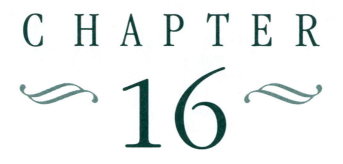

Principles of Working Capital Management

Learning Objectives

After reading this chapter, the student should be able to:

1. Explain how the Federal Reserve System can create money and credit.
2. Explain and measure the cash conversion cycle.
3. Explain the trade-off between the costs of liquidity and the costs of illiquidity.
4. Explain the basic principles of working capital management, as rooted in controlling opportunity costs.

Key Terms

Account receivable

Cash

Cash conversion
   cycle

Cash equivalent

Central bank

Federal Reserve
   System

Federal Open Market
   Committee (FOMC)

Inventory

Net working capital

Prepaid expenses

Working capital

The day-to-day work of financial management, the task of the treasurer, is most closely associated with the stewardship of working capital. **Working capital** refers both to current assets and to current liabilities. (Current assets are those assets that will be held for one accounting period or less; current liabilities are those liabilities that will be paid within the current accounting period; see Chapter 3). **Net working capital** refers to current assets *minus* current liabilities. An organization can cut its financing cost and enhance its value substantially by managing its working capital efficiently.

Consider the major classes of working capital: cash and cash equivalents, other (non-cash-equivalent) marketable securities, accounts receivable, inventory, and prepaid expenses. With the exceptions of cash equivalents and marketable securities, these are lazy assets; they do not pay any direct return. Accounts receivable age, and their collection becomes less likely the longer they are held. Inventories may corrode, expire, or be pilfered. Prepaid expenses simply go away. A major task of working capital management is to control the volume of resources committed to those classes of assets. Making do with small volumes of working capital (and financing working capital by the least costly means available) can allow one's organization to deliver the same amount of care at lower cost, or can allow an organization with a limited budget to deliver a greater amount of care.

This chapter explores some of the fundamental principles of working capital management. Among these are the control of opportunity cost and the net present value approach to working capital decisions. The chapter also presents, briefly, some important features of the market for short-term credit. The next three chapters discuss specific aspects of working capital management in greater detail. Chapter 19 closes Part Seven with a discussion of managing short-term liabilities. After reading this chapter, the reader will have a better sense of the opportunities and constraints inherent in working capital management and will be prepared for further study in the chapters ahead.

CURRENT ASSETS

Working capital consists of assets that are or can become available quickly to cover an organization's short-term needs. It is the lubricant that allows the organizations to function. Working capital comes in a dizzying variety of forms, some of which have become more complex than their names imply. **Cash** refers to currency and to checkable deposits. Once, under the Federal Reserve System's notorious Regulation Q, cash bore no interest and cash holdings carried large opportunity costs. With the lifting of Regulation Q, however, checkable deposits (bank accounts against which checks can be written) can pay interest. Now most organizations earn interest on all cash except the currency kept in the bursar's drawer, and the opportunity cost of holding cash has been reduced.

Cash equivalents are securities that are "cashlike" in two respects. They are so readily marketable that they can be converted into cash quickly (usually by the close of business on the day they are needed), and their market values are not affected by changes in interest rates. U.S. Treasury Bills and the commercial paper of major corporations are sufficiently marketable to meet the first condition, as are some other types of securities. The second requirement for cash equivalence *seems* to defy the inverse relationship between market value and interest rates that is central to asset valuation.

Assets that are sold at discounts (sold for the present values of their face values, paying no intermediate cash flows) have market values that rise, inexorably, to their face values as they mature. For example, a $5,000 90-day Treasury bill will sell, at auction, for about $4,938 if the effective yield is 5 percent. As the 90-day life of the bill passes, its market value will rise toward its par value ($5,000). On its expiration day, the bill is worth $5,000, the amount that is due the holder of the bill. Ten days before expiration, the bill is worth about $4,993, assuming the required interest rate is still 5 percent.

If those discount securities mature quickly enough, the momentum of their market values is such that only the widest possible swings in interest rates can affect their values. In effect, the increase of market value, from initial market value to par value, overrides any other factors. Securities maturing in 90 days or less have that feature and meet the second condition for cash equivalence. Cash equivalents provide market rates of return, and cash management consists in part of shifting assets into and out of cash equivalent form as needed.

Accounts receivable, or patient accounts, are generated in the normal course of business. They bear no interest for the provider (unless they have been converted into loans, with contractual interest rates), and their ultimate collection becomes less likely as they age.

Inventory consists of items held for resale and should be carefully distinguished from supplies. Inventory is a less important item for most health care providers than for manufacturing and retail organizations (the major exception being pharmacies). Nonetheless, inventory management offers interesting opportunities for improved efficiency in health care. Inventory stocks are remarkably nonmarketable (for some pharmaceutical inventories, resale may raise sticky legal issues), and many of the inventory items of health care organizations have short shelf lives.

Prepaid expenses are intangible assets that arise when an expense (a liability insurance premium, for example) is paid prior to the accounting period in which the expense is to be recognized (see Chapter 3 for a review of the accrual principle of accounting and the recognition of expenses). Once paid, prepaid expenses earn no interest and simply sit on the books waiting for the associated expenses to be incurred. One cannot, in any meaningful way, manage prepaid expenses once they are paid.

MONEY AND CREDIT: BANKERS' CONSTRAINTS

Any organization's ability to acquire and manage short-term assets depends on the availability of short-term credit. Also, the rates of return that can be earned on cash equivalents are determined in the market for short-term credit, the money market. The supply of money and credit is determined by the banking system. Crucial in that determination is the policy of the **central bank** (in the United States, the Federal Reserve System).

The **Federal Reserve System** (affectionately called "the Fed") is empowered to create money through several mechanisms (Melton, 1983). *Money* has several definitions in common usage and in economics, but the term means any generally accepted medium of exchange. The broad definition of money (M2) includes all currency in circulation and all checkable deposits. Checkable deposits are the overwhelming majority of the money included in M2, and it is the volume of such deposits that the Fed can control. Currency in circulation, to the surprise of many financial novices, is only a very small portion of the nation's money stock.

The Fed consists of 12 regional banks (in Atlanta, Boston, Chicago, Cleveland, Dallas, Kansas City, Minneapolis, New York, Philadelphia, Richmond, San Francisco, and St. Louis) and a Washington headquarters, presided over by a seven-member Board of Governors. The New York Fed plays a special role in the system, both as the clearinghouse for international transactions and as the site for the system's trading in Treasury bonds. Although the presidents of the other 11 regional banks rotate on and off of the **Federal Open Market Committee (FOMC)**, the president of the New York Fed is a permanent member of that crucial body (discussed below). All federally chartered banks must be members of the Federal Reserve System, and most large state-chartered banks choose to be members.

Because member banks must maintain a portion of their total deposits as reserves with their regional Federal Reserve banks (imposing a reserve requirement gives the system its name, *fractional reserve banking*), an increase in reserve balances allows member banks to create deposits by loosening their lending practices. Conversely, a decline in member banks' reserves forces them to be more restrictive in their loan creation. The leverage that reserve accounts have on the total money stock causes the total volume of reserves to be known as *high-powered money*. The FOMC meets monthly to determine whether the level of reserves in the system is appropriate and, if they believe it is not, to what extent that level should be adjusted. Following the directives of the FOMC, and operating through the bond trading desk at the Federal Reserve Bank of New York, the Fed can inject reserves into or remove reserves from the accounts of member banks. As the Fed injects reserves, it creates credit within the banking system, which in turn allows banks to create money by making loans.

As the Fed sells U.S. Treasury bonds to member banks ("open market operations") it absorbs their excess reserves. When reserves fall, banks must tighten their lending practices. They can accomplish that in several ways. They can be more restrictive in to whom and for what purposes they will lend ("We're sorry, Mr. McLean, we just can't justify a loan for your vacation on Majorca this year."), they can call in outstanding loans, and they can increase the interest rates at which they make loans. The Fed's influence over bank lending and interest rates echoes throughout the money market. Those who cannot obtain desired bank loans seek funds in short-term credit markets, putting pressure on those markets and causing interest rates to rise. When the Fed purchases U.S. Treasury bonds from member banks, it provides them with additional reserves for their accounts, allowing them to adopt less restrictive policies and to expand the stock of money, or to lower interest rates, or both.

It is ironic that Federal Reserve policy, intended to promote prosperity while controlling inflation, is, in an unintended way, health policy as well. Restrictive Federal Reserve policies impose constraints on the health care system but also offer opportunities for health care financial managers. Higher short-term interest rates make financing working capital more expensive but also create opportunities for gains in short-term investments. Those actions by the Federal Reserve's Open Market Committee make the task of working capital management one requiring constant vigilance and energy on the part of corporate treasurers.

THE CASH CONVERSION CYCLE

Working capital management, at its heart, is about conserving cash (to take advantage of short-term investment opportunities) while ensuring that the levels of accounts receivable and inventory that are necessary for day-to-day operations are available. Working capital managers are in the business of controlling the **cash conversion cycle**.

Figure 16–1 illustrates the cash conversion cycle. Every transaction ultimately depends on cash. Suppliers and employees want cash. Investors demand cash. Providers use their cash holdings to purchase inventory and supplies and to pay

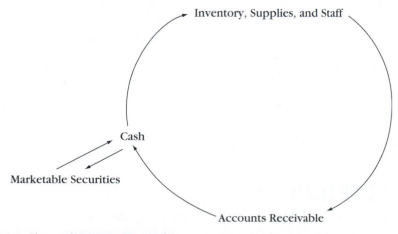

Figure 16-1 The cash conversion cycle.

staff. At any moment in time, a health care provider poised to deliver service represents a substantial commitment of cash to other short-term assets.

Providing health care services generates very little immediate cash. Most services are paid by third parties, who are notoriously slow in making cash payments. Other services are paid after a billing cycle ("I left my checkbook at home, can you send me a bill?") or by credit card (with cash coming only after periodic billing). The result is the accumulation of accounts receivable, or patient accounts.

Chapter 17 discusses patient accounts management in greater detail. For now, suffice it to say that patient accounts, although a lazy, non–interest-bearing, potentially wasting asset, are a necessary accompaniment to delivering health care. As the accounts are collected or sold, they are converted into cash and the cash conversion is complete.

There is a side flow (an appendix of sorts) to the cash conversion cycle. At any moment in time, an organization may have more cash than it needs to hold for operating purposes. The tool used to determine the presence of excess cash is the cash budget, discussed in the next chapter. Excess cash can be invested in cash equivalents and other marketable securities. Similarly, in times of inadequate cash, the organization can liquidate its reserves of cash equivalents or can tap a line of credit. Movement of cash into and out of cash equivalents and marketable securities is a potential source of significant gain and is an essential day-to-day function for the treasurer.

The cash conversion cycle can be measured in days. In some respects, it is like a garden hose. In equilibrium, the amount of water flowing out of a garden hose every second is equal to the amount of water flowing into the hose every second. The longer the hose, however, the greater is the amount of water tied up in it at any given time. Similarly, in a steady state, the amount of cash entering the cash conversion cycle every day will be equal to the amount of cash recovered from patient accounts every day. The longer the cash conversion cycle (in days), however, the greater is the volume of resources tied up in the cycle. Assets tied up in the cash conversion cycle earn little or no return and therefore incur substantial opportunity costs. Remember that opportunity costs are the returns forgone by having assets tied up in the cash conversion cycle rather than being used in operations or invested in marketable securities.

The length of the cash conversion cycle, measured in days, is the sum of two ratios. The first is the average inventory holding period, the average time that items are held in inventory. That ratio is ending inventory (or average inventory) divided by revenues per day. The second component is the collection period, the average time required to collect patient accounts. That ratio is equal to ending accounts receivable (or average accounts receivable) divided by revenues per day. Putting the two together, the cash conversion cycle is ending inventory plus ending accounts receivable all divided by revenues per day.

CONTROLLING LIQUIDITY

As discussed in Chapter 4, the extent to which an organization has current assets to cover its current liabilities is the extent to which that organization is liquid.

Working capital management is the management of liquidity. Figure 16–2 shows the relationship between liquidity and organizational costs.

As the organization's liquidity (its holding of current assets relative to its holdings of current liabilities, measured by the current ratio) rises, the costs of illiquidity fall. The costs of illiquidity are the additional short-term interest costs imposed by lenders to compensate for risk of default, the loss of ability to take advantage of trade credit (discounts available for paying within a specified billing period), and interest costs incurred by having to borrow to meet short-term obligations. Were the costs of illiquidity the only costs involved, one would wish to hold large stocks of working capital, especially cash and cash equivalents.

As the current ratio rises, however, the costs of liquidity also rise. The costs of liquidity are opportunity costs. Inventory and accounts receivable earn no rate of return. Cash in a bank account may earn interest, as do cash equivalents and other marketable securities, but the returns to real assets (physical assets used in the delivery of care) usually earn greater returns than financial assets. Holding assets in financial form incurs losses of potential returns.

Why must physical assets provide greater expected returns over time than financial assets? The returns to any security are based on cash flows generated by the users of funds (see Chapter 9). Ultimately, the returns to holding securities (financial assets) are based on the returns to physical assets. If some security promises to pay 8 percent return, the issuer must expect to earn more than 8 percent on the physical assets it would purchase with the proceeds.

It is tempting, when looking at Figure 16–2, to assume that the optimal current ratio is that at which the costs of liquidity equal the costs of illiquidity. That, however, is not the case. The optimal current ratio is that at which the sum of the costs of liquidity and the costs of illiquidity are minimized. Although that point may not be measurable before the fact, approximating it is how the treasurer can add considerable value to the organization.

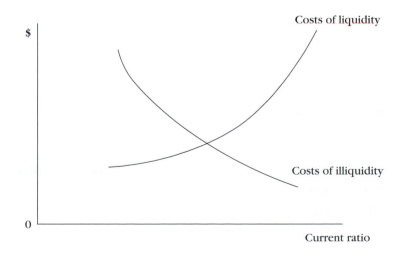

Figure 16-2 The volume of working capital costs.

A BASIC PRINCIPLE

Opportunity costs and interest costs are both real and both important. A little saving in interest cost, or a little interest gained, every day can amount to a substantial loss, or gain, over the course of the year. The purpose of managing working capital is the same as the purpose of any other aspect of financial management: to add value to the organization.

From the simple proposition flows a simple decision rule: undertake changes in working capital management practices that add value to the organization (that have positive net present values) (Sachdeva & Gitman, 1981). When faced with a choice between two or more possible means of managing current assets and current liabilities, select the alternative with the highest net present value (where cash flows may be actual inflows or may be cash outflows saved). Chapters 17 and 18 will illustrate the application of that rule to a variety of working capital situations.

Some working capital decisions, especially in the management of short-term liabilities (see Chapter 19), are not in themselves value adding. Rather, those decisions ought not to detract from the value of the organization and should reduce the unsystematic (uncompensated) risk borne by the organization's stockholders.

SUMMARY

Working capital refers to any asset or liability that will be "used up" within one accounting period. The management of working capital is important because of the possibility of earning interest on short-term funds and because of the need to pay interest on short-term funds borrowed. The cost of short-term funds, at any risk level, is given to the individual health care organization. It is determined in the interplay of supply (determined by the Federal Reserve System) and demand (determined by the potential users of funds) in the money market. Although the treasurer cannot affect the cost of money, without changing the organization's exhibited level of risk, she must balance the (higher interest) costs of illiquidity with the (opportunity) cost of excessive liquidity. Organizations that adopt a positive net present value rule can add substantial value by reducing interest and opportunity costs.

Discussion Questions

1. What constitutes working capital? Why is it called *working* capital? Doesn't all capital work?

2. How does the FOMC influence the banking system's ability to create credit?

3. In what sense is monetary policy also health care policy?

4. What are the advantages of a 10-day, rather than a 40-day, cash conversion cycle? What are the disadvantages?

CONTINUING CASE

Dr. Jackson and Janet Fowler were having a heated discussion about the future of PCI, Inc. Jackson's disappointment with the corporation's and the clinic's financial performance had grown over the past few months. Fewer beds were filled in the inpatient facility. Too much of the space in the clinic was rented, under long-term leases, at rates that barely paid for cleaning and utilities. Jackson blamed Fowler for the situation. He blamed her for the high short-term interest rates he paid at CCB Bank. He blamed her for failing to take advantage of the high interest rates of the 1980s by investing excess cash in long-term bonds. He and Henry Kirk had discussed firing Ms. Fowler, a move Kirk opposes strongly.

"Why must we pay 7 percent to borrow on a 90-day note? Just 20 years ago, I could get 90-day money for 4 percent. What has changed?" Dr. Jackson was in high dudgeon. "Why couldn't we put all of our cash into long-term bonds back in '84? I told you to do that, and you let me down."

"Dr. Jackson, I've reviewed all of our working capital policies and they are still the best for PCI and its shareholders." Ms. Fowler learned long ago that it was best to remain calm when dealing with Dr. Jackson. "If you'll just let me explain. . . ."

CASE QUESTIONS

1. What has changed to make short-term loans more costly now than in the mid-1970s?

2. Why was it not a wise decision to put all cash into long-term bonds in 1984 (or any other time)?

3. In what sense is a working capital policy "best" for the interest of any organization and its stakeholders? What criteria would one use to determine if a working capital policy is "best"?

REFERENCES

Melton, W.C. (1983). *Inside the Fed: Making monetary policy*. Homewood, IL: Dow Jones-Irwin.

Sachdeva, K.S. & Gitman, L.J. (1981). Accounts receivable decisions in a capital budgeting framework. *Financial Management, 10*(4), 45–49.

SELECTED READINGS

Brealey, R.A. & Myers, S.C. (2000). *Principles of corporate finance* (6th ed.). New York: McGraw-Hill.

Kalberg, J.G. & Parkins, K.L. (1993). *Corporate liquidity: Management and measurement.* Homewood, IL: Richard D. Irwin.

C H A P T E R

17

Cash, Marketable Securities, and Patient Accounts

Learning Objectives

After reading this chapter, the student should be able to:

1. Explain the role of the cash budget in working capital management.
2. Prepare a cash budget.
3. Design a corporate cash management system.
4. List and explain alternatives for speeding the conversion of patient accounts into cash.
5. Make decisions as to the adoption of new cash and patient accounts management policies.

Key Terms

Cash budget	Line of credit
Cash management agreement	Lock box service
Compensating balance	Money market mutual fund
Float time	Securitize

Chapter 16 explained the role of working capital management in avoiding interest and opportunity costs. This chapter expands on that theme by developing tools for the management of the most liquid types of working capital: cash and cash equivalents, marketable securities, and patient accounts. After reading this chapter, the reader should be able to design a cash management system, should be aware of the alternatives for converting patient accounts into cash, and should be able to make decisions about proposed changes in cash and patient accounts strategies.

CASH AND CASH EQUIVALENTS

Cash is the most liquid of assets, immediately available to meet obligations. The acceptability of cash (currency and checkable deposits) for payment is what makes it "money" in the economic sense. Every organization needs some cash on hand. Cash, however, earns little or no interest. Currency in the cash drawer just sits. Checking accounts may earn interest (since the Fed revoked its infamous Regulation Q, which forbade banks' paying interest on checking accounts) but always do so at less than market rates. Cash on hand, either currency or checking accounts, generates opportunity costs.

Managing cash holdings involves ensuring adequate liquidity while controlling opportunity costs. Putting excess cash to work, *even overnight*, can, in the course of a year, contribute significant value to the organization. Those overnight opportunities exist in modern money markets, and their exploitation is an important task.

Cash equivalents are those securities that are both easily converted into cash and of sufficiently short term to maturity that their market values are not affected by changing interest rates (see Chapter 16). These include 90-day U.S. Treasury Bills, 90-day commercial paper, short-term "jumbo" certificates of deposit, repurchase agreements, and bankers' acceptances. These are the instruments traded in the money market, the market for short-term funds.

Managing the opportunity cost of holding cash involves converting excess cash into cash equivalents and recovering cash from cash equivalents to cover cash needs. That type of management requires a plan: the cash budget.

THE CASH BUDGET

The **cash budget**, or cash forecast, is a spreadsheet representation of the expected cash inflows and outflows, and therefore of expected ending cash, of an organization for some planning period, usually a quarter, in advance. *Every* organization with cash flows should have a cash budget, whether it is as small as a Cub Scout pack or as large as a teaching hospital. The cash budget is the single most important tool for projecting one's ability to meet cash obligations.

Although treasurers have prepared cash budgets for many years, the development of the desktop computer and of spreadsheet software has greatly simplified the task. Table 17–1 shows the cash budget, for the first 4 months of some year (20XY), for a proposed clinic of the local health department of Clearwater County, the hypothetical county used in this text's continuing cases.

The clinic in question is operating under several conditions. It will provide services (vaccinations, prenatal and postnatal care under the Federal CHIPs (Children's Health Insurance Program), and some infectious disease care to its county residents. Those patients who have insurance must so declare (and some do) so that the clinic can bill their insurance carriers. The first row of the cash budget shows the monthly insurance claim filings. Insurance claims, like patient revenues, are not a cash inflow. Only when the claims are collected do they become cash inflows. The assumptions used here (a cash budget is based on a great many assumptions, usually based on experience) are that 50 percent of claims are collected 30 days after filing and that 45 percent of claims are collected 60 days after filing. The remaining 5 percent of claims go uncollected. Note that these percentages are for illustrative purposes only; they are not the assumptions one should automatically build into one's own cash budget. Every organization should examine its own collection experience in preparing its cash budget.

The rows marked as 30-day collections and 60-day collections represent cash inflows. For January, the 30-day collection amount ($1,437.50) is 50 percent of December insurance claims, and the 60-day collection amount ($1,575.00) is 45 percent of November insurance claims. Collected accounts are cash inflows. For any provider, it is collections, not revenues, that represents cash inflow. Note that, because claims in this example are paid as much as 2 months after filing, any cash budget must include at least 2 months of past claims information (hence the inclusion of November and December of 20XX in the cash budget for January through April of 20XY).

The next major item for each of the months under review is its beginning cash balance. Note that January's beginning cash balance is December's ending cash balance. Following the beginning cash balance are the clinic's monthly cash inflows. These include 30-day and 60-day collections, the county's appropriation in support of the clinic, and any interest earned during the month.

In this case, interest is assumed to accrue on excess cash balances at 5 percent per year. Thus the interest earned in January is $1/12$ of 5 percent of cumulative lending at the end of December ($9,000). That is, $9,000 \times 0.05 \times (1/12) = \$37.50$. Were there cumulative borrowing at the end of any month (as in March), the following month would see no interest earned, but interest paid out. On a spreadsheet, such a decision problem (earn interest at a 5 percent annual rate, paid monthly, if and only if cumulative lending is greater than zero) is easily modeled using the "logical if" statement (when cumulative lending or borrowing is in cell C28, the logical if statement, for determining interest earned is @IF[C28>0,C28*.05/12,0]).

Cash outflows follow inflows. These include rent, utilities, salaries, benefits,

Table 17–1 Clearwater County Health Department Central Clinic Cash Budget

	Nov. 20XX	Dec. 20XX	Jan. 20XY	Feb. 20XY	Mar. 20XY	Apr. 20XY
Insurance Claims Filed	$3,500.00	$2,875.00	$4,550.00	$5,230.00	$3,750.00	$3,250.00
Beginning Cash			12,500.00	8,350.00	4,238.96	1,954.54
Cash Inflows						
30-day collections			1,437.50	2,275.00	2,615.00	1,875.00
60-day collections			1,575.00	1,293.75	2,047.50	2,353.50
county appropriation			12,500.00	12,500.00	12,500.00	12,500.00
interest earned			37.50	20.21	3.08	0.00
Total Cash Inflows			15,550.00	16,088.96	17,165.58	16,728.50
Cash Outflows						
rent and utilities			1,800.00	1,800.00	1,800.00	1,800.00
salaries and benefits			15,400.00	15,400.00	15,400.00	15,400.00
supplies			2,500.00	3,000.00	2,250.00	1,875.00
interest paid			0.00	0.00	0.00	12.88
Total Cash Outflows			19,700.00	20,200.00	19,450.00	19,087.88
Net Cash Inflows			(4,150.00)	(4,111.04)	(2,284.42)	(2,359.38)
Ending Cash		12,500.00	8,350.00	4,238.96	1,954.54	(404.84)
Minimum Balance		3,500.00	3,500.00	3,500.00	3,500.00	3,500.00
Cumulative Net Lending (Borrowing)		$9,000.00	$4,850.00	$738.96	($1,545.46)	($3,904.84)

supplies, and any interest paid. In this example, interest expense is incurred at 10 percent per year ($\frac{1}{12}$ of 10 percent each month) on any cumulative borrowing. Supplies are assumed to vary seasonally, as cold and flu season hits its peak in the winter.

$$\text{Ending cash} = \text{Beginning cash} + \text{Cash inflows} - \text{Cash outflows}$$

Ending cash is the actual level of ending cash balance and the following month's actual level of beginning cash.

Many banks, however, require a minimum balance of their commercial customers. These are known as **compensating balances** and aid the bank in several ways. They both provide a cushion of security against defaults on loans and prevent the bank's reserve account with its regional Federal Reserve bank from being depleted (see Chapter 16). Under modern cash management agreements (discussed below) compensatory balances may be zero, with the bank's reward coming in the form of fees.

The difference between ending cash and the required minimum (compensating) balance is cumulative net lending or borrowing. That is excess cash (positive difference) that is available to lend. That lending rarely takes the form of simple loans. Rather, those are funds available to purchase cash equivalents. Purchasing a 90-day T-bill is the equivalent of making a 90-day loan to the U.S. government. Negative differences represent the need to take out loans to meet the bank's required minimum balance. Because it is the actual ending cash, not the minimum balance, that is moved to the top of the next column, the bottom row is, in fact, *cumulative* net lending or borrowing. That is, any cash over or under the minimum balance (any surplus or deficit) is moved to the top of the next month's column. Cash surpluses and deficits, then, are carried over on the cash budget, making the borrowing/lending row cumulative.

CASH MANAGEMENT SERVICES

Modern computing capability has made sophisticated cash management service available at relatively small cost to any organization with substantial cash flows. Commercial banks, in their search for non–interest-sensitive revenues, have developed these services for their customers, receiving monthly fees for their trouble. A **cash management agreement** involves several components. First is a simple checking account into which the organization agrees to make daily deposits. Second is the maintenance of a cash budget to project excess cash and borrowing needs for the months ahead. Third is a **line of credit**, whose size is determined by the forecasts in the cash budget. A line of credit is a potential loan to be tapped at will should the need to borrow arise.

Fourth is a **money market mutual fund**, managed by the bank for its own cash management customers only (not, to avoid regulatory nightmares, available to the public). A money market mutual fund is a fund in which investors purchase shares and that in turn purchases cash equivalent securities. Investment in such funds have been available to the public since the late 1970s. They differ from other mutual funds in that they purchase only money market securities. They are bound to that limitation not only by choice but also by the terms set forth in their prospectuses. Publicly available money market mutual funds are regulated, as are all mutual funds marketed in interstate commerce, under the Investment Company Act of 1940, administered by the Securities and Exchange Commission. By restricting access to their cash management customers, banks offering those services avoid regulation under the 1940 law.

Figure 17–1 illustrates the components of a cash management service. The clinic makes deposits with its commercial bank. Deposits go into the clinic's checking account, from which it can make regular withdrawals. If withdrawals place the balance of the account below its minimum level (which may be zero), the bank will automatically tap the clinic's line of credit. When loans are made via the line of credit, the clinic is assessed interest until it can repay the line of credit.

At the end of each business day, the bank "sweeps" any excess cash (checking account balance in excess of the minimum balance) into its proprietary money market mutual fund. That is, the clinic purchases shares in that fund, which then uses its assets to purchase short-term securities from money market dealers. These securities may be held for very short periods of time (sometimes literally overnight), but a little interest here and there on a large volume of assets can amount to a great deal of return over the course of a year. When the bank needs to raise cash to meet withdrawals from its customers accounts, it sells short-term securities back to dealers.

Cash management accounts (also called *sweep accounts* because banks sweep assets into their mutual funds) provide positive returns on excess cash without the customers' treasurers having to make any daily decisions. A large commercial bank's volume of money market purchases gives it some leverage with dealers. The banks also enjoy fee income for the service and collect interest when customers tap their lines of credit.

Where is the disadvantage for the client? The interest to be gained by participat-

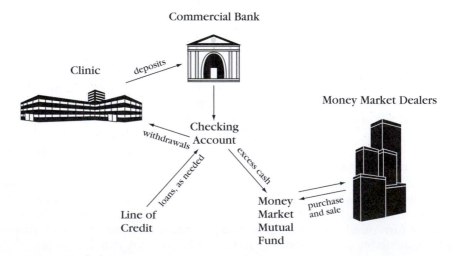

Figure 17-1 A cash management service in action.

ing in a cash management service may not justify the fees charged by the bank providing the service. The test is simple: is the expected monthly gain from participation at least as great as the monthly fee? If so, participation in the cash management service is justified.

Very large organizations have yet another decision to make. These organizations may fare better if they provide their own in-house cash management services. Setting up such a service involves some one-time cost (computing equipment) and some monthly costs (salaries, subscriptions to online securities quotation services). Again, the decision rule is simple: is the present value of all of the costs of in-house cash management service at least as great as the present value of the costs of perpetual use of the bank's service (assuming the two would perform equally well)? If so, use the bank's service.

MANAGING MARKETABLE SECURITIES

Chapter 12 discussed the management of the endowment, the securities and other assets held as long-term investments. In general, assets whose terms to maturity are longer than 1 year are not good vehicles for parking current assets. Asset values vary inversely with interest rates. Very short-term assets (90 days and less) move toward maturity so rapidly that the effect of changing interest rates on their values is negligible. For longer-term securities (all equity securities, all real estate, and debt securities of all but the shortest maturities), increases in interest rates cause losses in market value.

The interest sensitivity of capital market securities makes them inappropriate for current assets. Suppose one found $1 million in excess cash and used it to purchase 30-year corporate bonds. An unexpected increase in interest rates could make that bond investment less valuable very quickly. The effect is to diminish the amount of working capital available. If cash is to remain as working capital, it should not be subject to such interest rate risk.

PATIENT ACCOUNTS

Just as recent years have seen innovation in the field of cash management (the sweep account), the management of patient accounts has undergone great change, opening the possibility of enhanced value, in the past decade. Patient accounts (more generally, accounts receivable) arise in the course of doing business. It is not the case that the accumulation of patient accounts is a form of charity. Rather, willingness to extend credit to patients is a way of attracting business. Willingness to wait for an insurance carrier to pay the bill attracts that carrier's patients. It also leads to the accumulation of accounts receivable.

A key measure in the analysis of patient accounts management is the collection period (also known as days in accounts receivable). That ratio (see Chapter 4) is given by

$$\text{Collection period} = \text{Accounts receivable}/(\text{Net patient revenue}/365)$$

or accounts receivable divided by patient revenues per day. It answers the two questions, "How many days of revenue do we have tied up in accounts receivable?" and "How long, on average, does it take to collect our patient accounts?" The shorter the collection period, the smaller is the opportunity cost of assets tied up in accounts receivable. A zero collection period, however, means that the organization is demanding cash at the time of service and forgoing a great deal of business.

A health care provider's collection period is determined largely by the payment practices of its patients' insurance carriers. Hospitals with heavy Medicare and Blue Cross case loads typically have about 60- to 90-day collection periods. Their abilities to reduce that period are limited. Health maintenance organizations, and providers who accept capitated payments for their "covered lives," which accept premiums in return for providing whatever care is needed, have 30-day collection periods. The 30-day collection period is no surprise when one remembers how those premiums are paid: they are tied to enrollees payroll periods. Employers pay the HMO according to their own payroll schedule. Again, there is little the HMO can do to alter its collection period.

Technological progress has come to the aid of health care providers in accounts management. Most health insurance carriers provide electronic claims filing options for the providers who accept their payments (indeed, most carriers prefer electronic claims filing). Instead of using "snail mail," one can now file a claim at the speed of light. As a reward, most carriers will provide expedited processing for electronic claims.

What can one do to manage its receivables? One possibility is to engage a bank to provide **lock box service**. Commercial banks provide such services for a fee. The lock box is a post office box to which patients send their payments. An employee of the bank checks the box daily, taking all checks to the bank for immediate deposit. The result is a decrease in the **float time**, the time during which the check has been written but not credited to the provider's account. Lock box service can cut as much as several days from the usual float time, increasing the cash on hand for the provider, and, if combined with a cash management service, allowing several days of additional interest on each payment.

Organizations with widely dispersed payors (those who sell goods in the retail market through mail order catalogs, for example) often use lock box services in several cities, cutting their float times both by gaining immediate deposit and by reducing the time that any individual check is in the mail. It is not necessary to have geographically dispersed sales for a lock box system to make sense. Just reducing the time it takes checks to make it from the letter carrier's hand to the bank can often increase interest income substantially.

It is also important in managing patient accounts to have a posted, written credit and collections policy. It is not at all unusual to have a policy of "all copayments are due at the time of service." Patient accounts representatives, bookkeepers, and receptionists who must collect those accounts need clearly specified policies on credit, and patients need to be informed of those policies in advance. There is nothing that generates ill will more quickly than an unexpected demand for a large payment upon awakening from anaesthetic.

Several means are now available for speeding the conversion of receivables into cash, without altering patients' and insurers' payment patterns. First, one can accept payment via credit card. Banks offer credit card services to their customers to gain fee and interest income. Those banks also charge the businesses submitting credit card purchases a small fee, in the form of a discount from full reimbursement, for each transaction. These vary but are usually about 2 percent. In return for the discount, the provider receives its revenues quickly. A payment on-line capability, with patients charging to their credit cards through a web page, can further reduce the collection period.

Yet another means of turning patient accounts into cash is to sell them (Kincaid, 1993). Financial corporations stand ready to purchase accounts receivable for a discount from their face values. The advantage for the provider is in earlier receipt of cash. The disadvantage is in giving up some (negotiated) share of ultimate collections. If the purchaser of the accounts (the financial corporation) can borrow at lower rates than the provider (as is likely), then it is possible for the two to strike a deal that is mutually beneficial.

A more elegant way of turning patient accounts into cash is to **securitize** them. To securitize an asset is to sell securities that promise their holders payments, based on the cash flows from that asset. For example, the Government National Mortgage Administration (GNMA) securitizes pools of mortgages by selling bonds that promise to pay investors pro rata shares of the mortgage payments that GNMA collects from a specific pool.

Some large commercial banks purchase hospital receivables, act as bill collector, and sell receivables-backed commercial paper to investors (Pallarito, 1992). Such securitized patient accounts are relatively safe for investors, as third-party payors will eventually pay the underlying accounts. Large providers or managed care networks could also work with investment bankers to securitize their own receivables, collecting the accounts themselves, and passing the funds collected through to investors.

DECISIONS ON PATIENT ACCOUNTS

In contemplating any proposed change in patient accounts management, the simple but powerful net present rule should prevail. Will the present value of the cash flow gains from the change be at least as great as the present value of the cash outflows required to make the change? If so, then the change adds value to the organization and is worth doing. Even for those changes that require a monthly fee, it is the *present value* of the benefits and costs that should be compared. Benefits need not outweigh costs in every month in order to add value; only the present value of all future benefits must outweigh the present value of all future costs.

SOME EXAMPLES

Consider the choice of setting up or not setting up a lock box collection system, illustrated in Table 17-2. The clinic is facing a go/no-go decision on an 18-month trial program. The clinic whose decision problem is illustrated faces a growing number of monthly transactions (growing at 10 percent per year). The interest rate the clinic must pay is assumed to be 8 percent. On average, the instant deposit fea-

Table 17–2 Decision on a lock box collection system

Month	Number of Transactions	Average Days Saved	Average Transaction Size	Average Gain	Fee	Average Net Gain	Present Value @8% Per Year
1	1,015	3	$275.50	$183.87	$185.00	($1.13)	($1.12)
2	1,016	3	$275.50	$184.10	$185.00	($0.90)	($0.89)
3	1,017	3	$275.50	$184.25	$185.00	($0.75)	($0.73)
4	1,018	3	$275.50	$184.41	$185.00	($0.59)	($0.57)
5	1,019	3	$275.50	$184.57	$185.00	($0.43)	($0.42)
6	1,020	3	$275.50	$184.72	$185.00	($0.28)	($0.26)
7	1,021	3	$275.50	$184.88	$185.00	($0.12)	($0.11)
8	1,021	3	$275.50	$185.04	$185.00	$0.04	$0.04
9	1,022	3	$275.50	$185.20	$185.00	$0.20	$0.18
10	1,023	3	$275.50	$185.35	$185.00	$0.35	$0.33
11	1,024	3	$275.50	$185.51	$185.00	$0.51	$0.47
12	1,025	3	$275.50	$185.67	$185.00	$0.67	$0.62
13	1,026	3	$275.50	$185.83	$185.00	$0.83	$0.76
14	1,027	3	$275.50	$185.98	$185.00	$0.98	$0.90
15	1,028	3	$275.50	$186.14	$185.00	$1.14	$1.03
16	1,028	3	$275.50	$186.30	$185.00	$1.30	$1.17
17	1,029	3	$275.50	$186.46	$185.00	$1.46	$1.30
18	1,030	3	$275.50	$186.62	$185.00	$1.62	$1.44
							$4.13

ture of the lock box would reduce the collection float by 3 days. On average, each transaction is $275.50. The average gain per month is given by

Average gain = (Average number of transactions) × (Average days saved) × (Average transaction size) × (0.08/365)

That is, the interest gained in any period is equal to the dollars involved times the number of extra days those dollars are held times the daily interest rate.

In this example, the bank charges $185 per month for the lockbox service. In the early months of the contract, the service will add more cash outflow than it adds in cash inflow. One should, however, not look at any one month's net cash inflow, but at the present value of the net cash inflows over the life of the service. In this case, the decision to acquire the service has a positive net present value and is worth doing.

In considering any change in patient accounts management practice, one first finds what the benefits (in cash flow terms) will be. Next calculate what the cash outflows will be. The present value of the net cash inflows should be the determining factor in making or not making the change.

Another example is the decision to sell or not to sell one's accounts receivable. Consider an organization with $1,000,000 in patients accounts receivable from a reliable third-party payor (all of the numbers used in this example are hypothetical and used for illustration only). Past experience says that 95 percent of those accounts will be received in 45 days (5 percent of claims are denied). The organization could earn 7 percent on cash equivalents. Today, a financing company offers $975,000 for the accounts (the financing company will assume all collection responsibility). Is the sale worthwhile?

First calculate the benefits. The benefit is $975,000 of cash today. Next calculate the costs. The cost (an opportunity cost) is the amount of cash not to be received in 45 days. The relevant figure is the present value (at 8 percent) of 95 percent of $1,000,00 to be received in 45 days. In symbols,

Cash forgone = $1,000,000 × (0.95) × (1/{1+ [(0.08/365)*45]})

or

Cash forgone = $940,721.65

Because the benefit outweighs the present value of the opportunity cost, selling the patient accounts is a value-adding move.

Opportunities for such moves arise because the firms that purchase accounts receivable can often borrow at much lower rates than can the health care organizations that have accounts to sell. When those interest rate differentials obtain, the accounts are worth more to the purchaser than to the seller, and opportunities for mutual gain exists.

SUMMARY

Cash, cash equivalents, marketable securities, and patient accounts are the most liquid of any health care organization's current assets. Cash can be converted into cash equivalents quickly and vice versa. The cash budget, or cash forecast, is a useful planning tool for managing cash holdings.

The management of patient accounts has undergone great change in recent years. With growth in the extent of prepayment plans, patient accounts have become more "rationalized" than was once the case, with payments coming on a regular basis. Outstanding accounts can be held, sold, securitized, or turned over to collectors. The speed of collection can be improved, and the float reduced, by use of commercial bank lock box services.

In deciding on any type of change in working capital management, the net present value test should prevail. That is, a change adds value to the organization if and only if the net present value of the cash flows due to the change is positive.

Discussion Questions

1. What are the purposes of the cash budget? What organizations should prepare one?

2. How can the use of commercial banks' cash management services reduce opportunity cost and improve organizational performance? Explain.

3. What options are available for speeding the conversion of patient accounts into cash? Explain each.

4. What rule can one use in deciding whether or not to adopt an innovation in patient accounts management? Explain how to implement it.

CONTINUING CASE

The atmosphere at PCI, Inc., was unusually tense, and cash flow, as usual, was the topic of discussion. Henry Kirk explained to Dr. Jackson, "Our inpatient line is a mess. All of our patients carry insurance, which is good for avoiding bad debts, but bad for collection. Forty percent of our business is with one carrier, and that company doesn't pay for 90 days."

"We've tapped our line of credit until we can't tap anymore." Dr. Jackson was unusually worked up. "I have to borrow money [Jackson often personalized the corporation, even though there were 12 other shareholders] so that some health insurance leeches in Dallas can manage their assets. It's not fair and I won't stand for it."

Kirk asked Janet Fowler to explain the proposal that they had received from Keynote Capital Company. KCC would purchase all of Physicians' Clinic's current patient accounts (both KCC and Fowler estimated collection in 90 days) for 96 percent of their book value (charges minus expected uncollected accounts). The clinic, and therefore PCI, would receive cash flow by the close of business on the day the deal was closed.

"We're borrowing at 12 percent on our line of credit," Fowler went on. "Our experience is that our patients' insurance carriers pay 90 percent of the charges we submit." All three knew that Physicians' Clinic posted charges above anyone's usual, reasonable, and customary rates.

"It has to be up to you, Dr. Jackson; we've never sold our patient accounts before." Kirk didn't want responsibility if the deal went sour, or if KCC's collection practices hurt the clinic's standing in the community.

"Dammit, Kirk, I'm a doctor, not an accountant!" Dr. Jackson really did not know what to do.

CASE QUESTIONS

1. Is the deal offered by KCC in the best interest of PCI, Inc.?

2. How, if at all, should PCI evaluate the possibility of adverse effect if KCC uses heavy-handed collection practices?

REFERENCES

Kincaid, T.J. (1993). Selling accounts receivable to fund working capital. *Healthcare Financial Management, 47*(5), 27–36.

Pallarito, K. (1992). Receivables financing continues to evolve. *Modern Healthcare, 22*(45), 40–42.

SELECTED READINGS

Brealey, R.A. & Myers, C.S. (2000). *Principles of corporate finance* (6th ed.). New York: McGraw-Hill.

Kalberg, J.G. & Parkins, K.L. (1993). *Corporate liquidity: Management and measurement.* Homewood, IL: Richard D. Irwin.

CHAPTER

18

Inventory Management: Mathematics and Judgement

Learning Objectives

After reading this chapter, the student should be able to:

1. Recognize inventory control as a key element of supply chain management.
2. Determine optimal order quantities and reorder points for inventory and supply items.
3. Determine upon which inventory and supply items to concentrate one's attention and which to ignore.
4. Develop plans for working with suppliers to develop just-in-time inventory and supply delivery schemes.

Key Terms

ABC inventory
   system
Economic order quantity
   (EOQ)
Holding cost
Just-in-time
   inventory management
   (JIT)

Safety stock
Stock-out
Supply chain management

Strictly, inventory consists of items held for resale. Inventory, narrowly defined, is not a significant asset for most health care organizations (pharmacies being the most obvious exception). Health care providers, after all, provide care; they do not sell *things*. The methods developed for the management of inventories, however, are equally applicable to the management of supplies, an asset category that is significant for most providers. This chapter develops methods and rules of conduct that can enable managers to add value to their organizations through appropriate management of inventory and supplies. This is an important element of a critical field of modern management: **supply chain management**.

Supply chain management is not, strictly, a financial function. Materials managers, industrial engineers, operations research specialists, and floor nurses all have much more to do with inventory management than does anyone who reports to the Chief Financial Officer. Personnel from operating departments use inventory and supplies and route reorder forms through "materials" or "purchasing," not through the budget office. The goal of supply chain management, minimizing system-wide costs, is every manager's concern. The only task for the CFO in the inventory and supply process is to approve and pay the invoice. Some financial models can, however, serve as guides in inventory (and supply) management. These models, like those in earlier chapters, are based on opportunity cost control and value maximization. Because inventory and supplies are considered current assets, these methods are appropriately included in this section.

This chapter explains some useful techniques for the management of inventory and supplies. After completing this chapter, the reader should be able to design systems for managing and monitoring inventory and supplies. Compared to most of the other chapters in this volume, Chapter 18 is unusually brief. In part, this brevity is due to inventory management's relying on a few mathematical expressions. Mathematics is a particularly compact language. Good judgment, however, is also a component of inventory management. It makes little sense to spend $10,000 monitoring an item whose annual cost to the organization is only $7,500.

WHY BOTHER?

Why is inventory management an issue at all? Why not simply hold as much inventory as possible? Because inventory is a notoriously lazy asset. It earns no returns and no rate of interest. Inventory on hand incurs opportunity cost. The assets tied up in inventory could otherwise be invested in short-term securities. Further, especially in health care, inventory (and supplies) can be wasting assets. They not only generate opportunity costs; they also lose their own value (monetary *and* therapeutic) over well-defined (often short) shelf lives.

Inventory and supplies also impose **holding costs**. Their temperatures must be controlled (many drugs require refrigeration; most cannot be exposed to extremes of heat or cold). They must be kept clean. For many items, their presence must be monitored to ensure that they are not misused (as simple and common an item as a syringe can be greatly abused in the wrong hands). Inventory imposes costs (Scherr, 1989).

Why, then, not carry as little inventory as is possible? **Stock-outs** occur when an organization's inventory of some item falls to zero. For pharmaceuticals, losses due to expiration and contamination are as likely causes of stock-outs as are sales and in-house usage. A sporting goods store will find stock-outs of baseballs to be very inconvenient, resulting in unhappy customers and losses of sales. A hospital, however, finds stock-outs to be totally unacceptable, as they can result in unnecessary death and substantial legal liability. Stock-outs (at least of critical items) in most health care settings must be avoided at all costs. The management of inventory and supplies in health care organizations is a balancing act, balancing the opportunity costs and holding costs of having assets on hand against the probability of the enormous costs that a stock-out could impose.

THE TIME PATH OF INVENTORY USE

Inventory and supplies are used over time, often in predicable patterns. Figure 18–1 shows a caricature of one such pattern, constant daily use.

In Figure 18–1, the passage of time, measured in days, is shown on the horizontal axis, and units of the supply item are shown on the vertical axis. Imagine that the units represent some commonly used supply item, such as 1-cubic-centimeter disposable syringes with 27-gauge needles attached. A **safety stock** level, below which this organization may not allow units on hand to fall, is shown by S. Why keep safety stocks? Because in real health care settings, demand has a large random component. A hospital's average daily occupancy rate may be 45 percent, but that average will mask a wide variation in day-to-day experience. Because it is impossible to predict exactly how many syringes will be needed on Tuesday morning, some minimum level (S) must always be on hand. The maximum amount that is ever to be held is given by **EOQ**, an abbreviation explained below.

A delivery of syringes is received at time 0. It is logged in, checked for agreement with the order, and taken to storage. Over time, the syringes are used, with daily usage being the negative of the slope of the descending "units on hand" function.

When to Order?

At some point, a reorder must be processed. If it is processed too soon, too many syringes will be on hand on delivery day ("the supply bins are overflowing") and

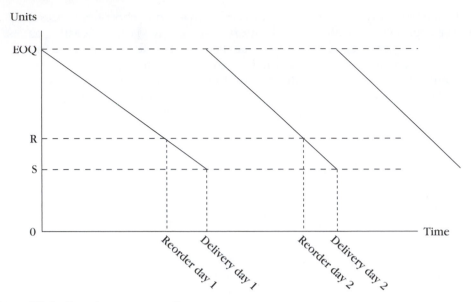

Figure 18-1 Supply usage over time.

the opportunity cost of holding syringes will be too great. If the reorder is processed too late, the number of units on hand will fall below the safety stock level (*S*).

The task of the purchasing director or materials manager is to solve a Goldilocks problem: not too soon, not too late, but just right. To determine the appropriate reorder point, one must know the necessary delivery and processing times. How much time will elapse between telling the materials management director that more syringes are needed and the moment those syringes are available in the supply bins? Call that delivery and processing time *D*. Optimal supply management dictates that the new delivery should arrive exactly when the number of units on hand reaches S. That is, the new stocks of syringes should be present at the moment that the stock on hand reaches the safety stock level. At that point, the unit's nurses become anxious, knowing that the next injection will place them below safety stock level. They will greet the arrival of the new shipment with a chorus of cheers.

For the new syringes to arrive at exactly the right moment, one must reorder when the amount on hand just equals the safety stock level plus the amount that will be used in *D* days. Thus reorder when

$$\text{Amount on hand} = S + [D \times (\text{Average daily usage})]$$

The reorder point is shown by the amount *R* on the vertical axis in Figure 18–1.

Note that, by reducing the delivery time, *D*, one can reorder later; carry, on average, smaller supplies; and reduce the assets tied up in inventory. Delivery times are to some extent determined by suppliers and are beyond the control of health care providers. Using on-line order systems and improving internal materials handling processes are ways that one can reduce the effective delivery time.

Pharmaceutical wholesalers have been very successful, with continuous on-line monitoring of retailers' stock on hand, and automatic reorders.

How Much to Order?

The next question is equally interesting and important: how much should one reorder? That amount is generally known as the **economic order quantity (EOQ)**. As shown below, it would be better known as the "optimal amount to have on hand after processing an order." The EOQ model, however, assumes that the safety stock level is zero (or, equivalently, that safety stocks must be replaced, due to wasting, with each order). In determining the EOQ, one should minimize the sum of two types of costs: the cost of making an order and the cost of having material on hand. The former consists of telephone and mailing costs and any incremental cost (*not overhead* cost) of materials handling. The latter consists of two parts: the opportunity costs of having assets tied up in inventory or supplies rather than earning interest, and any incremental cost of having the material on hand (including, perhaps, expected losses due to spoilage, theft, and other forms of wasting).

Let A be annual usage, C be the cost of making an order, H be holding costs, r be the opportunity cost of capital, and p be unit price of the item in question. In a year, the organization will make A/EOQ orders. That is, the number of orders to be made in a year is annual usage divided by how much is to be ordered each time. Over time, the average amount on hand (the average holding), assuming a constant rate of use, is $\text{EOQ}/2$. Expressing the two types of costs on an annual basis,

$$\text{Ordering costs} = C \times (A/\text{EOQ})$$

and

$$\text{Holding costs} = (\text{Interest rate} \times \text{Price per unit} \times \text{Average holding}) +$$
$$(\text{Holding costs per unit} \times \text{Average holding})$$

or, after substituting and rearranging,

$$\text{Holding costs} = (rp + H) \times (\text{EOQ}/2)$$

The total costs of ordering and holding inventory over the year is the sum of ordering costs and holding costs, or

$$\text{Total inventory cost} = (C \times A/\text{EOQ}) + [(rp + H) \times \text{EOQ}/2]$$

The manager's task is to find the value of EOQ that *minimizes* that total inventory cost function. The problem is a familiar one to readers who have studied differential calculus. Taking the first partial derivative of total inventory cost with respect to EOQ and setting that function equal to zero yields the optimal value of EOQ to be

$$\text{EOQ} = \sqrt{[2CA/(rp + H)]}$$

The square root function, although not intuitively obvious, falls out of the minimization process. Mathematically sophisticated readers may wish to verify that the result is, in fact, a global minimum. The optimal amount to order, if there is a non-zero, non-wasting safety stock level, is $\text{EOQ} - S$.

The formula for EOQ reveals several important points. First, the greater the cost of making an order (*C*), the larger should be the amount ordered, and therefore the fewer the number of orders per year. Second, the larger the annual usage (*A*), the larger the amount in each ordered. The size of the order varies inversely, however, with the prevailing interest rate and price per unit (opportunity cost) and with holding cost. None of these results is surprising given the trade-off to be made between ordering costs and holding costs.

It is very difficult for any organization to put explicit numbers on some of the items in the EOQ formula. The formula does, however, provide a way of organizing one's thinking about inventory and supply orders and management. It is a guide to managing those items that deserve the most attention.

THE ABCs OF GOOD JUDGEMENT

The EOQ formula is sufficiently complex to suggest that one ought not to bother calculating it for every item one carries as inventory and supplies. A hospital, for example, uses so many tablets of nonprescription pain reliever, each of them so inexpensive, that little is to be gained from carefully monitoring their usage and their delivery time. It does not add value to spend $10,000 on the analysis required to save $1,000 in opportunity cost over the course of a year.

To focus attention on those items from whose management value can be added, inventory specialists have devised the **ABC inventory system**. Each inventory or supply item is categorized as belonging in one of three groups: A, B, or C. Group A consists of those items that are very costly, either per unit or as a share of total inventory and supply cost. It is on these items that attention is concentrated, calculating the EOQ explicitly and monitoring use carefully. Group A items might include very expensive pharmaceutical items or radioactive trace elements. Digital monitoring and automatic reordering are justified for Group A items.

Group C items, on the other hand, are those items that represent very little cost, either per unit or as a share of total inventory and supply cost. These items can be all but ignored. Materials management specialists need only be told, "Don't let us run out." Group C items might include bottles of nonprescription pain relievers, adhesive bandages, or casting materials for setting broken bones.

The intermediate category, Group B, consists of all other items. For these, one should monitor use and apply the EOQ model in an implicit way, changing order quantities (and therefore stocks on hand) as interest rates and unit prices vary. The implication of an ABC inventory system is that most items go into category C, and attention can be applied where it can add value.

OPPORTUNITIES FOR VALUE ENHANCEMENT

As one seeks to exercise good judgment in an ABC/EOQ framework, one can often find opportunities to reduce the organization's opportunity costs. For example, when markets for supplies are competitive, vendors will often offer discounts from their usual wholesale prices. The EOQ model suggests that when unit price falls, the optimal order quantity will rise. That is, when a discount is offered, increase the amount ordered. Such a rule is no surprise, but following it is often a way to reduce supply costs substantially.

In urban areas, suppliers can offer such short delivery times that the supplier's warehouse can, in effect, become the provider's storeroom. Sometimes such "quick delivery, small order" service comes at the expense of an exclusive contract. The expected savings from such a contract need to be balanced against the lost opportunity for saving from other vendors. Providers in rural areas, who do not have such opportunities for quick delivery, suffer from their absence.

Japanese automobile manufacturers pioneered many techniques for cutting costs. Among those is **just-in-time (JIT) inventory management**. Under JIT inventory (and supply) management, supplies are delivered just as they are needed rather than in advance. The manufacturer need never hold a stockpile of supplies. JIT management requires a solid working relationship with suppliers and precise calculation of needed supplies.

JIT supply management can, however, be applied to a limited number of items by health care providers, all of them Group A items. When diagnostic procedures are scheduled in advance, radioactive trace materials can be ordered for delivery just before test time. Near-JIT delivery can be accomplished for other items, such as sterile surgical packs for prescheduled procedures. The trick to obtaining the desired results from JIT supply management is in working with suppliers to plan deliveries to coincide with scheduled activities.

SUMMARY

Management of inventory and supplies provides opportunities to add value to the organization by reducing holding costs, wasting costs, and opportunity costs. Health care providers hold substantial amounts of costly "stuff," much of which merely wastes if not used soon after its arrival. Pharmacies hold expensive inventories, which have limited shelf lives and which must be carefully managed. Among the methods that can add value through inventory management are optimal timing of reorders, EOQ analysis, ABC inventory management, and delivery management. For items that are costly on a per-unit basis and for items that constitute a large portion of supply and inventory cost, attention to detail can add substantially to the organization's worth.

Discussion Questions

1. Given the following data, what is this hospital's economic order quantity for urinary catheters?

Opportunity cost of capital	0.05
Holding cost per year	$ 2.00
Price per unit	$25.00
Annual use (365 days)	1,460
Cost of placing an order	$50.00

2. Using the data in Question 1, if the safety stock level is zero and an order requires 2 days, what is the reorder point?

3. What sorts of arrangements must one work out with a supplier in order to use just-in-time inventory and supply management?

4. For what sorts of inventory and supply items is just-in-time management a reasonable goal? Explain.

CONTINUING CASE

Billy Bob Ferguson was looking at the bill from Central Texas Pharmaceutical Supply Company, the Waco-based firm that shipped drugs and sterile solutions to LSHHS on a weekly basis. He paid special attention to the items for several varieties of insulin. Home care for elderly diabetics had become one of LSHHS's steadiest lines of business. Two nurses now made daily visits to 23 patients to check on diet, monitor blood glucose, and to administer (in 17 cases) insulin injections. For several of those patients, the visits were more than once per day.

Insulin had become a large item in LSHHS's supply room. Three types of insulin (regular, NPH, and Ultra-Lente), distinguished by the speed with which each is used in the body, were always on hand. The overwhelming majority of the insulin used was of the Ultra-Lente (Latin for "very slow") variety. Ferguson thought that the volume of assets tied up in that one drug was, if not huge, at least worth examining.

Billy Bob had some figures on a legal pad. "Two hundred vials of ultra-lente insulin per year (including some shelf expirations), each vial wholesaling for $20. We go through almost a full vial of Ultra-Lente almost every day." The realization was startling. "We could earn 5 percent interest if we could leave that money in the bank. It costs us about $50 per year to log in and refrigerate the insulin." Billy Bob had no idea where he came up with the last figure, but he liked to sound precise about such things. "It costs us a $2 phone call to Fort Worth to make an order, and an order takes 2 days to arrive."

Alice Ferguson, as a nurse, had administered thousands of doses of insulin in her time and thought the whole exercise was silly. "Just order the stuff, Billy. The clients have to have it, we're providing a valuable service [Alice's mother was among those receiving both regular and Ultra-Lente insulin], and it doesn't cost much. What will you gain by worrying over those numbers?"

CASE QUESTIONS

1. Is Alice correct in that the cost of the insulin supplies is too small to merit such concern? Explain fully.

2. Assuming that the safety stock of NPH insulin must be three vials, what is the optimal order quantity? What is the optimal number of orders per year?

REFERENCE

Scherr, F.C. (1989). *Modern working capital management*. Englewood Cliffs, NJ: Prentice Hall. (out of print)

SELECTED READINGS

Scherr, F.C. (1989). *Modern working capital management*. Englewood Cliffs, NJ: Prentice Hall. (out of print)

Simchi-Levy, D., Kaminsky, P., and Simchi-Levy, E. (2000). *Designing and managing the supply chain*. New York: McGraw-Hill.

CHAPTER

19

Current Liabilities:
Short-Term Financing

Learning Objectives

After reading this chapter, the student should be able to:

1. Explain the role of the matching principle in controlling overall financial risk.
2. Explain the role of the yield curve in determining the relative costs of short-term and long-term financing.
3. List possible sources of short-term financing and explain the characteristics of each.
4. Make decisions as to whether or not to accept discounts for early payment.

Key Terms

Bank note   Trade credit
Commercial paper   Yield curve
Matching principle
Term structure of
   interest rates

The other side of working capital management is the management of current liabilities, those obligations that will be paid within the current accounting period. Most large organizations carry substantial amounts of current liabilities, and failing to understand the implications of those short-term debt burdens can lead to financial disaster.

Short-term financing is needed for a variety of reasons. It is essential to the conduct of operations. No going concern can issue paychecks to its employees every hour or to pay all of its suppliers at the moment of delivery, as would be necessary to avoid carrying accounts payable. Short-term financing is also a necessary component of cash management. The sweep accounts discussed in Chapter 17 have two aspects. One is the short-term investment of excess cash. The other is the ability to draw, for short periods, on a line of credit. No health care provider can count on being in a cash surplus position at all times.

Yet another reason for using short-term borrowing is to take advantage of low interest rates. At most times, the **yield curve** (the relation between yield and term to maturity for debt securities) is upward sloping. That is, loans with longer terms to maturity carry higher interest rates than otherwise equivalent loans with shorter terms to maturity. Short-term liabilities, then, *usually* involve lower costs of capital than do long-term liabilities.

Finally, short-term liabilities are sometimes incurred to deal with emergencies. When organizations are in financial distress, they may find banks willing to lend for 90 days but no creditors willing to extend long-term loans.

One word of clarification is in order here. Short-term financing is not, strictly speaking, the mechanism for financing short-term assets. Unless tied to specific assets (as in the case of mortgage bonds or equipment bonds) all of the organization's liabilities and equities finance all of the organization's assets, both in the legal and the economic senses. There are reasons, however, discussed below, for matching the volumes of current liabilities and current assets, but the former do not specifically finance the latter.

This chapter develops some rules for managing short-term liabilities. After completing the chapter, the reader should be able to distinguish among the various types of short-term financing, to assess the appropriateness of each for his organization, and to manage a short-term financing program.

THE MATCHING PRINCIPLE

Short-term liabilities (current liabilities) are debt obligations that require repayment within the current accounting period (usually 1 year). These include accounts payable (of all types), short-term debts, and that part of long-term debt whose principal must be repaid within the current year. Equity claims are never current liabilities. Although short-term liabilities are usually low cost, they expose the organization to substantial *refinancing risk*, the risk that interest rates will rise in the short run and that refinancing will require a higher cost of capital.

Short-term liabilities must be rolled over, refinanced, each time they mature. Ninety-day notes must be refinanced (or repaid) every 90 days. One cannot know today what short-term interest rates will be in 3 months. Typically, outstanding short-term debt is repaid with funds raised by issuing new short-term debt (the volume of short-term debt outstanding seldom falls). Thus, by undertaking short-term financing, one exposes one's organization to the vicissitudes of the money market frequently.

Long-term financing, on the other hand, is usually expensive. Long-term interest rates within any risk class are usually higher than short-term rates within that risk class. Long-term financing is low-risk financing, however, as it locks in interest rates for as long as 30 years. Rollover risk is essentially eliminated when one uses long-term debt.

Short-term assets are usually low risk. They are assets (cash, cash equivalents, marketable securities, accounts receivable) that either are unlikely to lose their market values or can be unloaded easily. Long-term assets (property, plant, and equipment) are assets whose value in the future is highly uncertain and that may be difficult to sell.

An organization that is attempting to control the extent of its overall risk will, then, wish to match (low risk/low return) short-term assets with (high risk/low cost) short-term liabilities and (high risk/high expected return) long-term assets with (low risk/high cost) long-term financing. The control of risk by coordinating financing with the expected lives of assets is called the **matching principle**. It is not true that short-term financing raises the money for short-term assets, only that overall risk is reduced when the volumes of those assets and liabilities are matched (Scherr, 1989).

An organization with 90 percent of its assets in property, plant, and equipment ought not to have 90 percent of the claims on the right-hand side of its balance sheet in short-term liabilities. If it did, a sudden increase in short-term interest rates (remember the volatile rates of the early 1980s) could jeopardize its financial viability.

Consider a clinic that, rather than taking out a 30-year mortgage, finances a $5 million expansion with 90-day notes. During the planning stages and during construction, 90-day commercial rates are, say, 7 percent, well below mortgage rates of, say, 10 percent. The clinic's management believes it has done its stakeholders a great service. As the expansion opens its doors, rates begin to rise. The expectation of rising rates pushes both long-term and short-term rates up, with short-term rates temporarily above mortgage rates. At the next refinancing, the 90-note requires 11 percent while mortgage rates are 10.5 percent. Now management doesn't look so good.

Over time, those 90-day rates, renegotiated between borrower and lender every 3 months, can continue to rise. Short-term rates are usually much more volatile than are long-term rates. The clinic is at constant risk of higher costs of capital and of possible inability to meet its varying debt-service requirements. Had mortgage financing been used at the outset, the cost of capital for the expansion would have been locked in at 10 percent for the life of the mortgage (up to 30 years).

A NOTE ON SHORT-TERM INTEREST RATES

Observers often speak of *the* interest rate, as if there were one and only one. This text has presented interest rate differentials based on risk, liquidity, tax treatment of interest, and term to maturity. Interest rates, within risk/liquidity/tax treatment classes, have a term structure at any moment in time. The **term structure of interest rates**, described by the yield curve within the risk/liquidity/tax treatment class, describes how interest rates vary as yield to maturity varies. Figure 19–1 shows one possible yield curve for AAA-rated corporate bonds.

Short-term securities involve less risk of default than do long-term securities, everything else equal. For long-term securities, there is just more time for things to go wrong. Usually, then, short-term rates, having lower risk, display lower yields. The term structure of interest rates is a complex and controversial subject, and the interested reader should consult the technical literature on the subject (McEnally & Jordan, 1991).

Because, in a world without arbitrage profits (a world with efficient markets), the existing rate on a 5-year bond must be the geometric average of expected 1-year rates over the life of that bond, some unusual things can happen to the yield curve. The rate on a 5-year bond in a given class is

$$r_{5,0} = [(1 + r_{1,0}) \times (1 + r_{1,1}) \times (1 + r_{1,2}) \times (1 + r_{1,3}) \times (1 + r_{1,4})]^{1/5} - 1$$

where $r_{5,0}$ is the rate prevailing at time = 0 on a 5-year security, and $r_{1,4}$ is the rate now expected to prevail on an otherwise equivalent 1-year security at time = 4.

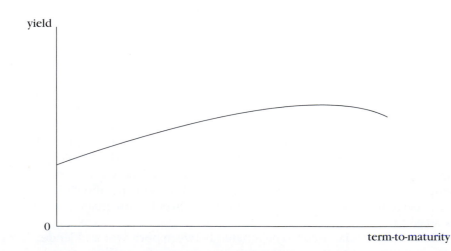

Figure 19-1 Typical yield curve for AAA-rated corporate bonds.

What would make $r_{5,0}$ be greater than $r_{1,0}$ (what would make the yield curve upward sloping)? If *expected* 1-year rates for future years are above the current 1-year rate ($r_{1,0} < r_{1,1}, r_{1,2}, r_{1,3}, r_{1,4}$) the yield curve will slope upward. With a little experimentation, one can see that long-term rates will vary less in percentage points than will short-term rates. One can also see that if short-term rates are expected to fall substantially in the future, long-term rates *can* be lower than short-term rates. Although an upward-sloping yield curve is considered "normal," flat and downward-sloping yield curves are quite possible.

SOURCES OF SHORT-TERM FINANCING

Organizations can use a wider variety of short-term financing vehicles. More such vehicles are available than most managers realize (Stigum, 1990). Although some of these, bankers' acceptances, for example, are not routinely available to health care organizations, the choices that are possible are quite varied. The most commonly used type of short-term financing is the account payable (or its cousins, benefits payable, dividends payable, interest payable, salaries payable, and wages payable).

Accounts Payable

Accounts payable are financing vehicles because they represent short-term loans extended, in the normal course of business, by vendors and employees. Those individuals, rather than requiring payment at the moment of service, allow some time to elapse between delivery (or service) and payment. In the intervening time, the organization has the advantage of the supply or service. The effect, for the borrower, is identical to taking out an *interest-free* loan and paying at the moment of delivery.

Trade Credit

Yet another source of short-term credit is **trade credit**. Trade credit is the extension of time for repayment by vendors. For example, most suppliers do not expect payment at the moment of delivery; to do so would impose a substantial burden on their delivery personnel. Rather, they expect invoices to be paid at the end of some defined period, usually 30 days. Trade credit amounts to a loan of up to 30 days.

The trade credit loan may not, however, be interest free. Often the terms of trade credit are quoted as "2/10, net 30," or "two-ten, net 30." The meaning is, "a 2 percent discount if paid within 10 days, otherwise the full amount is due in 30 days." Other terms, "1/10, net 30," for example, are also possible. When such terms are granted, the effect is to place an opportunity cost on trade credit. By not paying the invoice in 10 days, one is giving up the discount, which is the opportunity cost of waiting until the end of the 30-day period to pay.

Consider terms granted as "2/10, net 30." If one pays within 10 days, one saves 2 percent. That is, paying 20 days early yields a 2 percent discount. There are 18.25

(365/20) 20-day periods in a year. Thus, in a year, there are 18.25 opportunities to save 2 percent per period if one is offered terms of "2/10 net 30." The result is that terms of "2/10, net 30" provide an opportunity cost of 36.5 percent (2 percent per period x 18.25 periods per year) if one waits until the end of the 30 days to pay. Similar calculations make the opportunity cost embedded in "1/10, net 30" equal to 18.25 percent.

Short-Term Bank Note

A more obvious source of short-term financing is the short-term (usually 90-day) **bank note**. A short-term loan from a commercial bank carries an interest rate and is payable in full, principal plus interest, on the specified maturity date. Rolling over the debt consists of paying the interest and borrowing enough to repay the principal at the end of the loan period. Doing so provides, in effect, permanent financing at short-term rates (usually less than long-term rates). On the other hand, rolling over short-term debt exposes the borrower to the risk that interest rates will rise during the 90-day life of the loan. Borrowing at a new, higher rate may not seem the bargain that was anticipated at the beginning of the loan program.

Similar to taking out 90-day notes is the practice, discussed in Chapter 17, of using a line of credit. The line of credit is set up in advance with a participating commercial bank. Whenever cash balances fall below a preset level, the line of credit is automatically tapped. Alternatively, one can establish a standby line of credit for use on demand. Interest is charged on the outstanding balance of the loan. Establishing a standby line of credit is a prudent action, whether as part of a cash management program or independently.

Commercial Paper

Large organizations, within the health care sector and without, can establish programs of borrowing via issuing **commercial paper**. Commercial paper is a publicly tradable, short-term certificate of indebtedness, much like a U.S. Treasury bill. Usually issued for 90 days, commercial paper sells, like T-bills, at a pure discount; there is no coupon. Thus a 90-day issue offering a 10 percent interest rate, with a par value of $1,000,000, would sell for $975,000,000. That is, for 90/360 (yes, 360, not 365) of a year, the purchaser is earning 10 percent. Thus the discount is 2.5 percent of par value (Stigum, 1990, p. 542).

The commercial paper market is huge, dominated by some of the largest American corporations. Commercial banks are the agents through which corporations sell these instruments, acting as pure agents, without any underwriting responsibilities. Only the largest health care corporations will be able to offer commercial paper in sufficient amounts to make this form of short-term financing feasible.

SUMMARY

This chapter has explained the role of short-term financing in the organization's capital structure. Short-term liabilities do not, except in unusual cases, finance short-term assets. Rather, short-term liabilities provide a means of tapping (usually) low-cost money market funds. The use of short-term financing also exposes the organization to periodic refinancing risk. To control overall risk, the volume of short-term debt should approximate the volume of the organization's short-term assets.

A wide variety of short-term financing vehicles are available. Some of these, accounts payable and trade credit, arise from the normal course of business. Others, such as bank notes, lines of credit, and commercial paper, require planning. In any case, organizations should develop *programs* of short-term finance that are consistent with their overall financial plan and their overall risk tolerance.

Discussion Questions

1. If the yield curve is usually upward sloping, why don't more organizations finance themselves exclusively with short-term debt?

2. Why ought one not match long-term assets with rolling 90-day financing?

3. In what sense is the accumulation of accounts payable a form of short-term financing? In what sense is it a particularly desirable form of short-term financing?

4. What prevents most health care organizations from initiating commercial paper programs for short-term financing?

5. Remember the possibility of securitizing patient accounts that was discussed in Chapter 17. Develop a framework (a set of procedures) for using collections of patient accounts as the basis for a program of borrowing via issuing commercial paper.

CONTINUING CASE

Roger Jackson, Henry Kirk, and Janet Fowler were nervous as they waited in Tom Land's office at CCB Bank. Kirk had pressed Land for months to grant a larger line of credit to PCI. The sale of accounts receivable to Keynote Capital Corporation had fallen through (see the Continuing Case for Chapter 15) and PCI needed cash and needed it now.

This was about PCI's last chance. As the meeting began, Dr. Jackson tried his usual bluster. "Tom, I've been one of this bank's best customers for years. You owe me. If I don't get a bigger line of credit, I'll take my business to one of those Dallas banks that call me all the time." Dr. Jackson didn't mention that it had been some time since a Dallas banker had paid a call.

Janet Fowler provided an analytical balance. "Tom, we have the cash budget you wanted. We anticipate that, with a larger line of credit, we can finance some modest improvements, and we'll be able to service all of the debt easily. This would be a good move for you."

Land had already explored the situation. He was leery of PCI and wanted some reassurance. "Janet, Roger, I want to help you, but you've got to work with me. I want you to outline all of your sources of short-term finance. Where does it come from? How can you get more? I don't want an increase in your standby line of credit to replace other sources of short-term finance. Besides [his voiced dropped a little at this point], Mr. Land [Tom always spoke of his uncle, the president of the bank's holding company, in very formal terms] says any more credit to PCI will have to be in the form of a note, not a larger line of credit."

Leaving the meeting, Roger Jackson was both furious and frustrated. "I need to know what we're going to do *now*. Who does that kid think he is, calling me 'Roger'?"

Kirk asked Fowler to do some exploring. "We've always paid all of our accounts at the end of 30 days. Should we pay earlier and take the discounts? If a bank note would cost us 10 percent, what are the implications of the '1/10, net 30' terms our suppliers quote us? We've had all of our employees on a 2-week payroll cycle. Does that hurt us? Can you run up some more numbers, Janet?"

CASE QUESTIONS

1. What are the answers to the questions Kirk posed to Fowler?

2. Why does Dr. Jackson prefer the line of credit to a bank note?

3. Why does the bank prefer to extend credit in the form of a note rather than as a line of credit?

4. Is a commercial paper program feasible for PCI, Inc.?

REFERENCES

McEnally, R.W. & Jordan, J.V. (1991). The term structure of interest rates. In F.J. Fabozzi (Ed.), *Handbook of fixed income securities* (3rd ed., pp. 1245–1295). Homewood, IL: Business One Irwin.

Scherr, F.C. (1989). *Modern working capital management*. Englewood Cliffs, NJ: Prentice Hall. (out of print)

Stigum, M. (1990). *The money market* (3rd ed.). Homewood, IL: Dow Jones-Irwin.

SELECTED READINGS

Brealey, R.A. & Myers, S.C. (2000). *Principles of corporate finance* (6th ed.). New York: McGraw-Hill.

Stigum, M. (1990). *The money market* (3rd. ed.). Homewood, IL: Dow Jones-Irwin.

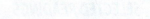

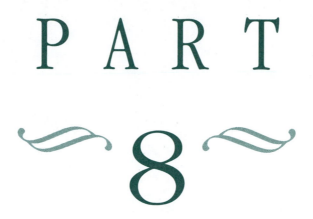

PART

8

Frontiers of Health Care Financial Management

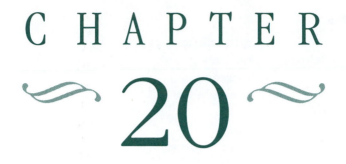

CHAPTER 20

Beyond Bean Counting

Learning Objectives

After reading this chapter, the student should be able to:

1. Explain the financial approach to strategic planning and to participate effectively in that process.
2. Advise senior management on financial restructuring possibilities, including mergers, acquisitions, joint ventures, and joint operating agreements.
3. Evaluate and advise senior management on the acceptance of capitated contract proposals.

Key Terms

Acquisition	Joint operating agreement
Actuarially expected cost of	Joint venture
care	Leveraged buyout
Actuary	Limited partnership
Antitrust regulation	Load
Capitation	Merger
Economies of scale	Per member per month
Economies of scope	(PMPM)
Financial planning	

This is a book about making certain types of decisions according to a certain type of decision rule. That is what financial management is all about. In years past, the managers and trustees of many health care organizations viewed financial criteria as being much less important than is now the case. Health care financial managers, almost all trained as accountants, often referred to themselves, in mock self-derision, as bean counters. The financial management of health care organizations in virtually every setting has moved far from bean counting. Decisions about financing, capital structure, cash management, pension and endowment management, asset choices, and capitated contract negotiation now dominate the field of health care financial management and are primary concerns for all health care executives.

As the role of the health care financial manager has expanded, it has come to include not only the financial functions just listed but also some areas within the domain of strategic management (Pallarito, 1993). The tools of financial decision making can be applied to such strategic issues as which services to pursue and which to drop, whether or not to enter a merger, how best to structure the organization (partnership, corporation, not-for-profit, or investor owned), and whether or not to enter into a proposed managed care contract. The modern chief financial officer is not just a bean counter but an important member of the senior management team.

Similarly, nonfinancial managers (the career destination of most of the readers of this textbook) will use financial decision methods in their own work. In making strategic decisions, managers use discounted cash flow analysis, knowledge of financial market processes, and other financial tools to add value to their organizations and to their communities. This final chapter is about the use of financial methods in making strategic decisions. It also presents the critical decisions involved in at-risk, capitated contracting as financial and strategic choices. After completing the chapter, the reader should understand the application of financial tools to those problems and recognize the potential role of the financial manager in solving them.

STRATEGIC FINANCIAL PLANNING

Strategic planning (and its implementation, strategic management) is usually taught by behavioral scientists and, in health care organizations, is often assigned to marketing staff. Although there may be good reasons for such assignments, financial decision models can play an important role in the strategy-making process. Decisions to accept lines of service, to delete lines of service, and to construct and staff new facilities are all strategic; they are all important to an organization's carrying out its mission and to its long-term prosperity. Those decisions are also straightforward applications of the same net present value rule used throughout this text.

Brealey and Myers (2000) describe **financial planning** as the process of (1) analyzing the financing and investment opportunities available to the organization, (2) anticipating the future consequences of current decisions, (3) selecting among alternatives, and (4) measuring performance and comparing it to anticipations. The process they describe can be applied to decisions to refinance an issue of debt, choices among lines of service, or decisions of whether or not to establish for-profit subsidiaries. The process is essentially the same as the capital budgeting process discussed in Chapters 10 and 11, with two differences.

The first difference is that, in strategic financial planning, few decisions are independent. The logic of capital budgeting becomes fuzzy when decisions have interdependent consequences. If the choice of A over B influences the cash flows from C, then those changes in C must be accounted for in the choice of A or B. In making strategic choices, most, if not all, decisions are interdependent. The cash flows from the existing imaging facility will be affected by the choice of the site of the new facility.

The second difference between strategic financial choices and "simple" capital budgeting decisions is that the strategic options (see Chapter 11; Magiera & McLean, 1996) become paramount. It is the option to establish an outpatient ophthalmic surgery service that makes a contract with an ophthalmological group valuable. When one discusses strategic decisions, it is the possibilities for the future, as much as the cash flows in the next year, that create value for stakeholders.

Brealey and Myers (2000) describe a complete financial plan as a *super-budget*. It incorporates all of the elements of a single year's budget (projected financial statements, capital investment plans) but forecasts these items out for several years into the future. The plan also includes a financing plan, indicating where the money will come from. The choice of debt and equity financing percentages (discussed in Chapter 13) should be projected into the future alongside the investment plan.

Just as there are many alternatives for the current year's investment, there are many more alternatives for a strategic financial plan. Finding the set of investments and service lines to pair with the best means of financing to optimize stakeholder value requires looking at a host of combinations. Although spreadsheets can be used to ask a multitude of "What if?" questions, specialized software models for financial planning, most based on linear programming models, are available to perform the task more efficiently.

FINANCIAL STRUCTURE AND RESTRUCTURING

Modigliani and Miller (1958) showed that, under some conditions, financial structure does not matter, that the organization's value depends on its assets and the cash flows they produce, not on the way the organization is financed (see Chapter 13). In the 1980s, however, one saw many changes in corporate financial structure that seemed to do nothing more than to change financial structures. Some of these seemed to provide substantial returns for their architects. Examples were the **leveraged buyout** of Hospital Corporation of America (HCA) in 1988 and HCA's later decision to offer its stock to the public once again.

Such purely financial changes (which are quite distinct from mergers, acquisition, and divestitures, which involve actual changes in assets) usually are efforts to take advantage of frictions in the financial markets. For example, in the United States interest payments are tax-deductible expenses. Therefore not only is debt less costly than equity because of its higher standing in bankruptcy, it is *much* less costly than equity because interest payments to debt holders are tax-deductible expenses. There is, then, a strong incentive for tax-paying corporations to issue as much debt as they can service.

Leveraged Buyout

In the 1980s a large number of corporations (including American Medical International and Hospital Corporation of America) took advantage of the tax-deductibility of interest payments by becoming almost all-debt financed organizations. The process, called a leveraged buyout, is extremely simple. Consider a hypothetical firm, MedCorp. A group of investors, perhaps members of management, incorporate a shell, MedCorp Holdings (note that MedCorp Holdings is distinct from MedCorp). MedCorp Holdings finds a cooperating bank (or other lending institution) to provide "mezzanine" (interim) financing sufficient to allow it to acquire all of the shares of MedCorp. Once holding all of the shares of MedCorp, MedCorp Holdings issues bonds sufficient to pay back its mezzanine financiers. In the end, MedCorp Holdings has all of the shares of MedCorp. The holding corporation has assumed all of MedCorp's debt and has issued a large amount of new debt. The only equity in MedCorp Holdings company is the (small) amount of equity that the organizers of MedCorp Holdings put up to incorporate their shell.

How did MedCorp Holdings obtain all of the shares of MedCorp? It may have made a tender offer to MedCorp's shareholders. The offer was similar to "We will purchase any and all shares of MedCorp that are tendered (offered up) to our agent (a commercial bank) on or before a cut-off date. In return, we will pay $X per share." $X, to induce the shareholders to tender their shares, is always greater than the current market price of a share of MedCorp. Alternatively, MedCorp Holdings may have approached the board of directors of MedCorp with an offer. If the board of MedCorp is satisfied with the offer, it can vote to accept and the deal is done. Note the presence of agency problems if the boards of MedCorp and MedCorp Holdings overlap. The board of the original corporation has a legal obligation to obtain fair value for all of its stockholders, but the "business judgment rule" says that the courts will intervene only when the fleecing of stockholders is egregious.

What is the advantage to the investors in MedCorp Holdings? They can use the cash flows from MedCorp to service and, ultimately, to retire the debt used to purchase MedCorp. They can enjoy the leverage benefits of debt, perhaps making an extraordinary rate of return on their own, small, initial investment. They also enjoy a very low weighted average cost of capital due to their small use of equity financing and the tax-deductibility of debt. Some leveraged buyout firms (including Hospital Corporation of America and American Medical International) have found the financial pressure imposed by their heavy debt service requirements to have other benefits. Pressured to maintain healthy cash flows, they reduce fixed costs and develop leaner, more efficient organizations. After a period of such cost cutting, and after paying off some of their debt burdens, they sell the stock of the original corporation to the public once again. The investors in the holding company then reap the benefits of their efficiency moves in the form of capital gains on the stock of the original firm. It is interesting to note that, since reissuing shares to the public, both AMI and HCA have ceased to exist. AMI acquired National Medical Enterprises, and the new organization became known as Tenet. HCA was subsumed in the giant firm Columbia-HCA. For public relations purposes, Columbia-HCA later became "HCA, the Healthcare Company."

Why do lenders go along with such arrangements? Jensen (1988) developed the notion of free cash flow (cash flow in excess of all debt service obligation and of that necessary to finance all positive net present value projects) to explain the willingness of lenders to put funds into leveraged buyouts. Firms that throw off a lot of cash provide their managements with the opportunity to profit at shareholders' expense (agency problems enter the scene once again). Firms in mature industries (in which there are few obvious investment opportunities) and that produce a high level of cash flow offer managements the opportunity to consume a lot of perquisites rather than disbursing those cash flows to shareholders. Leveraged buyouts are a way of requiring management to pay out almost all of the organization's cash flow in the form of debt service. Lenders' willingness to loan money to leveraged buyout firms is a demonstration of their desire to obtain firms' free cash flows.

Where is the downside in a leveraged buyout? As in any highly leveraged organization, the debt in a leveraged buyout requires servicing. Inability to repay the interest obligations due to lenders means the bankruptcy of the organization. It is not for nothing that the bonds used to finance leveraged buyouts are known as junk. Perhaps another negative feature of a leveraged buyout is the nature of the projects that a firm so structured must undertake. Due to the high degree of financial leverage risk involved in the buyout structure, it is possible that these firms will be undesirably risk averse, rejecting projects and activities that would be in the public's interest to undertake.

Not-For-Profit to For-Profit

Another paper-shuffling reorganization is the not-for-profit to for-profit conversion. Once rare, a large number of such transitions have occurred for a variety of reasons (Young, 1986). Some organizations, such as the former U.S. Public Health

Service hospitals (originally charged with caring for merchant seamen), underwent such conversions in order to privatize public facilities (a conscious, mission-changing move). Others have "gone for-profit" because participation in lines of business they wanted to enter would have cost them their tax-exempt status anyway.

One privatizing move that has had powerful effects on health care delivery in a few cities (Wichita, Kansas, after the sale of Wesley Medical Center, for example) has been the purchase of a not-for-profit facility by an investor-owned organization. Consider a fictitious organization, Beneficial Hospital. Beneficial's physical plant is aging, its board of trustees sees no way to raise the funds to renovate it adequately, and its cash flows have been consistently negative. An investor-owned organization (HosCorp, also fictitious) has decided that it would like to purchase, renovate, and operate Beneficial.

Beneficial's board needs to reconstitute the organization as Beneficial Health Foundation, whose principal asset is the hospital. HosCorp can then contract with the foundation to purchase its hospital. The cash raised from the sale of the hospital becomes the corpus of the foundation's endowment. The income from the endowment can be used to serve a variety of desirable ends, including paying for care that indigent patients receive at the hospital (now renamed Beneficial-HosCorp). The effect is to inject capital, for health care purposes, into the community. The hospital is still operating (HosCorp did not want to purchase it just to shut it down). The change in ownership, in fact, may have kept the facility from shutting down. On the other hand, the new owners may pursue policies to which patients, physicians, and employees are unaccustomed. If the old operating rules were leading Beneficial Hospital to ruin, it is virtually certain that new owners will institute new policies and procedures.

MERGERS AND ACQUISITIONS

Most corporate restructuring is not purely financial but involves changes in the organization's assets and activities. The most visible of these changes are **mergers** and **acquisitions** (Gaughan, 1991). In a merger, two organizations unite to form a new organization. In an acquisition, one preexisting organization becomes part of another preexisting firm. Neither of these two actions is confined to the investor-owned sector; there have been not-for-profit mergers and acquisitions as well.

Motivations for Mergers and Acquisitions

Why do firms engage in mergers and acquisitions? Often for reasons one might not expect, and never for some reasons the general public believes in (Finkler, 1985). When acquiring an existing organization, firms often talk of the need to diversify, much like an investor acquires new stock to diversify his portfolio. Pure diversification, however, is not a valid motivation for an acquisition. Investors can diversify their own portfolios without any help from corporate management. When managements diversify firms' holdings purely to smooth cash flows, they are creating an agency cost, sacrificing returns to investors to make their own positions more secure. One may wish to acquire another organization in order to enter a new line of business inexpensively, but to do so purely to smooth cash flows is an inappropriate motive.

Also, one may wish to acquire another organization to achieve **economies of scale** or **economies of scope**. Economies of scale are reductions in unit costs due to spreading fixed costs over greater numbers of units of output. When fixed costs are great, and variable costs per unit are relatively small, economies of scale can be achieved by expanding capacity and output. An example exists in hospital networks. Most hospital costs are fixed costs. Almost all of the costs of operating the central office of a hospital network are fixed. Bringing 10 more hospitals into the network sometimes achieves economies of scale. By including the newly acquired sites in the management information system, the group purchasing system, and the existing financing arrangements, one can often lower costs per bed-day.

Economies of scope are reductions in cost per unit that are achieved by including under one organization and management (and hence under one umbrella of fixed costs) distinct, but related, activities. This is the source of cost savings that laymen often call *synergy*. The same management expertise, the same marketing strategy, and some of the same types of supply purchases will support a group medical practice that support inpatient care. Thus some savings in unit cost can, sometimes, be obtained when hospitals (or hospital holding companies) purchase group practices. Similar savings can be achieved through the mergers of medical suppliers and launderers.

Another reason for acquisition in the investor-owned sector is the "throw the rascals out" motivation. Sometimes management's egregious imposition of agency costs on shareholders lowers stock values sufficiently that another firm, or a "corporate raider," realizes that, without the incumbent management, the organization would be worth more. In such cases an acquirer can purchase a majority of the shares of the target firm, replace the management, increase the value of the outstanding shares, and resell her shares on the open market. Such acquisitions are always known as "takeovers" in the news media and are viewed with great suspicion by the general public. The threat of such takeovers, however, is the only effective deterrent to management's behavior.

One additional reason for mergers and acquisitions lies in the United States Tax Code. Investor-owned firms pay tax on their reported profit. In years when those firms suffer losses, however, there is no negative income tax. Firms may, however, carry their losses in one year forward to future years (to offset profits in those years) or backward (by filing amended tax documents) to offset profits earned in previous years. Firms with strings of losses, year after year, have no opportunity to use their "tax loss carry-forwards." Those unused carry-forwards are valuable to firms that have positive earnings (and therefore tax liabilities) in the present. Profitable firms are often willing to pay to acquire unprofitable ones to obtain their tax loss carry-forwards.

Whatever the motive, the analysis of a merger or acquisition should be a straight-forward exercise in valuation analysis (see Chapter 6). Is the present value of all of the benefits acquired at least as great as the cost (including investment banker, lawyer, and accountant fees) of doing the acquiring? If so, the merger or acquisition is in the shareholders' interest and should be undertaken. If not, the restructuring is not worth doing and should be abandoned.

Empirical analysis of a large number of acquisitions suggests that many were not in the interest of the acquiring firm's shareholders. It is most often the shareholders of acquired firms that realize above-market prices for their shares, whereas the shareholders of acquiring firms often see their shares decline in value (Jensen, 1988).

One cautionary note is due in any discussion of mergers and acquisitions. In the United States, statute law and an enormous body of complex case law exist governing such actions. **Antitrust regulation** seeks to preserve competition and to limit the acquisition of market power by private parties. Proposed mergers of hospitals (not-for-profit or investor-owned) and of corporations must pass review of the U.S. Federal Trade Commission and the U.S. Department of Justice (which have overlapping jurisdiction in such matters).

Joint Venture

If the merger of two organizations is like a marriage, a **joint venture** is akin to cohabitating without benefit of clergy (Kaufman, Hall, & Higgins, 1986; Snook & Kaye, 1987). There are as many ways to organize joint ventures as there are joint ventures to organize. In every case, however, two or more organizations, remaining otherwise independent, enter into an arrangement to carry out some purpose together. In the 1980s one veteran health care manager told the author, "We've been joint ventured to death." The current enthusiasm for physician-hospital organizations (PHOs) is a resurgence of that joint venturing.

Limited Partnership

A common organizational vehicle for joint ventures is the **limited partnership**. Limited partnerships are like partnerships in that income and tax advantages flow directly to the partners (there is no "double taxation" of profits, as there is in a corporation). They are like corporations, however, in that the limited partners are liable only for the money they have invested. Only the general partner (who alone can have a role in management) has unlimited liability. Corporations (such as hospitals) can act as general partners, so long as they are not shells set up for that purpose.

Some joint ventures are set up to erect and operate facilities (such as physicians' office buildings). Limited partners put up a small amount of the initial capital, with the partnership, as an organization, taking out a mortgage for the remainder of the needed funds. The general partner manages the facility, charging a fee from the partnership. The real gain for the hospital is the referral base (an adjacent building is a better source of referrals than a dispersed medical staff). The limited partners enjoy tax advantages, as the interest paid on the mortgage is a deductible expense flowing through to the partners.

In other joint ventures, the hospital puts up capital, with a medical practice operating (under contract or under a lease) the facility. Operation of an imaging center by a radiology practice is an example. The radiologists obtain a facility they could not otherwise afford. The hospital receives cash from the operation of the facility, as well as referrals. In any case, joint ventures are most likely when one party has differentially good access to capital while the other has a differentially good ability to bear operating risks or to manage a facility.

Joint Operating Agreements

A relatively recent form of cooperative venture is the **joint operating agreement**. In a joint venture, two or more existing organizations form a common offspring. Under a joint operating agreement, however, two existing organizations agree to be governed by a newly created common parent. Consider the case of Hospital A and Medical Center A, each with a significant market share and a loyal clientele in a metropolitan area. A and B agree, under a joint operating agreement, to be affiliates of Metro Health Services, which will have a new governing board, and the power to borrow on its own behalf. Metro Health Services might build new facilities, and as the new "parent," might change the nature of operations in the two original organizations. The agreement might have an escape clause, exercisable at the option of either A or B; or exercisable at some fixed review date.

Why have so many organizations opted for such an arrangement? It is a way that two organizations can merge without merging. They can enjoy the benefits (purchasing power, access to capital) of a larger organization without losing their individual identities and customer bases. They also cease to compete with one another, and can rationalize and consolidate their product lines (raising, in some cases, anti-trust concerns).

AT-RISK CONTRACTING

For as long as anyone can remember, the mainstream of health care delivery in the United States has worked like this: providers waited for patients to "present" with conditions. Upon completion of patient encounters (or inpatient stays), providers sent bills to their patients (or the patients' insurance carriers), the charges on which were based on the care delivered. The more patients who presented at one's door, the greater was one's revenue.

Managed care, especially delivery of care under **capitation** agreements, changes this scenario. Under capitation, some entity contracts with the patient to provide whatever services the patient needs for a fixed periodic payment (the capitation rate, or the **per member per month**, **PMPM**, fee). Whatever party is at risk has an incentive to keep enrollees away from health care providers, especially away from hospital, where the cost of an encounter is greatest.

Managed care organizations take many forms, the description of which is beyond the scope of this book (Kongstvedt, 2000). In open-panel health maintenance organizations (HMOs), an insurance carrier is at risk for patients' costs of care, and members of the panel of physicians agree to provide services to enrollees. The members of the panel receive an incentive if the costs of care for their enrollees do not exceed a specified annual cap, and may or may not be at risk for excess costs of care.

In closed-panel HMOs, such as the Kaiser Permanente Health Plan, a physician group and an insurance carrier jointly contract with enrollees. The medical group serves only the HMO's enrollees, and its income is dependent, under a contract, on the cost of care for the enrollees. The plan may contract out hospital and subspecialty services, or may include them in the plan.

The proportion of the population under some form of managed care has exploded in recent years, although the percent in pure HMOs seems to have leveled off. Under cost pressure, employers have encouraged their employees (in some cases required their employees) to enter managed care plans. The provider who does not have a managed care strategy will find itself either losing patients or acting in ignorance in the new competitive environment.

The managed care arrangements of the future will ever more often involve providers' acceptance of some portion of the financial risk of caring for the members of the covered population. Figure 20–1 depicts one such possible arrangement.

Purchasing groups (usually employers) sign a contract with a managed care organization, also known as a managed care network. The network may be organized by an insurance carrier, a hospital, a group practice, or some independent body, such as an organization of employers. Under the contract, the purchasers agree to pay the network a fixed monthly fee per covered life (the capitation fee). The network agrees to provide all of the needed care, within included categories, for all of persons whose lives are covered. The network has the advantage of a

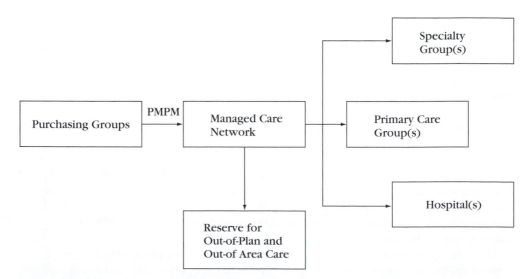

Figure 20-1 A managed care plan with providers at risk. (Adapted from Jennings, Ryan, & Kolb, 1994)

steady, fixed stream of cash flows, without the need to worry about collecting accounts receivable.

The network is, however, at risk for the cost of all of the care for its covered lives (within the included categories). One approach networks might take is to accept that risk and to purchase care as it is needed. More and more often, however, networks will seek out providers to share the financial risk of care with them. That is, the network will sign contracts with providers under which the providers accept covered lives and agree to provide services, within their specialties, for a predetermined share of the PMPM. Some services may still be purchased as needed (arcane subspecialty services and services required when an enrollee is traveling outside the service area, for example), but some member of the network is now at risk for most types of care.

Success Under Capitated Payment

Under competitive pressure, many medical groups and hospitals have signed on with managed care networks, often without analyzing carefully the consequences of their actions. The "tricks" to success under capitated payment are few in number. First, one must know one's costs. As discussed in Chapter 7, that is not as simple as it seems. One must know the full cost of providing a unit of service, for each type of service for which one is responsible, because the PMPM payment must, if managed care contracting is to be feasible, cover the full cost of providing care to the covered lives for which one is responsible.

It is not enough just to know the cost of a unit of service, however. The second trick to success in managed care contracting is projecting how much of each type of service one will be called on to provide. What is the expected utilization of each type of service for each covered life? That type of analysis is the job of the **actuary** (Sutton & Sorbo, 1993). Actuaries are experts in the estimation of the expected cost involved in assuming financial risks and in ensuring financial viability given those risks, and insurance companies have long been their primary employers. During a long process of certification (usually following one or more university degrees in mathematics, statistics, or actuarial science), actuaries can qualify for the title of Fellow of the Society of Actuaries (FSA). Every organization contemplating undertaking risk under a managed care contract should begin with an actuarial analysis, conducted by a staff or consulting actuary.

One's actuary will consider the age, race, education, and sex distribution of the population of lives to be covered to determine expected utilization rates for the services for which the organization is responsible (note that one may be responsible, under the contract, for services other than those one actually offers). Those expected utilization rates, coupled with unit cost information, provide information on the **actuarially expected cost of care** for a covered life in the population under review. The managerial question that remains is whether or not the PMPM offered by the managed care network is adequate to cover that actuarially expected cost of care.

The provider, under managed care, then, must evaluate an insurance product, health care provision under a capitated fee, from the standpoint of the insurer. If the PMPM exactly equals the actuarially expected cost of care, the provider will go bankrupt. That is because a string of months in which the actual cost of care exceeds the actuarially expected cost (and there will be such strings) will leave the provider without resources. A cushion, or **load**, must be maintained between the PMPM and the actuarially expected cost of care both to cover administrative costs and to provide a reserve against adverse experience.

The larger the population of covered lives, the closer, on average, will be the actual cost of care to the actuarially expected cost (that is the effect of the familiar "law of large numbers"). Thus managed care plans that cover 100,000 lives can charge lower loads and have a competitive advantage over plans that cover 10,000 lives. The evolution of managed care plans and at-risk contracting may be one of the factors that will cause small providers to unite into larger organizations.

It is worth noting that under managed care, all of the providers in the network have very different incentives than those that obtain under fee-for-service medicine. In order to keep the largest possible proportion of the PMPM, the network will act to restrain utilization, especially utilization of the most costly types of care (inpatient services and subspecialty care). Under managed care, the hospital is a cost center in a larger organization, and the principal role of the hospital administrator is to constrain costs, not to expand services, and certainly not to keep the beds full.

Consider the implications of the hospital's being (or of any other provider's being) a cost center in a managed care network. Now there is no direct link between any asset and cash inflows, because there is no direct link between any one service and cash inflows. The only providers who still have such asset-to-service-to-cash linkages are those outside the network who contract to provide services for fees. Inside the network, other bases must be established to justify capital spending.

Will the breakdown of the service-to-cash connection lead to reductions in hospitals' (and other providers') capital spending? Although only time and empirical analysis will tell, it seems likely. What basis will those providers use to justify investment? One possibility is options analysis. Acquisition of an MRI device provides options to the organization: the option to provide services in-house (rather than contracting providers), and the option to bid to provide imaging services for other plans and providers. Managed care networks may be the first to use options analysis extensively in their capital budgeting analyses.

INTERNATIONAL HEALTH CARE FINANCIAL MANAGEMENT: THE FRONTIER BEYOND THE FRONTIER

Once, health care services, like haircuts, were consumed where they were produced, and health care organizations operated from single facilities in single cities. Modern technology, and modern corporate finance, have made it possible for health care providers to operate on an international scale (McLean, 1997). This aspect of globalization introduces new opportunities for value enhancement, but also presents new problems for health care managers to solve.

The simplest way for health care organizations to offer international services is to recruit patients overseas for treatment in the United States. Although the recruitment may require contacts, language fluency, and special knowledge of visa requirements, this form of internationalization presents no special financial management problems. Indeed, as most international patients pay their own bills, this activity may reduce the organization's overall collection period and enhance its cash position.

There are also ways to offer services in settings outside the United States. Information technology, for example, makes it possible for a physician in Cleveland to diagnose a patient in Budapest. "Telemedicine" makes the international sale of services possible, even if it is not yet common. U.S.-based organizations can also operate facilities abroad, treating patients on-site and receiving payment from the patient or his insurance carrier in host county currency.

It is when a U.S.-based provider receives payment in a currency other than U.S. dollars that a financial issue arises. Exchange rates between currencies vary continuously. If an American provider has a patient account denominated in euros (the currency circulating within the European Union), it is constantly at risk that the value of the euro relative to the dollar will fall. One way to avoid that risk is to demand payment in U.S. dollars. Doing so, however, may limit the very business that the provider has gone abroad to generate.

Another way to mitigate foreign currency risk is to hedge one's foreign currency exposure in the currency futures market. Hedging strategies are beyond the scope of this text (McLean, 1987), but corporations that have substantial foreign currency risk exposure use them daily.

SUMMARY

The changes taking place in financial management in health care spring from several causes. One cause is the competitive pressure to hold down costs. The result is the growth of managed care contracting and the need to evaluate capitated contracts for their financial feasibility. Another cause is the need to raise financial capital to acquire and to maintain the technology of modern health care. The result is the plethora of forms and cases of joint ventures and joint operating agreements.

The presence of a highly developed financial system in the United States provides both challenges and opportunities for American health care. With all of the financing opportunities available to corporations in the United States, it was inevitable that health care organizations would seek out capital (at the lowest obtainable cost) in previously unfamiliar ways. Over time, that search for low-cost financing has given rise to hospital revenue bonds, joint ventures, and the sale of (and the securitization of) patient accounts. It was also inevitable that health care organizations, especially in the investor-owned sector, would come into play, their identities and controls being bought and sold. The result may be greater efficiency (although that is not yet proven), but it also generates disquietude in communities accustomed to stable, locally controlled health care organizations.

Financial management in health care organizations has progressed far from its roots in accounting. Today financial managers are important members of the senior management team, participating fully in strategy determination as well as assuming responsibility for obtaining the funds that enable acquisition of technology and organizational survival.

It is not only financial management professionals who need to understand the financial approach to problem solving, however. Every manager, from the department level to the executive suite, needs to understand and to use some basic financial tools: cost analysis, budgeting, and decision making based on opportunity cost and the time value of money. Like their organizations, those who use those financial tools will prosper; those who fail to learn and to use them will falter.

Discussion Questions

1. What roles should financial professionals play in the strategic planning process in health care organizations? Do those roles vary according to organizational type (government owned, private not-for-profit, investor-owned)?

2. What may have motivated National Medical Enterprises' acquisition of American Medical International (to form Tenet Healthcare Corporation)? List and discuss several possible motives.

3. Consider a merger of health care organizations that has taken place in your area. Have economies of scale or of scope actually been achieved?

4. What information does a medical practice need to have in order to decide whether to accept or to reject a proposed capitated contract? Where (from whom) can it obtain that information?

5. Consider some management positions typically found in health care organizations. Under what circumstances and how might individuals in those positions use financial tools?

> Chief Executive Officer
>
> Chief Operating Officer
>
> Chief of the Medical Staff (or Medical Director)
>
> Director of Risk Management
>
> Director of the Laboratory

CONTINUING CASE

"I've never liked Roger Jackson, and I certainly don't think he's trying to do us a favor with this offer," Billy Bob Ferguson complained to his wife, Alice, over breakfast. He and the board of Lone Star Home Health Services (LSHHS) were facing a new kind of challenge. "How did I ever get involved in the home health business?"

The Jackson Group (Dr. Roger Jackson's practice and the largest tenant of Physicians' Clinic) had negotiated a contract to act as the primary care provider in Clearwater County for Health Connection (HC), a Dallas-based managed care network. The Jackson Group would serve as gatekeeper and primary care provider for all of HC's covered lives in the county. Jackson, at first, thought the $145-per-member-per-month capitation payment was manna from heaven. The revenue would bolster his practice's income, and, in a real coup, PCI, Inc., became a participating hospital in the plan, drawing $45 per adult member per month (separate from the Jackson Group's allotment) for the county's covered adults for nonsurgical inpatient stays.

It was only later that Jackson realized that the Jackson Group was responsible for other services, covered in the enrollees' contracts but not provided by his practice. Surgical services were capitated separately, but medical specialities (cardiology, gastroenterology, nephrology, pulmonology) were Jackson's responsibility. The Jackson Group would have to pay out of its own pocket for all of their referrals to nonsurgical specialists. Also, the group's responsibility included two covered nonmedical services, physical therapy and home health care. Instead of paying charges for these services, Roger Jackson was trying to line up cooperating providers to accept part of the capitated risk.

Jackson wanted to cover his home health services needs by negotiating a contract, in advance of any referrals, with LSHHS. Because this was a Jackson Group matter, Henry Kirk and Janet Fowler of PCI were not involved.

Dr. Jackson proposed the following to Ferguson at their first meeting. LSHHS would provide as many as 10 post-hospital home visits for any enrollee released from surgical or medical inpatient stays, and would provide other home services (monitoring of home-bound diabetics, some infusion services), as prescribed by Jackson Group primary care physicians, for $15 per member per month. If any enrollee needed more than 10 post-hospital visits, or more than 50 covered home visits per year, those would be reimbursed according to a fee schedule (Dr. Jackson just happened to have one with him). Jackson explained that the Jackson Group would take out stop-loss insurance against those possibilities.

"$15 PMPM is chicken feed, Roger," Billy Bob complained. "You'll have a population with heavy home health needs and primary care 'docs' prescribing home care for everybody they see. LSHHS will lose its shirt."

Dr. Jackson liked neither the use of his first name nor the rejection of his offer, but agreed to entertain a counteroffer at a subsequent meeting. Didn't Ferguson know that $15 was coming straight out of *his* PMPM? He did not consider the possibility that LSHHS would say no to his proposal (forcing the Jackson Group to *buy* home health services).

"All right, Billy Bob, do your analysis and see what *you* can come up with." Jackson was frustrated and annoyed.

> Once again, Billy Bob had more calculating to do, and once again he was navigating uncharted waters. This capitation stuff wasn't what he intended to be doing when he took on a job with a charity. "Where do I begin? What information do I need? Why don't I just retire?"

CASE QUESTIONS

1. What information does Ferguson need to analyze Jackson's offer?

2. What are the minimum requirements for any reasonable counter offer?

3. If LSHHS says no, what sort of noncapitated arrangement might it seek to make with the Jackson Group? Is it feasible for a subcontracting provider to operate on a fee-for-service basis while the gatekeeping provider remains at risk?

REFERENCES

Brealey, R.A. & Myers, S.C. (2000). *Principles of corporate finance* (6th ed.). New York: McGraw-Hill.

Finkler, S.A. (1985). Merger and consolidation: The motives behind healthcare combinations. *Healthcare Financial Management, 39*(2), 64–74.

Gaughan, P.A. (1991). *Mergers and acquisitions*. New York: HarperCollins.

Jennings, Ryan, & Kolb. (1994). Capitation and risk sharing. Paper presented at a Dec. 8-9, 1994 Regional Seminar of the Healthcare Financial Management Association.

Jensen, M.C. (1988). Takeovers: Their causes and consequences. *Journal of Economic Perspectives, 2*(1), 21–48.

Kaufman, K., Hall, M., & Higgins, D. (1986). Joint ventures revisited: We're all in this together. *Healthcare Financial Management, 40*(3), 25–32.

Kongstvedt, P.R. (Ed.). (2000). *The managed care handbook* (4th ed.). Rockville, MD: Aspen.

Magiera, F.T. & McLean, R.A. (1996). Strategic options in capital budgeting and program selection under fee-for-service and managed care. *Health Care Management Review, 21*(4), 7–17.

McLean, R.A. (1987). Futures markets provide risk-shifting options for providers. *Healthcare Financial Management, 41*(4), 80–87.

McLean, R.A. (1997). Opportunities in the international health services arena. *Healthcare Financial Management, 51*(8), 60–64.

Modigliani, F. & Miller, M.H. (1958). The cost of capital, corporation finance, and the theory of investment. *American Economic Review, 48*(3), 261–297.

Pallarito, K. (1993). A change in focus for CFOs. *Modern Healthcare, 23*(26), 65–74.

Snook, J.D., Jr. & Kaye, E.M. (1987). *A guide to health care joint ventures*. Rockville, MD: Aspen.

Sutton, H.L., Jr. & Sorbo, A.J. (1993). *Actuarial issues in the fee-for-service/prepaid medical group.* Englewood, CO: Center for Research in Ambulatory Health Care Administration.

Young, D.W. (1986). Ownership conversions in health care organizations: Who should bene-fit? *Journal of Health Politics, Policy and Law, 10*(4), 765–774.

SELECTED READINGS

Brealey, R.A. & Myers, S.C. (2000). *Principles of corporate finance* (6th ed.). New York: McGraw-Hill.

Gaughan, P.A. (1991). *Mergers and acquisitions*. New York: HarperCollins.

Kongstvedt, P.R. (Ed.). (2000). *The managed care handbook* (4th ed.). Rockville, MD: Aspen.

Glossary

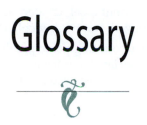

ABC inventory system: management system that concentrates attention on the A category of items, which are few in number but have high costs per unit.

Accelerated depreciation: a method of determining depreciation to increase depreciation expense in turn lowering tax liabilities in the early years in the life of an asset.

Accept/reject: capital budgeting decision problem in which one chooses to acquire or not to acquire a single asset, there being no alternative assets under consideration.

Accounting cycle: the process of recording, summarizing, and reporting financial transactions.

Accounts receivable: current asset, created in the course of doing business, consisting of revenues recognized, but not yet collected as **cash**.

Accrual principle: the accounting principle that requires that revenues are recognized at the time the associated service is provided (rather than when cash is collected) and that expenses are recognized at the time the associated service is received (rather than when cash is disbursed).

Acquisition: purchase of one organization (the acquired) by another (the acquirer); the acquired is subsumed within the acquirer.

Activity-based costing: cost accounting system that identifies cost drivers, activities that produce costs, and allocates indirect costs on the basis of associated cost drivers.

Actuarially expected cost of care: the expected cost of providing health care to an individual or to a population based on prices of health care inputs, customary treatments, and risks to health status.

Actuary: one trained in the use of quantitative methods to assess risks of hazard and to estimate expected losses due to those risks.

Adjusted book value: the approach to valuation that uses the values of assets as recorded in the organization's financial statements.

Agency cost: reduction in the value of an organization due to the presence of **agency problems** within it.

Agency problem: an opportunity, arising from an **agency relationship**, for an agency to benefit at the expense of the principal in whose interest he or she is supposed to act.

Agency relationship: a relationship in which one party (the agent) acts on behalf of another (the principal).

Annuity: a stream of equal payments, equally spaced over time.

Antitrust regulation: body of American law forbidding combinations in restraint of trade.

Appraisal: the process and any of several methods for establishing the market values of assets.

Arbitrage Pricing Theory (APT): model of **security** pricing that uses securities' sensitivities to multiple factors as the bases for returns.

Arbitrage profit: profit that is possible when the **law of one price** is violated; one can buy in the low-price market and simultaneously sell in the high price market, earning a profit with no commitment of resources.

Asset: an item owned by the organization.

Asset/equity ratio: ratio of total assets to owners' equity (or to net assets).

Auditors: those practicing the branch of accounting that verifies that financial statements have their bases in verifiable fact, and that they accurately reflect the position of the organization, according to **generally accepted accounting principles**.

Auditor's opinion: a statement that guarantees Generally Accepted Accounting Principles were used to prepare the audit.

Balance sheet: financial statement showing the equality between the organization's **assets** and its **liabilities** and **owners' equity** at the end of the accounting period.

Bank note: short-term (usually 90 days) loan from a commercial bank; principal and interest are due on the maturity date.

Bankruptcy costs: reductions in the total value of the firm due to bankruptcy proceedings; reductions in value that cause claimants to be able to recover less than the prebankruptcy value of the organization.

Basic accounting equation: assets equal liabilities plus owner's equity.

Best efforts basis: agreement between an investment bank and an issuer of securities in which the bank agrees to do its best to sell the securities for their par value, but makes no guarantee that it can (it declines to **underwrite** them).

Beta: the sensitivity of **returns** for an individual **security** to changes in the market's **return** premium over the risk-free rate of interest.

Bond: a security sold to a lender, promising regular interest payments and repayment of principal, in exchange for the loan in the present.

Bond counsel: law firm that certifies, to the best of its knowledge, that an issue of municipal bonds is in fact tax-exempt.

Bond covenant: the contract specifying the obligations of a **bond's** issuer to its purchasers.

Bond insurance: insurance contract that guarantees that the bond holders will receive their scheduled payments, even if the issuer defaults.

Bottom-up budgeting: budget process in which a great deal of information flows from responsibility centers to the Chief Financial Officer.

Broker: an individual or institution making **securities** purchases and sales as an agent for members of the public.

Budget: a plan for revenues and expenditures for a **budget period**; coverts goals and objectives into targets for revenue and spending.

Budgeting: the process of converting the organization's operating plan into revenue, expense, and cash flow projections.

Budget period: the period of time for which a **budget** is prepared, often one fiscal year.

Capital: assets whose expected useful lines are longer than 1 year; also, funds for the purchase of such assets.

Capital Asset Pricing Model (CAPM): model of **security** pricing that uses securities' sensitivities to the market's **return** premium over the risk-free rate as the basis for **returns**.

Capital budget: the plan for expenditures for assets whose expected useful life is longer than 1 year.

Capital budgeting: process of selecting long-lived assets according to financial decision rules.

Capital market: the **market** for long-term (more than 1 year to maturity) funds.

Capital market line: the ray, in **risk-return** space, extending from the risk-free rate of interest through the **risk-return** coordinates of the market portfolio and beyond.

Capital rationing: capital budgeting problem in which the best subset of possible projects is to be selected for the expenditure of a fixed amount of money.

Capital structure: the organization's mix of sources of funding.

Capitation: agreement under which a health care plan collects a **per member per month** premium in exchange for providing any of a set of contractually specified services on demand.

Cash: current asset, consisting of currency on hand plus bank deposits against which checks can be written.

Cash budget: the forecast of cash inflows and cash outflows associated with the revenue and spending plans incorporated in the **budget** as a whole.

Cash conversion cycle: the process through which **cash** finances operations that generate **accounts receivable**, which are collected in the form of **cash**; measured in days.

Cash equivalent: current asset, consisting of those marketable securities that (1) can be converted into cash quickly and (2) whose values are not sensitive to the rate of interest.

Cash flow: increase in cash holdings over a period of time.

Cash flow coverage: ratio of available cash flow to debt payment obligations.

Cash flow statement: document showing the flow of cash into and out of the entity over the course of the reporting period.

Cash management agreement: an agreement between an organization and a commercial bank, in which the bank agrees, for a fee, to open a line of credit and to manage the short-term investing needs of the organization.

Central bank: a nation's bankers' bank; controls the supply of money and credit.

Certainty equivalent: an amount, to be received with certainty, that a risk-averse person accepts as being just as good as participating in a lottery with a known, but risky, expected pay-off.

Certified Healthcare Finance Professional (CHFP): professional designation, conferred by the Healthcare Financial Management Association, earned by completion of continuing education and examination. It is an intermediate step toward achieving **Fellow of the Healthcare Financial Management Association (HFMA)**.

Chief Financial Officer (CFO): corporate officer responsible for the entire financial management function.

Chief Information Officer (CIO): corporate officer responsible for all information, technology systems.

Collection period: the average time required to convert accounts receivable into cash; accounts receivable divided by revenue per day.

Commercial paper: short-term security, sold to the public by a corporation, as a source of short-term financing.

Common-size statement: financial statements reconstructed to show all entries not in dollar terms, but as percentages of total revenues (income statement) or of total assets (balance sheet).

Common stock: equity claim against the organization, not entitled to any fixed dividend, but (usually) with a voting right.

Compensating balance: a minimum balance required of organizations having loans from or **cash management agreements** with a commercial bank.

Compound: the accumulation of money through the earning of interest on interest.

Comptroller (or controller): officer responsible for financial record keeping and reporting; reports to the **Chief Financial Officer**.

Conservation: attempts to maintain the value of the organization and its assets.

Contra-asset: an adjustment to an asset, entered as a negative debit.

Correlation: the statistical relationship between the movements of two variables, varying from 0.00 (no relationship) to 1.00 (exactly the same proportional movement).

Cost: cost of production; the market value of the goods and services used to produce a good or service.

Cost allocation: the distribution of costs from cost centers to other cost centers and to revenue centers, in order to determine the total cost of producing goods or services.

Cost center: responsibility center charged with controlling its own cost, but without responsibility for generating revenue.

Cost of goods sold (CGS): the historical cost of the items sold to consumers, as calculated by the **inventory** valuation method used.

Cost/volume/profit analysis: method of determining at what level of volume the production of a good or service will **break even**.

Coupon payment: one of the periodic payments of cash to the holder of a bond.

Coupon rate: the percent of **principal paid** to a bond holder, via **coupon payments**, during a year.

Covariance: a statistical relationship between the variances of two variables, defined as the product of the standard deviations of the two variables multiplied by their **correlation**.

Credit: a right-hand-side accounting entry; used to record liabilities, owners' equity, and revenues.

Current assets: Assets that will cease to exist within one accounting period.

Current liabilities: Liabilities that are due within the current accounting period.

Current ratio: ratio of all current assets to all current liabilities.

Dealer: an individual or institution making **securities** purchases and sales for his (or its) own account.

Debenture: a bond that is not secured by a claim on any particular asset or group of assets.

Debit: a left-hand-side accounting entry; used to record assets and expenses.

Decision tree: a pictorial representation of the possible net present values, for some investment, given the possible annual cash flows and their probabilities.

Deferred tax liability: a liability representing the difference between the income tax liability actually incurred and the income tax liability that would have been incurred had the same method of depreciation been used for income tax and corporate reporting purposes.

Depreciation: the process of matching the historical cost of an asset to expenses in the periods in which it is used. May be **straight line** (taking equal amounts of depreciation expense in each year) or **accelerated** (taking greater amounts of depreciation expense in earlier years).

Diagnosis-related group (DRG): any of the broad categories into which patients are classified on admission to a hospital; DRG classification is the basis for hospital payment under Medicare.

Direct allocation method: cost allocation method that allocates the costs of each cost center directly to **revenue centers**, without any intermediate allocations to other cost centers.

Direct cost: costs directly associated with the production of the good or service in question.

Discount rate: the interest rate used to reduce a **future value** to its **present value**.

Discounted cash flow: the approach to valuation that uses the present values of the organization's expected future cash flows.

Discounting: reducing an expected future amount to its **present value**.

Dividend discount model: the approach to the valuation of common stock that uses the present value of expected future cash dividends as the basis for value.

Double distribution method: cost allocation method that allocates cost from cost centers to revenue centers with intermediate steps, as in the **step-down method**, but that does not close cost centers until the second round of cost allocations.

Due diligence: process of determining that the assertions made in financing documents are true and accurate.

EBITDA: Earnings Before Interest, Taxes, Depreciation, and Amortization; a measure of cash flow.

Economic order quantity (EOQ): optimal amount to have on hand after delivery of each new order.

Economies of scale: reductions in average total cost due to increases in the size of the organization.

Economies of scope: reductions in average total cost due to increases in the number of services offered by, and the number of functions performed within, the organization.

Efficiency: the degree to which **securities'** prices reflect available information.

Efficient frontier: the set portfolios representing the highest attainable expected **return** at all levels of **risk** and the lowest attainable **risks** for all given expected **returns**.

End-of-period assumption: the assumption, on which most tables of present value and future value are based, that cash flows are made or received only at the end of each period of time.

Endowment: assets invested to provide a cash flow subsidy for the organization.

Equilibrium: the stable price/quantity relationship toward which any **market** tends to move.

Equivalent annual amount: the annual cash flow, for an annuity, that has the same net present value as that of some project whose anticipated cash flows are not themselves an annuity.

Equivalent annual cost: the annual cash outflow, for an annuity of cash outflows, that has the same present value as that of some cash outflow only project whose anticipated cash outflows are not themselves an annuity.

Expense budget: that component of the **budget** forecasting expenses for the **budget period**.

Feasibility study: part of the **full disclosure** documentation for an issue of hospital revenue bonds; indicates what the bonds would finance, what the level of utilization of the funded project is likely to be, and what the financial statements of the organizations with the new project in place.

Federal Open Market Committee: committee of governors of the **Federal Reserve System** and presidents of regional banks, meeting regularly to determine the need to inject or to withdraw money and credit from the economy.

Federal Reserve System: the **central bank** of the United States; 12 regional banks and Washington headquarters.

Fellow of the Healthcare Financial Management Association (FHFMA): professional designation, earned through continuing education and examination, signifying a high level of proficiency and experience in the financial management of health care organizations.

Financial accounting: the branch of accounting that deals with recording, summarizing, and reporting the transactions of the organization.

Financial Accounting Standards Board (FASB): group, chartered by the United States Congress, charged with developing and publishing the standards under which the accounting reports of corporations (not-for-profit and investor-owned) are to be constructed.

Financial engineering: development of securities and contracts that offer unusual cash flow patterns.

Financial leverage: the use of debt by an organization; includes the degree of indebtedness (capital structure) and the degree to which the organization can meet its debt obligations (coverage).

Financial management: the process of selection, financing, and stewardship of the assets of any organization.

Financial market: a set of institutional arrangements for purchase and sale of short-term or long-term funds.

Financial planning: process of analyzing financing and investment opportunities, anticipating their consequences, and selecting among them.

Financial reporting: the process of converting bookkeeping entries into useful **financial statements**.

Financial statement analysis: the study of an organization's periodic financial statements in order to diagnose the organization's strengths and weaknesses.

Financing cash flow: cash flow associated with payments to the suppliers of capital.

First in-first out (FIFO): method of valuing **inventory** that assumes that goods sold are the oldest in stock.

Fixed budget: an **expense budget** in which responsibility centers have expenditure targets that do not vary with service volume.

Fixed cost: cost that does not vary as volume varies.

Flexible budget: an **expense budget** in which responsibility centers have expenditure targets that vary with service volume.

Float time: the time that elapses between a payor's writing a check and the time that the associated funds become available to the payee.

Footnotes: explanatory notes attached to **financial statements**.

Free cash flow: cash flow above that which is necessary to pay debt service obligations and that required to invest in any positive net present value projects.

Full disclosure: the requirement that **financial statements** disclose all material information, whether favorable to the organization or not.

Fund accounting: accounting method employed in some government-owned and not-for-profit organizations to ensure proper stewardship of assets.

Future value: an amount to be received in the future; the amount to which some present value would grow if invested at some assumed interest rate for some specified period of time.

General obligation bond: debt obligation issued by a municipal bond authority that is guaranteed by the full faith and credit of that authority.

Generally accepted accounting principles (GAAP): the rules developed and published by the Financial Accounting Standards Board that govern the recording and summarizing of financial transactions.

Geometric mean: the nth root of the product of n values.

Going concern: the accounting convention that requires that all entries be made on the assumption that the organization will continue to exist beyond the current period.

Goodwill: the accounting entry that records the difference between what was paid to acquire an organization and the value of the assets that the organization showed on its balance sheet prior to the acquisition.

Government Accounting Standards Board (GASB): group, chartered by the United States Congress, charged with developing and publishing the standards under which the accounting reports of units of government and of government-owned organizations are to be constructed.

Healthcare Financial Management Association (HFMA): organization of professionals in health care financial management and accounting; awards the **Certified Healthcare Finance Professional** and **Fellow of the Healthcare Financial Management Association** designations.

Historical costs: the original cost of property, goods, or services without showing market value.

Holding cost: annual cost to hold an item in stock.

Hospital revenue bond: debt obligation issued by municipal bond authority on behalf of government-owned or private not-for-profit health care providers, guaranteed only by the revenues of the entity for which issued.

Income statement: financial statement showing the organization's revenues, expenses, and net income for an accounting period.

Incremental budgeting: budget process in which the budgets for succeeding **budget periods** are based on those for earlier **budget periods**.

Indirect cost: a cost that is not directly associated with the production of the good or service in question.

Initial cash outflow: the cash flow required to bring an asset into use.

Insider trading: securities purchases or sales by corporate officers (or by those who have received information from corporate officers) on the basis of information that is not available to the public; prohibited under U.S. securities law.

Interest: payments made in return for the use of money.

Internal auditing: branch of accounting activity that provides internal scrutiny of the bookkeeping processes and reporting activities of the organization.

Internal auditor: staff member charged with ensuring that financial records are properly documented and maintained, adhering to generally accepted accounting principles.

Internal rate of return: the rate of discount that makes the **net present value** of an asset or project equal to zero; the rate of return earned by the asset or project.

Inventory: current asset consisting of items held for resale.

Investment banker: specialist in bringing newly issued securities to market.

Joint Commission on Accreditation of Health Care Organizations (JCAHO): entity that accredits hospitals and other health care organizations; some third party payments are conditioned by such accreditation.

Joint operating agreement: a contractual agreement in which two or more previously existing organizations agree to become subsidiaries of a newly created, mutual parent organization.

Joint venture: cooperative arrangement between two organizations, each of which continues to exist as an independent entity.

Journal entry: the original entry of debit and credit amounts, recording a financial transaction.

Just-in-time inventory management (JIT): delivery of items occurs at the moment at which they are to be used.

Last in-first out (LIFO): method of valuing **inventory** that assumes that goods sold are the newest in stock.

Law of one price: two identical items for sale in the same location must sell for the same price (until there are barriers to the flow of information); if the prices differ, they must quickly move toward equality.

Least common multiple: method of comparing assets and projects of unequal expected lives, considering replications of the projects not for one expected life but for the least common multiple of their lives.

Leveraged buyout: financial restructuring involving issuing large quantities of debt in order to purchase all outstanding equity claims.

Liability: a financial obligation of the organization.

Limited partnership: organizational form combining the limited liability of the corporation with the pass-through of income and tax deductions of the partnership.

Line of credit: a standby loan; an amount that a borrower can borrow on demand.

Linear programming: procedure for finding values that maximize a linear function, subject to a set of linear constraints.

Liquidity: in the study of financial statements, ratios that show the ability to meet short-term financial obligations out of short-term assets.

Load: difference between the insurance premium charged to a client and the client's **actuarially expected cost of care**.

Lock box service: collection service by a commercial bank; checks are sent to a post office box, the bank retrieves them several times daily and immediately deposits them into the client's account.

Long-term debt to equity: ratio of long-term (more than 1 year to maturity) debt to owners' equity (or to fund balance).

Managed care: any of a large variety of arrangements for organizing and financing health care in which the insured individual has an incentive (or, in the extreme, a requirement) to use the services of a designated primary care physician (PCP), and incentives to use the services of those specialists to whom the PCP refers the insured.

Managerial accounting: branch of accounting responsible for taking information about the costs of doing business from the financial records; also known as the cost accountant.

Mandatory registration: requirement that securities offered to the public be registered with the U.S. Securities and Exchange Commission (corporate issues only) and with the state securities commissioners of the states in which they are to be sold (corporate and municipal issues).

Market: any set of arrangements for bringing buyers and sellers together to effect transactions.

Market maker: dealer who maintains an inventory of some **security** and who stands ready to make purchases for and sales from that inventory.

Market value: the approach to valuation that uses the prices at which comparable organization or assets have recently been sold.

Matching principle: the volume of short-term (low-risk) assets should be matched by the volume of short-term (high-risk) liabilities.

Maximizing behavior: individuals' attempts to seek the highest wealth possible at the risk levels they have chosen.

Merger: combination between two preexisting organizations in which a new organization is formed and the two merging organizations cease to exist.

Mezzanine financing: short-term loan to provide financing until the necessary long-term securities can be issued.

Modified accelerated cost recovery system (MACRS): method of accelerated depreciation mandated by the U.S. Internal Revenue Code.

Monetary terms: accounting priciple requiring that all assets, liabilities, expenses, and revenues be measured in units of money.

Money market: the **market** for short-term (less than 1 year to maturity) funds.

Money market mutual fund: an entity in which investors purchase shares and that uses the proceeds of those sales to purchase money market securities.

Mortgage bond: debt obligation guaranteed by a claim on some specific asset or assets.

Mutually exclusive choice: decision problem in which one selects one and only one asset from a menu of alternatives.

Net advantage of leasing: present value of the periodic benefits from leasing, rather than purchasing, an asset.

Net assets: In a not-for-profit or government-owned organization, the difference between total **assets** and total **liabilities**; the **owners' equity** claim.

Net present value: the sum of the present values of the **initial**, **operating**, and **terminating cash flows**; the project's addition to the value of the organization.

Net working capital: current assets minus current liabilities.

Net working capital commitment: the additional current assets (cash, inventory, supplies, accounts receivable) that must be acquired in order to bring an asset or project into service.

Operating cash flow: periodic cash flows associated with the use of an asset or project in place.

Opportunity cost: the value of some benefit forgone in order to produce some good or service.

Option: right to purchase (call) or sell (put) an asset at some predetermined price at some time, or over some time interval, in the future.

Ordering cost: cost of making an order and of receiving shipment of an inventory or supply item.

Owners' equity: the difference between the organization's **assets** and its **liabilities** (known as **fund balance** in government-owned and not-for-profit organizations).

Par value: the **principal** amount (or face value) of a bond.

Pecking order theory: theory that organizations have a preferred order for obtaining external financing, preferring retained earnings to new debt and new debt to new equity.

Per member per month (PMPM): amount collected each month for each person enrolled under a **capitated** contract; covers all contractually specified health care.

Per-unit contribution margin: revenue per unit minus **variable cost** per unit.

Performance (or asset utilization): class of financial ratios that indicate how effectively the organization uses its assets to generate revenues and cash.

Portfolio: a collection of **securities**.

Post: process of transferring **journal entries** to the organization's accounts.

Preferred stock: equity claim against the organization, entitled to a fixed annual dividend, but (usually) without any voting right unless the promised dividend is not paid.

Prepaid expenses: current asset consisting of the value of future periods' expenses paid in the current period.

Present value: the amount that, if invested today at some specified rate of **interest**, would generate a specified **future value** at a specified time in the future.

Price variance: that part of the **total variance** due to price's being different from that which was planned.

Principal: an amount borrowed.

Profitability: any of several ratios that compare profit (or net income or excess of revenues over expenses) to some measure of organizational size.

Profitability index: the present value of **operating cash flows** from use of an asset divided by the absolute value of the required **initial cash flow**; the project's gain per initial dollar invested.

Prospective payment system: system for making Medicare payments to hospitals, introduced in 1983, in which compensation is predetermined, based on each patient's diagnosis upon admission.

Pure play: a firm engaged solely in a single activity, said activity duplicating the project whose riskiness is being assessed.

Quantity variance: that part of the **total variance** due to quantity sold or purchased's being different from that which was planned.

Rating agency: a firm specializing in assessing the riskiness of **securities** and of their issuers.

Ratio analysis: analysis of financial statements via the construction of ratios; using one number taken from the financial statements to normalize another number taken from the financial statements.

Reciprocal cost allocation method: cost allocation method that allocates **cost** from **cost centers** to **revenue centers** via flows that run both from cost center to revenue center and from revenue center to cost center.

Responsibility center: an organizational subunit, usually with its own budget, assigned responsibility for management or one or both of its cost and revenue.

Return: terminal price minus initial price, plus cash flows received, divided by initial price.

Return on assets (ROA): sometimes called return on investment (ROI); ratio of profit (or net income or excess of revenues over expenses) to total assets.

Return on equity (ROE): ratio of profit (or net income or excess of revenues over expenses) to owners' equity (or fund balance).

Revenue budget: that component of the **budget** forecasting receipt of revenues for the budget period.

Revenue center: responsibility center charged with generating revenues.

Risk: variation in possible **returns**.

Risk-adjusted discount rate (RADR): project-specific discount rate raised or lowered from the firm's **weighted average cost of capital**, due to the differential riskiness of the project under review.

Risk aversion: the almost universal characteristic of preferring a given **return** with certainty to participating in a lottery with the same expected outcome.

Safety stock: amount of an inventory or supply items below which one's holding should not be allowed to fall.

Secondary market: market for securities previously issued.

Securitize: to convert an asset's promised cash flows into the periodic cash flows of an associated security; to convert an asset promising cash in the future into a lump sum of cash (the proceeds from the sale of the security) in the present.

Security: contract entitling the owner to future cash flows.

Security Market Line: ray, in **beta-return** space, emanating from the risk-free rate of interest, through the market's expected **return** and beyond.

Senior: (adjective) the order in which claims are to be paid; security A is senior to security B if the holders of A are paid their promised cash flows before the holders of B; especially important in cases of financial distress.

Sensitivity analysis: comparison of forecasts under different basic assumptions.

Set of feasible solutions: in a **linear programming** problem, the set of values of the decision variables that satisfy all of the linear constraints.

Shadow cost center: cost center identified for analytical convenience, but in which there is no actual organization.

Simplex theorem: theorem for the solution of **linear programming** problems; requires that the optimal solution to such a problem be at a "corner," where one variable takes a zero value, or where at least two constraints are binding simultaneously.

Specialist: in auction-based stock exchanges, a member of the exchange that makes an orderly market in a listed stock; trading on the exchange occurs when brokers and dealers place orders with the specialist.

State-preference theory: theoretical approach to risk adjustment in capital budgeting; requires that utilities be attached to all possible cash flow outcomes.

Statement of cash flows: financial statement that converts the **accrual**-based income statement into a statement of the flow of cash into and out of the organization during the accounting period.

Statistics budget: that component of the **budget** forecasting service volume and resource use for the **budget period**.

Step-down allocation method: cost allocation method that allocates **cost** from **cost centers** to **revenue centers** with intermediate steps, and that closes cost centers as soon as all costs have been allocated from them.

Step-fixed cost: cost that is constant over some range of output but that rises in a discreet increment as output exceeds the upper limit of that range.

Stock: a security guaranteeing an equity claim.

Stock-out: condition in which one's holding of an inventory or supply item has fallen to zero.

Straight line depreciation: beginning with the full historical cost of the asset then subtracting the expected salvage value at the end of the asset's useful life divided by the number of years in the asset's useful life.

Systematic risk: the risk associated with holding any risky security; cannot be eliminated through diversification.

Systems design: the branch of accounting that deals with the design of accounting systems and the flow of financial information within the organization.

Tax-exempt revenue bonds: debt instruments, backed by organizational revenues, issued by municipal authorities and, therefore, paying interest that is not subject to Federal income tax.

Tax shield: cash flow that would otherwise have been required for payment of taxes, but that is saved due to depreciation (or some other factor).

Term structure of interest rates: description of the relationship between term to maturity and market yield for securities within some risk class.

Terminating cash flow: cash flows recovered, through salvage value or release of net working capital commitment, upon the sale of an asset or the termination of a project.

Time value of money: preference for some amount of money today over today's riskless promise of the same amount of money at some time in the future.

Times interest earned: ratio of earnings before interest and taxes to interest expense.

Top-down budgeting: budget process in which a great deal of information flows from the chief financial officer (or other senior management official) to responsibility centers.

Total asset turnover: ratio of revenues to total assets.

Total margin: ratio of profit (or net income or excess of revenues over expenses) to revenues plus nonoperating gains.

Trade credit: suppliers' willingness to defer payment (usually for periods of up to 30 days).

Treasurer: officer charged with stewardship of the organization's financial assets.

Trial balance: step in the accounting cycle, following posting, in which debit balances are compared to credit balances to ensure their equality in the aggregate.

Trustee: commercial bank representing the holders of an issue of bonds; ensures that the issuer of the bonds meets its contractual obligations.

Underwrite: agreement between an investment bank and an issuer of securities in which the bank guarantees a percentage of the par value of the securities to the issuer, retaining any remaining proceeds for itself.

Underwriter's spread: the difference between the selling price of an issue of new securities and the proceeds that the investment bank guaranteed to the issuer.

Unsystematic risk: the risk associated with holding a specific security; can be eliminated through diversification.

Valuation: the process of estimating the market value of an organization or asset, when no record of active trading is available to establish such a value.

Variable cost: cost that varies continuously as volume varies.

Variance: difference between a forecast amount and the amount actually realized; budget variances should not be confused with statistical variances.

Variance analysis: the accounting activity that evaluates the differences between budgeted amounts and the amounts actually realized.

Weighted average cost of capital (WACC): the cost (in percentage terms) of an additional dollar of funding, given some capital structure.

Working capital: current assets and current liabilities (but *not* their sum).

Working capital management: process of managing current assets and current liabilities.

Yield curve: graphical representation of the relationship between term to maturity and market yield for securities within some risk class. (See **Term Structure of Interest Rates**)

Zero-base budgeting: budget process in which the budgets for succeeding budget periods are unrelated to those of earlier budget periods, but are justified on their own merits, as if no previous budgets have ever been prepared.

Answers to Selected
Discussion Questions

Chapter 1

1. The comptroller (or controller) is responsible for accounting functions: bookkeeping, financial reporting, and cost accountings. The treasurer is responsible for obtaining and safeguarding financial assets: long-term financing, commercial bank relations, and cash management. In small organizations, the same person may perform both sets of duties.

3. Cash is immediately available, unambiguous and necessary to meet obligations. Profit (computed according to generally accepted accountings principles), although not without use, is subject to several resources of ambiguity, depending on choice of accounting convention, and is not available to meet obligations.

5. The law of one price can be violated (even for long periods) when there are impediments to the free flow of information or of goods and services. Equivalent bonds can offer different yields (at least in the short run) if there is insufficient trading in them to provide investors with information about the discrepancy.

Chapter 2

1. An agency relationship exists when one party (the agent) is authorized to act on behalf of another (the principal). In health care organizations, manager and owners, physicians and patients, and insurers and their clients are all involved in agency relationships.

3. The more closely the principal can monitor the agent's activities, the less ability the agent has to impose costs on the principal. In health care settings, such monitoring is often difficult, as the agent (managers, for example) may have expert information that the principal (boards of trustees, for example) needs in order to monitor but does not have.

5. Corporations that generate substantial cash flows provide the opportunity for managers (agents) to benefit at the expense of inventors (principals) by taking excessive perquisites for themselves. Because inventors realize that such possibilities exist, the market values of such firms are lower than they need to be. Substituting debt (which requires regular cash payment) for equity has proven to be a way of solving this agency problem as of increasing the values of those firms (see Chapter 20).

Chapter 3

1. Most accountants agree that the accrual basis is superior for large organizations. The accrual basis measures the flow of resources (not just cash) through the organization. For example, expenses, under accrual, are recognized when they are incurred (when resources are used) rather than when cash is disgorged.

3. Accrual accounting introduces several ambiguities. Asset values are affected by the choice of depreciation method (depreciation is necessary only under accrual accounting). The prediction of a collection rate, to determine the value of net accounts receivable, is necessary only under accrual accounting. The calculation of inventory expense, affected by choice of FIFO or LIFO, is necessary only under accrual accounting.

5. For many nonaccountants, *credit* has a positive connotation, as in "I'll credit your account." *Debit*, not used as often in everyday speech, is assumed to have a negative connotation, being the opposite of *credit*. In accounting, however, *debit* only means a left-hand-side entry, used to increase an asset or an expense. *Credit* only means a right-hand-side entry, used to increase liabilities, owners' equity, or revenues.

Chapter 4

1. Liquidity measures ability to pay debts only in cases of bankruptcy. It is better understood as a measure of the organization's riskiness. Debt service coverage (cash flow coverage), on the other hand, measures the organization's ability to meet its debt obligations out of the cash flows generated by operations.

3. Most analysts believe ROA (return on assets) in the more important. It measures the organization's ability to use its assets to generate profits.

Chapter 5

1.

$$V_5 = \$1,250 \times \text{FVF}_{7\%, \ 5 \text{ yrs}}$$

$$= \$1,250 \times 1.4236$$

$$= \$1,753.25$$

$$V_{10} = \$1,250 \times \text{FVF}_{7\%, \ 10 \text{ yrs}}$$

$$= \$1,250 \times 1.9672$$

$$= \$2,459.00$$

$$V_{20} = \$1,250 \times \text{FVF}_{7\%, \ 20 \text{ yrs}}$$

$$= \$1,250 \times 3.8697$$

$$= \$4,837.13$$

2. 12% per year is (approximately) 1% per month.

The present value of the New Year's Eve value (valued 1 month prior to the first deposit, but 13 months prior to New Year's Eve) is

$$V_{-1} = V_{12} \times PVF_{1\%, .8787}$$

$$V_{-1} = V_{12} \times 0.8787$$

The present value of the annuity of payments (valued 1 month prior to the first payment) is

$$V_{-1} = \$50 \times PVFA_{1\%, \text{ 12 mos}}$$

$$V_{-1} = \$50 \times 11.2551$$

Set $V_{-1} = V_{-1}$ to obtain

$$V_{12} \times 0.8787 = \$50 \times 11.2551$$

$$V_{12} = \$640.44$$

3.

$$5\%: V_0 = \$250,000 \times PVF_{5\%, \text{ 15 yrs}}$$

$$V_0 = \$250,000 \times 0.4810$$

$$V_0 = \$120,250$$

$$10\%: V_0 = \$250,000 \times PVF_{10\%, \text{ 15 yrs}}$$

$$V_0 = \$250,000 \times 0.2394$$

$$V_0 = \$59,850$$

$$20\%: V_0 = \$250,000 \times PVF_{20\%, \text{ 15 yrs}}$$

$$V_0 = \$250,000 \times 0.0649$$

$$V_0 = \$16,225$$

4.

$$V_0 = \$500,000 \times PVF_{\text{cont., } 10\%, \text{ 15 yrs}}$$

$$V_0 = \$500,000 \times 0.2231$$

$$V_0 = \$111,550$$

5.

$$V_0 = \$45,000 \times \text{PVFA}_{6\%,\ 15\ \text{yrs}}$$

$$V_0 = \$45,000 \times 9.7122$$

$$V_0 = \$437,049$$

6.

$$V_0 = (\$45 \times \text{PVFA}_{3\%,\ 20\ \text{per}}) + (\$1,000 \times \text{PVF}_{3\%,\ 20\ \text{per}})$$

$$V_0 = (\$45 \times 14.8775) + (\$1,000 \times .5537)$$

$$V_0 = (\$669.49) + (\$553.70)$$

$$V_0 = \$1,223.19$$

7. Under quarterly compounding, interest is compounded more often and begins to accrue earlier than under annual compounding.

8. Contract B is exactly 8 percent more valuable, because each payment can earn interest for one additional period. It represents an "annuity due," whereas contract A is an "annuity in arrears." To turn Table 5-4 into factors for annuities due, multiply each entry by $(1 + r)$.

9. Present value of the debt is $150,000.

Present value of the payments are

$$V_0 = X \times \text{PVFA}_{12\%,\ 8\ \text{yrs}}$$

$$150,000 = X \times 4.9676$$

Solving:

$$X = \$30,195.67$$

10.

$$V_0 = \frac{D_1}{r\text{-}g}$$

$$V_0 = \frac{\$12}{0.80 - 0.02}$$

$$V_0 = \frac{12}{0.06}$$

$$V_0 = \$200$$

Chapter 6

1.

Approach	Strengths	Weaknesses
Rules of thumb	- Easily applied	- No basis in theory - No fixed relation to market value
Adjusted book value	- Consistent with accounting rules - Data easily obtained	- No relation to market value
Market value	- Approximates market value	- Requires data on value of similar organizations
Discounted cash flow	- Consistent with theory - Consistent relation with market value - Data easily obtained	- Requires projection of cash flows - Requires selection of a discount rate

3. As a not-for-profit organization, Charity Hospital pays no income tax on its net earnings, enjoys no tax shield from interest or depreciation, and, in most jurisdictions, pays no property tax. Charity Hospital may also enjoy low interest rates from issuing tax-exempt hospital revenue bonds. ABC should recalculate Charity's cash flows taking into account these changes in tax shield.

Chapter 7

1. The quote provided is a paraphrase of Arthur Thomas's conclusion on "the allocation problem." There are, of course, unreasonable bases for allocating costs (allocating the cost of the CEO's office on the basis of each department's share of brown-eyed employees). There are, however, many reasonable bases for allocating indirect costs, and many are equally viable. The CEO's office cost might be allocated on a percentage of payroll, percentage of headcount, or percentage of square feet basis. Be careful, however, not to allocate fixed cost items on a percentage of sales basis, as doing so treats it as a variable cost.

Chapter 8

1. Even the most authoritarian organization seeks information from first-level supervisors. The use of those data varies from reading but denigrating it to using it as the role impact for planning. Even the U.S. Congress seeks information from operating personnel.

3. Zero-base budgeting forces the careful consideration of every planned expenditure. The effort required to implement it, to prepare a budget package, and to justify every item is beyond what most organizations are willing to expend on an annual basis.

Chapter 9

1. Early in a household's lifetime, in the years of home purchase and furnishing and childbirth, it is likely to be a user of funds. Later, as retirement looms, it is likely to be a supplier of funds, actively investing. Still later, after retirement, it will be a supplier of funds, reaping promised cash flows.

3. The lowest level of risk achievable is that of systematic risk, the risk level inherent in participation in the market for risky securities.

5. Analysts use the interest rate prevailing on 90-day U.S. Treasury bills. Those securities are free (or virtually free) of default risk and interest rate risk. A portfolio of T-bills, however, is subject to rollover risk, the variability in yield introduced at the (frequent) reinvestment dates.

Chapter 10

1. Follow the NPV rule when it conflicts with IRR in mutually exclusive choice situations. The alternative with the highest NPV is that which will add the most to the organization's value.

5. Sources of ambiguity:
   Cash flow projections
   Discount rate choice
   Degree of risk assumed

Chapter 11

1. Linear programming is a powerful computational tool, but that is all it is. It cannot evaluate the reasonableness of a solution, only its numerical optimality. The analyst needs to specify constraints if she wishes to avoid such solutions as "Repeat project I over and over until the budget is exhausted" or "Build 5 percent of the clinic in year 1, 0 percent in year 2, and 95 percent in year 3."

3. Most health care organizations neither adjust their discount rates for project risk nor use discounted cash flow methods for project selection. The reasons include ignorance of the methods and belief that they are unimportant. Those organizations would have better guidance as to what projects and assets would add value if they used appropriate methods appropriately.

Chapter 12

5. The wisdom of any investment strategy depends on the investor's unique goals and constraints (including degree of risk aversion). The strategy of investing only in U.S. Government Securities is very conservative and may be appropriate for very risk-averse organizations. For only a little additional risk assumptions, however, one can achieve substantially higher expected return.

Chapter 13

1. Investor-owned health care organizations can gain external financing through bank lending or by issuing commercial paper, common stock, preferred stock, or corporate bonds. Not-for-profit organizations have access to external financing through bank loans, philanthropy, and issuing hospital revenue bonds or other bonds.

3. The optimal capital structure for an organization is the one that minimizes its weighted average cost of capital, thereby maximizing its value.

5. A 100 percent debt capital structure is probably not optimal, given the bankruptcy costs that would be present. The factors that favor heavy use of debt, however, are its lower cost (when compared to equity) and the tax-deductability of interest payments.

Chapter 14

1. Issuing securities to the public is a troublesome and expensive process. Funds can be obtained from public offerings of securities, however, at lower costs of capital than from commercial banks. Therefore, when the amount of funds needed is large enough to justify the high fixed costs of selling securities, that is the preferred way to access external financing.

3. Purchase bond insurance if an only if the premium for the insurance is no greater than the present value of the expected interest rate savings due to being insured.

5. An *effective* prohibition of inside trading would mean that corporate insiders could not profit at the expense of an uninformed public. It would also, however, remove one source from which effective managers could be compensated. How one feels about prohibiting insider trading depends on which of these two factors (fairness to the public and compensation for managers) one values more.

Chapter 15

1. The quotation is from a former colleague of mine. Organizations that don't survive, however, cannot perform their missions. Failed organizations deliver no health care.

3. Probably not. In the capital market, charitable organizations compete with all others. Government-owned and not-for-profit health care providers may, however, enjoy a lower cost of capital on average than investor-owned organizations.

4. The imaginary world of no external financing for health care organizations is much like the real world of many emerging countries' health care systems. Average age of plant is higher than in the United States, use of new technology spreads less rapidly, and much of the equipment is older.

Chapter 16

1. Working capital consists of current assets and current liabilities. It is *working* capital in that it facilitates the conduct of current operations. Cash, for example, is necessary to pay current obligations. Accounts receivable and accounts payable are generated in the normal course of business.

3. Monetary policy influences the availability of credit for all potential users of funds in the capital market. Federal Reserve decisions, then, determine what acquisitions and projects will be feasible (financiable) for health care organizations. Thus monetary policy affects the public's access to health care technology.

Chapter 17

1. The cash budget forecasts cash inflows, cash outflows, ending cash, and cumulative short-term borrowing (or lending). *Every* organization should have a cash budget.

3. a. Lock box system: payments are mailed to a post office box; a bank representative collects payments several times daily; payments are immediately deposited.
   b. Selling patient accounts to third parties.
   c. Hiring collection agencies.
   d. Securitizing receivables: issuing commercial paper promising a share of future collections to each paper holder.

Chapter 18

1.

$$EOQ = \sqrt{\frac{2CA}{(rp + H)}}$$

$$= \sqrt{\frac{2(50)(1460)}{[(.05)(25) + 2]}}$$

$$= \sqrt{\frac{146,000}{3.25}}$$

$$= \sqrt{44{,}923.08}$$
$$= 211.95, \text{ or } 212 \text{ catheters}$$

3. The supplier must agree to be responsive to calls and to maintain inventories of the necessary items. The purchaser must agree to make orders sufficiently far in advance ("We need 10 sterile surgical packs at 7:00 AM tomorrow"), which requires advance scheduling. The supplier and materials handling staff must have a good working relationship and agree to keep one another informed.

Chapter 19

1. Although the yield curve is usually upward sloping (short-term debt is less expensive than long-term debt), the use of short-term debt involves substantial risk. Short-term debt must be refinanced, at prevailing market rates, frequently. As a result, most organizations (being risk averse) match the volume of their long-term assets to long-term financing.

3. One could pay cash for goods and services at the moment of delivery. When vendors allow time to pass before payment (allow accounts payable to accrue); they are granting short-term credit. Trade credit (as the accumulation of accounts payable is called) is a particularly desirable form of short-term financing because it is interest free.

5. a. Through a commercial bank sell commercial paper promising cash flows based on collection of *specified* blocks of patient accounts (the paper must be registered with the SEC and state reputation).

   b. Engage a third party to accept collections and to dispense payments to lenders.

   c. The commercial paper is retired as all of the associated accounts receivable are collected.

   d. At every step, sell commercial paper based on only the highest-quality patient accounts (accounts due from the most reliable payors).

Chapter 20

1. The roles of financing professionals can vary from providing advice on cash flows and the cost of capital to establishing the criteria for making strategic decisions. In many not-for-profit organizations they will take a role such as the former. In many investor-owned organizations they will take a role such as the latter.

Index

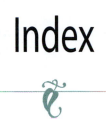

A